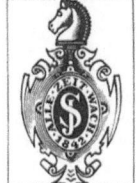

K. Tabuchi A. Nishimoto

Atlas of Brain Tumors

Light- and Electron-Microscopic Features

With 258 Figures

Springer-Verlag
Tokyo Berlin Heidelberg New York London Paris

KAZUO TABUCHI, M.D.
Professor and Chairman
Department of Neurosurgery
Saga Medical School
Saga, 840-01 Japan

AKIRA NISHIMOTO, M.D.
Professor and Chairman
Department of Neurological Surgery
Okayama University Medical School
Okayama, 700 Japan

ISBN-13: 978-4-431-68065-9   e-ISBN-13: 978-4-431-68063-5
DOI: 10.1007/978-4-431-68063-5

Typesetting: Asco Trade Typesetting Ltd., Hong Kong

Foreword

In the many years since the electron-microscopic observation of surgical specimens first began, countless papers on the subject have been published. Because of the large number of the papers and the fact that they are to be found in all kinds of publications, it is difficult fully to keep abreast of them all. To remedy this situation, Drs. Tabuchi and Nishimoto have put together a superb book on the light- and electron-microscopic features of brain tumors. Despite being restricted to human material, the quality of the photographs is excellent, and it will surely be constantly used by clinicians as well as clinical investigators. This volume is clearly the result of detailed and careful study. It is a great achievement.

Isehara, Japan   Paul K. Nakane

To our patients

Foreword

It is a pleasure to introduce both to the general reader and to the specialist this attractively and meticulously illustrated Atlas of Brain Tumors by Profs. Tabuchi and Nishimoto. The information provided by the light-microscopic appearance of these neoplasms, obtained both with traditional staining techniques and the more recently developed immunohistochemical approaches, is harmoniously blended with a detailed, up-to-date survey of their principal fine-structural features. This combination reflects the extensive experience of the authors in the different morphological aspects of brain tumors. The high quality of the illustrations adds considerable esthetic appeal to the scientific value of this work.

This atlas will, therefore, prove to be a reliable source of reference for the pathologist confronted with these diagnostic problems as well as a most useful aid in the day-to-day practice of neuropathology. It is greatly welcome, and I wish it all the success that it so clearly deserves.

Charlottesville, VA, USA   L. J. Rubinstein

Preface

This atlas is planned as a guide for those studying the pathology of tumors arising from the central nervous system. As the title implies, it is concerned mainly with the light- and electron-microscopic features of brain tumors and should prove useful to pathology residents, neurologists, neurosurgeons, neuroradiologists, and senior medical students who are confronted with a variety of brain tumors.

Recently, the innovations in neuroradiology, including computed tomography (CT), magnetic resonance imaging (MRI), and positron emission tomography (PET), have greatly contributed toward the precise localization of brain tumors; the ultimate diagnosis, however, is still based on the histopathological findings from tumor specimens obtained at surgery. Although brain tumors are generally diagnosed by ordinary light- and electron-microscopic examination of the specimens, the recently developed immunoperoxidase methods have added a new dimension to the histopathology of brain tumors by enabling different types of proteins or peptides, such as immunoglobulins and hormones, to be localized. We believe that accurate diagnosis is essential for the appropriate management of patients with brain tumors.

The material in this atlas represents approximately 700 brain tumor specimens collected mainly in our clinics but also derived from other sources. In the majority of cases, we present both light- and electron-microscopic images of the same case since the two are essentially complementary.

Unless otherwise indicated, all the material was processed according to routine procedures for diagnosis. Biopsy tissues of each tumor were placed in 10% formalin and processed for conventional light microscopy. The tissue samples for electron-microscopic examination were cut into small blocks of about 1 mm^3, fixed in 2.5% glutaraldehyde, and embedded in Epon after dehydration with ethanol. Ultrathin sections were stained with metals and observed and photographed in the electron microscope.

With regard to nomenclature, we have tried to follow the classification of brain tumors recommended by the World Health Organization in the series of publications "International Histological Classification of Tumours, No. 21: Histological Typing of Tumours of the Central Nervous System, 1979."

Saga, Japan

K. Tabuchi
A. Nishimoto

Acknowledgments

This atlas could not have been compiled without the courtesy and support of many friends and colleagues. We are especially indebted to Mr. Hideki Wakimoto, who expertly processed most of the biopsy tissues and prepared innumerable prints from which those that appear in this atlas were selected. Several colleagues have been most helpful in supplying us with specimens or blocks of tissues from which some of the illustrations in this atlas were derived; they include Prof. emeritus Katsuo Ogawa, Prof. Yasuyuki Kawarai, Drs. Hajime Fujita, Kazuo Hamaya, Makoto Motoi, Akihiro Doi, Yasuto Kawakami, Shoji Asari, and Kenji Shibata. Thanks are due to Drs. Yoshio Moriya, Tomohisa Furuta, Rinkichi Ohnishi, Takahiro Tsuchida, and Takashi Tamiya for their collaboration in the immunohistochemical examination of brain tumors at Okayama University Medical School. We wish to express our special gratitude to Profs. Lucien J. Rubinstein and Paul K. Nakane for writing the foreword. Our thanks also go to Mrs. Chihoko Ideguchi for her secretarial assistance.

Contents

1. Fibrillary Astrocytoma. 1

2. Pleomorphic Xanthoastrocytoma. 9

3. Subependymal Giant Cell Astrocytoma 13

4. Anaplastic Astrocytoma 17

5. Oligodendroglioma 23

6. Ependymoma 41

7. Choroid Plexus Papilloma. 49

8. Glioblastoma 59

9. Medulloblastoma 75

10. Ganglioglioma 87

11. Central Neurocytoma 93

12. Cerebral Neuroblastoma. 109

13. Olfactory Neuroblastoma (Esthesioneuroblastoma) 115

14. Primitive Neuroectodermal Tumor (PNET) 121

15. Pineocytoma. 127

16. Germinoma. 131

17. Teratoma and Teratoid Tumor 139

18. Schwannoma. 149

19. Pituitary Adenoma and Oncocytoma 157

20. Meningioma 185

21. Meningioangiomatosis. 195

22. Hemangioblastoma 199

23. Hemangiopericytoma. 203

24. Melanoma. 209

Contents

25. Malignant Lymphoma.................................. 213

26. Craniopharyngioma.................................. 221

27. Chordoma.. 229

28. Metastatic Tumor................................... 235

References.. 239

Subject Index 245

1. Fibrillary Astrocytoma

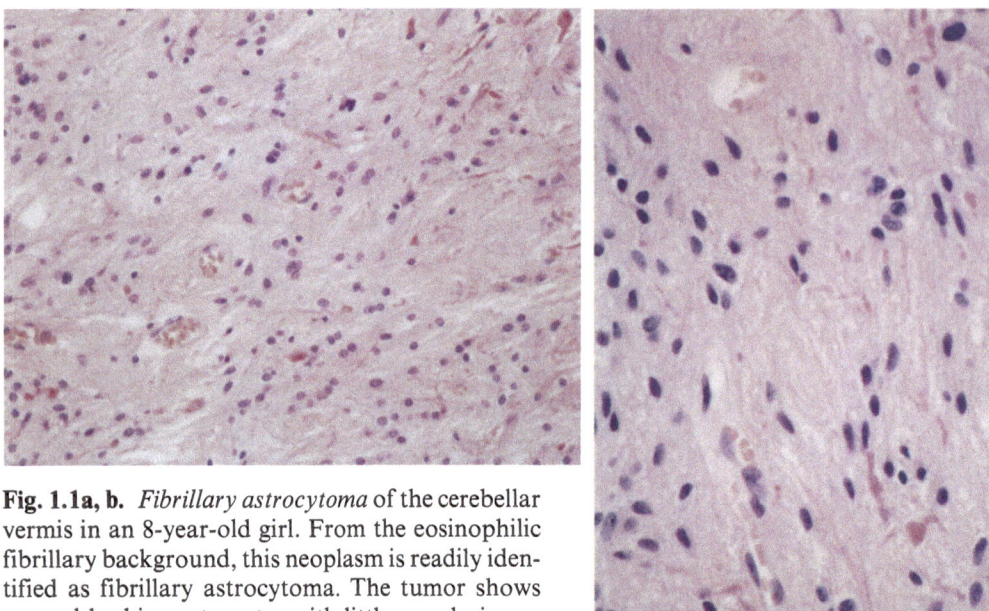

Fig. 1.1a, b. *Fibrillary astrocytoma* of the cerebellar vermis in an 8-year-old girl. From the eosinophilic fibrillary background, this neoplasm is readily identified as fibrillary astrocytoma. The tumor shows normal-looking astrocytes with little anaplasia, no mitotic figures, and thin-walled vessels filled with erythrocytes. The Rosenthal fibers tend to stain bright red and are variable in configuration. H and E; **a** × 90, **b** × 180

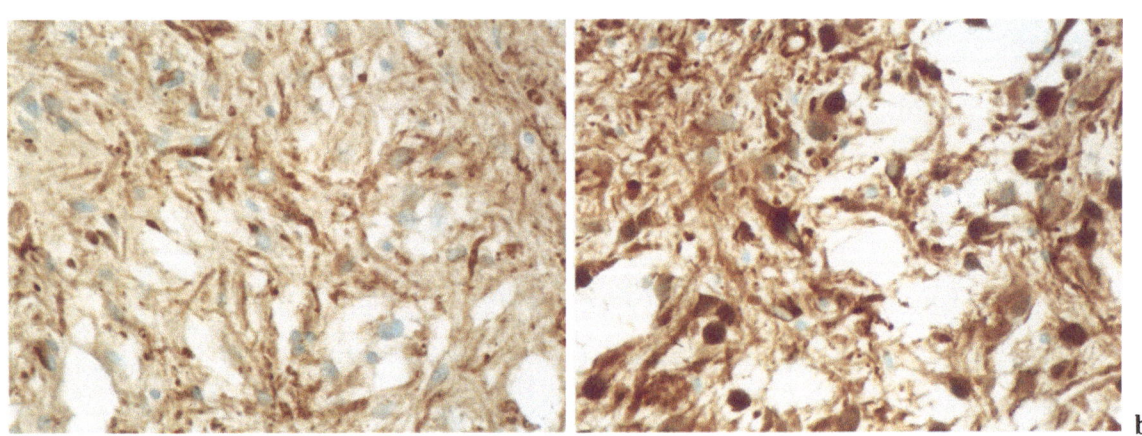

Figs. 1.2a, b. *Fibrillary astrocytoma* (the same case as in Fig. 1.1). Immunohistochemical demonstration of glial fibrillary acidic protein (GFAP, Fig. 1.2a) and S-100 protein (Fig. 1.2b) in fibrillary astrocytoma. A dark-brown reaction product of diaminobenzidine, which indicates positive staining for GFAP, is prominent in the astrocytic processes of the tumor cells. An intensely positive reaction for S-100 protein is observed both in the cytoplasmic processes and nuclei of most tumor cells. There are multiple small cysts in the tumor. Indirect immunoperoxidase method counterstained with methyl green, × 160

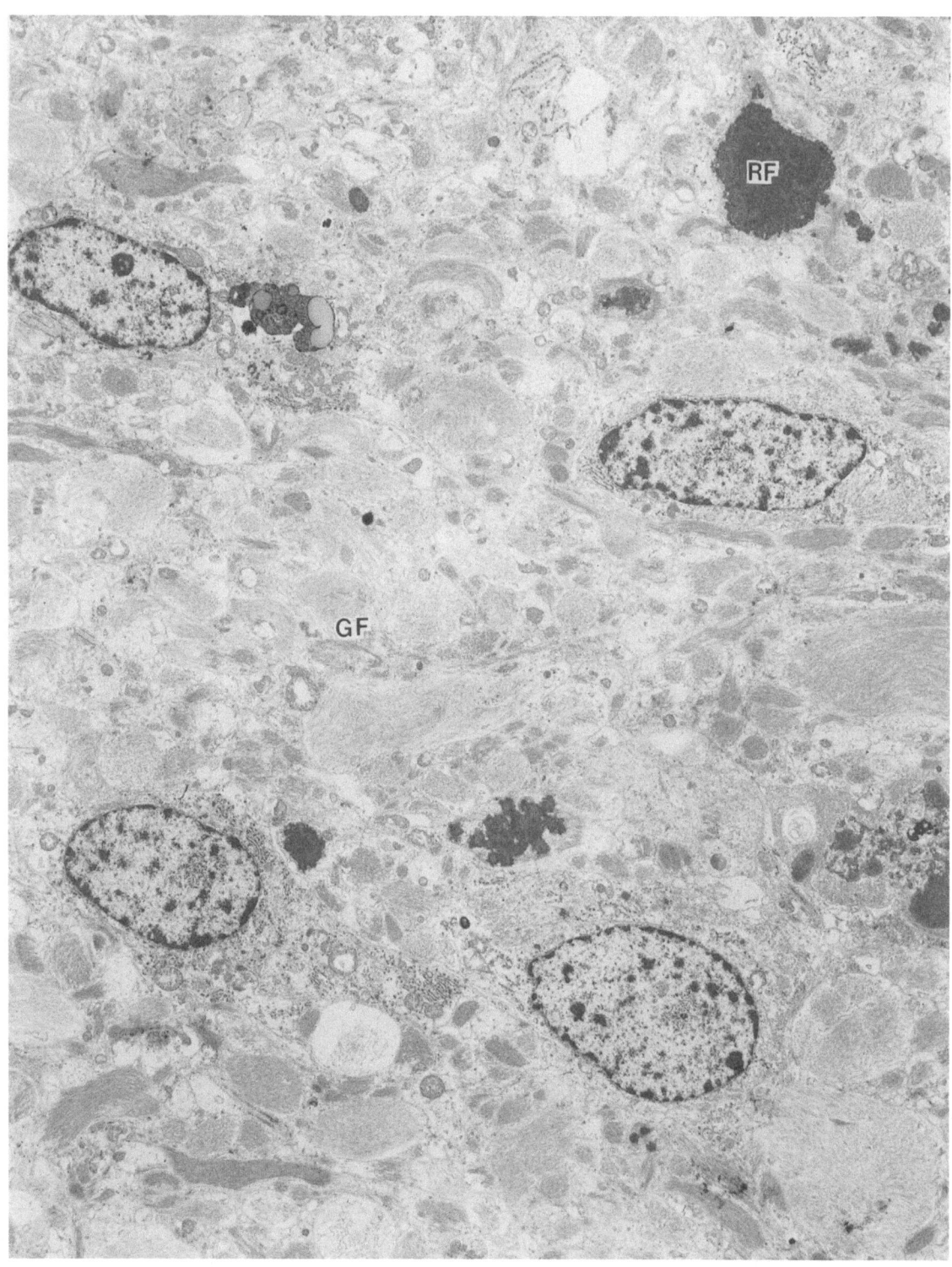

Fig. 1.3. *Fibrillary astrocytoma* (the same case as in Fig. 1.1). At a lower magnification, the tumor cells appear to be similar and the nuclei, with or without nucleoli, are uniform in size. The tumor is characterized by many intermingled glial filaments (*GF*). The Rosenthal fibers (*RF*) are revealed as electron-dense amorphous masses. × 5400

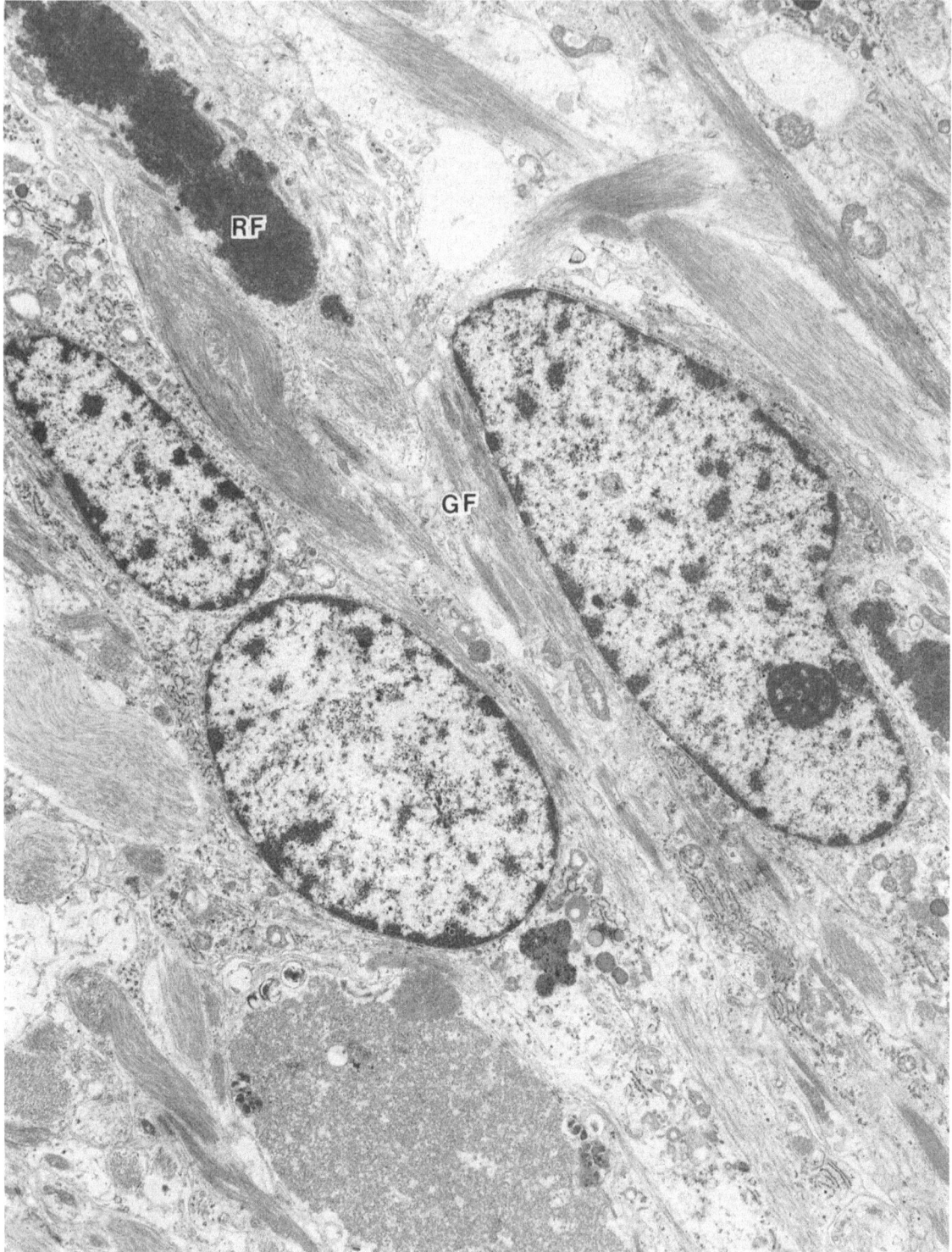

Fig. 1.4. *Fibrillary astrocytoma* (the same case as in Fig. 1.1). The cytoplasm of the tumor cell is filled with bundles of glial filaments (*GF*) and organelles are few. *RF* Rosenthal fiber. × 9000

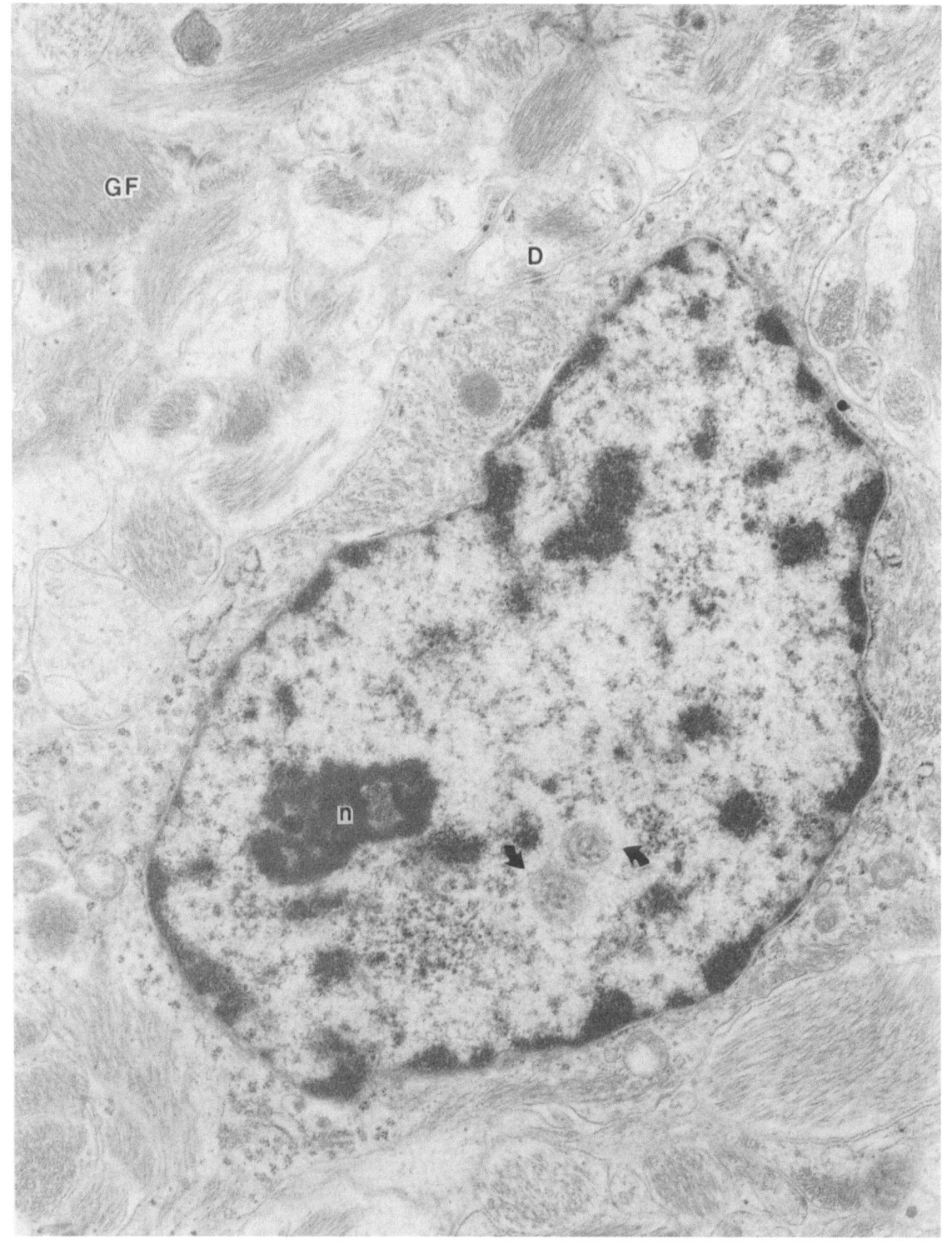

Fig. 1.5. *Fibrillary astrocytoma* (the same case as in Fig. 1.1). The tumor cell with a few organelles has many bundles of glial filaments sectioned either longitudinally or transversely. Nuclear bodies (*arrows*) surrounded by clear halos are present. *GF* glial filaments, *D* desmosome, *n* nucleolus. × 20 000

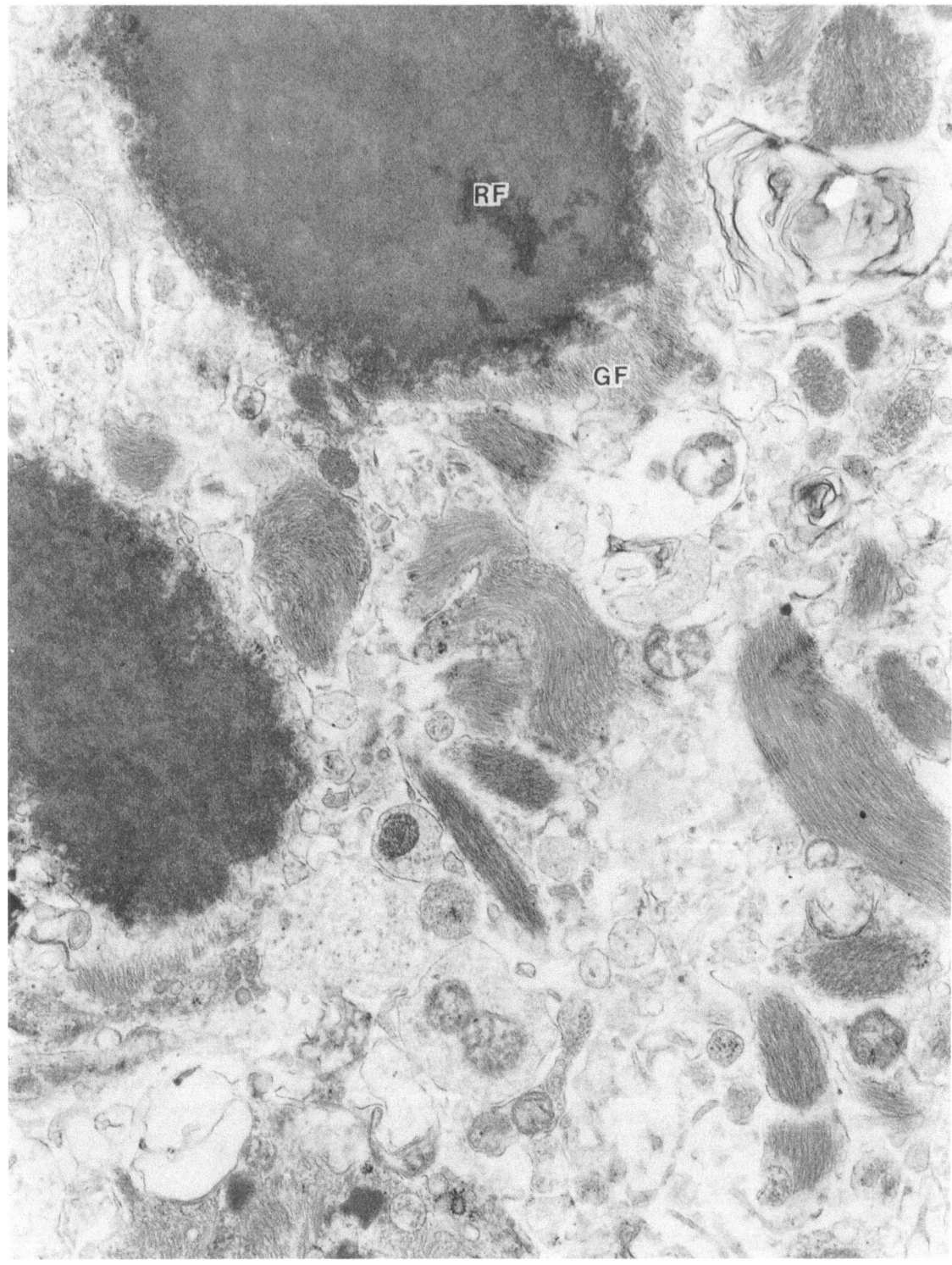

Fig. 1.6. *Fibrillary astrocytoma* (the same case as in Fig. 1.1). At a higher magnification, the amorphous electron-dense Rosenthal fibers (*RF*) seem to be closely associated with glial filaments (*GF*) measuring 7–9 nm in diameter. × 24 000

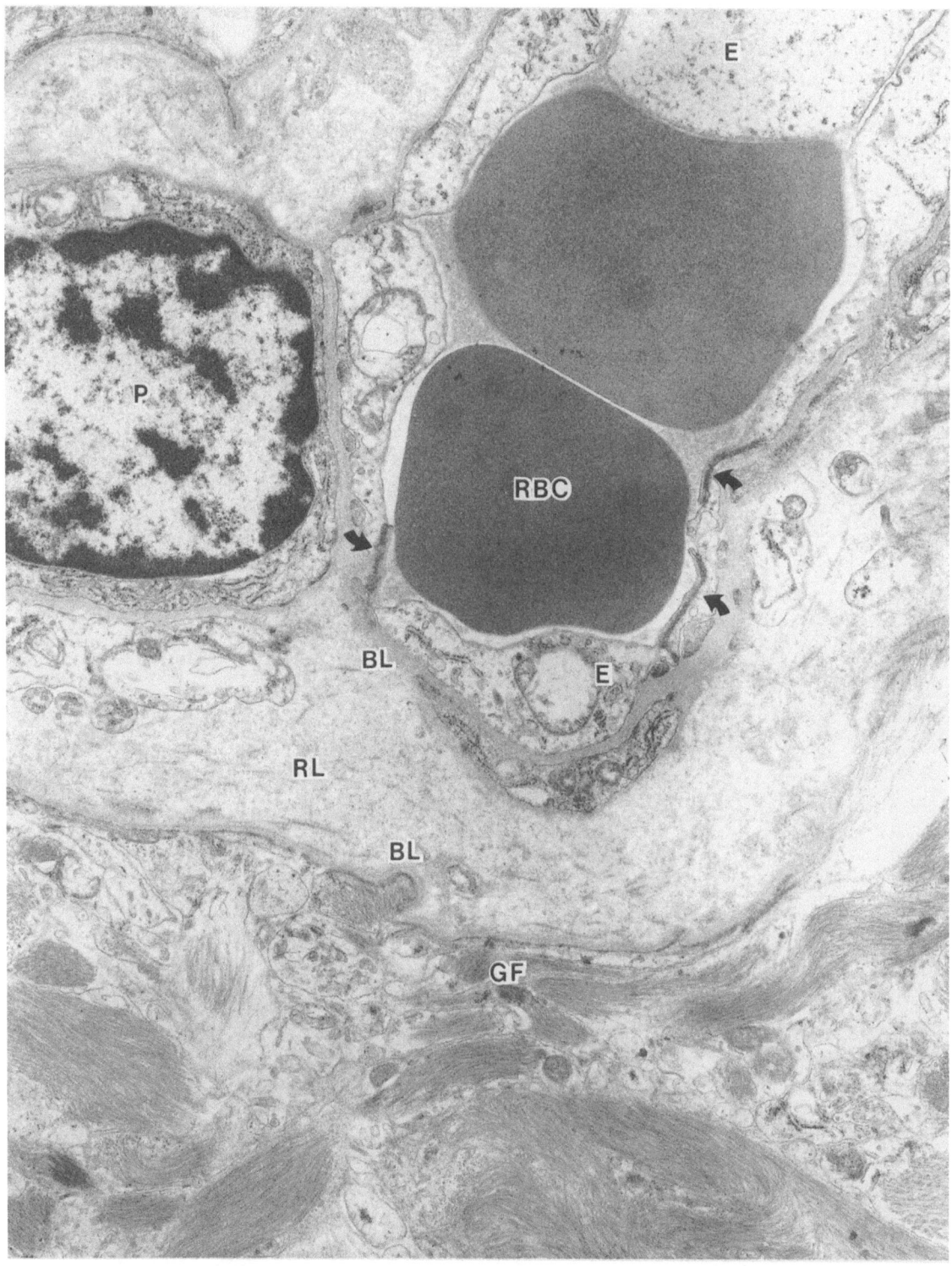

Fig. 1.7. A capillary in *fibrillary astrocytoma* (the same case as in Fig. 1.1). The basal laminae (*BL*) and reticular lamina (*RL*) lie between capillary endothelial cells (*E*) and astrocytic processes of tumor cells filled with glial filaments (*GF*). Tight junctions (*arrows*) are seen between the endothelial cells. *P* pericyte, *RBC* erythrocyte. × 9000

2. Pleomorphic Xanthoastrocytoma

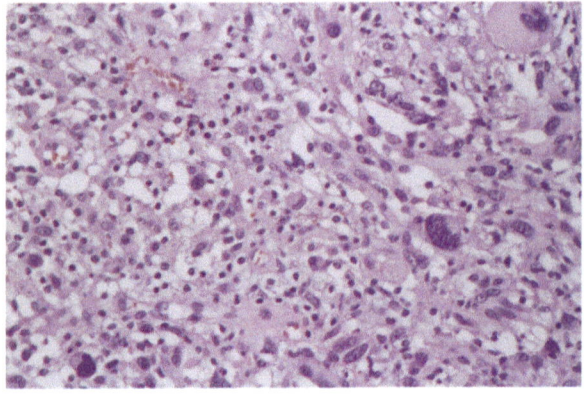

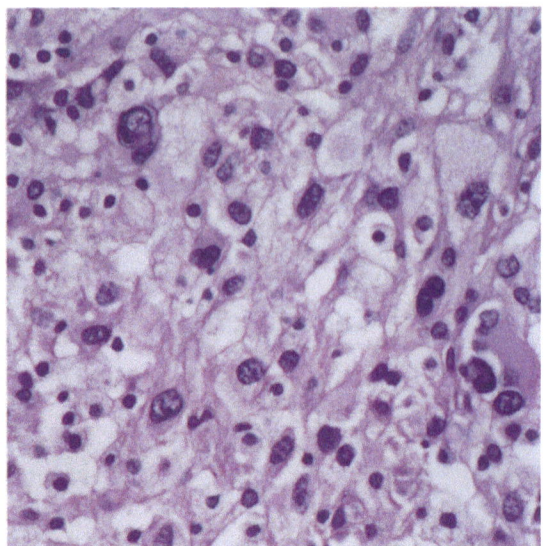

a

b

Fig. 2.1a, b. *Pleomorphic xanthoastrocytoma* of the left temporal lobe in a 14-year-old girl. Pleomorphic turmor cells are characterized by intracytoplasmic vacuoles. Neither necrosis nor mitotic figure are observed. H and E; **a** × 90, **b** × 360

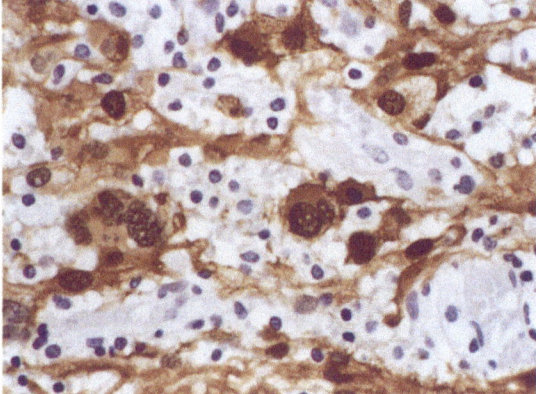

Fig. 2.2. *Pleomorphic xanthoastrocytoma* (the same case as in Fig. 2.1). Many tumor cells reveal strong positivity for glial fibrillary acidic protein (GFAP) restricted to the cytoplasm. Indirect immunoperoxidase method counterstained with hematoxylin, × 320

Fig. 2.3. *Pleomorphic xanthoastrocytoma* (the same case as in Fig. 2.1). The large tumor cells show intensely positive staining for S-100 protein both in the cytoplasm and nuclei. Indirect immunoperoxidase method counterstained with hematoxylin, × 320

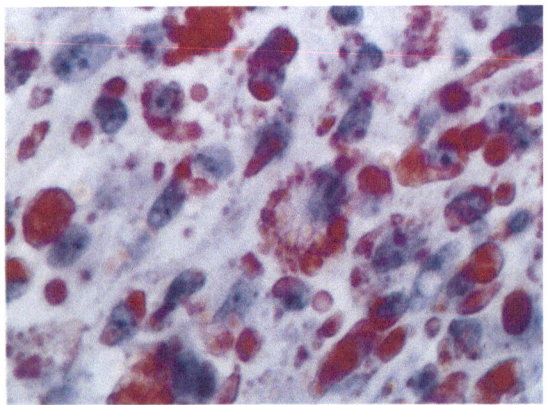

Fig. 2.4. *Pleomorphic xanthoastrocytoma* (the same case as in Fig. 2.1). Pleomorphic tumor cells with lipid-filled cytoplasm. Sudan III, × 320

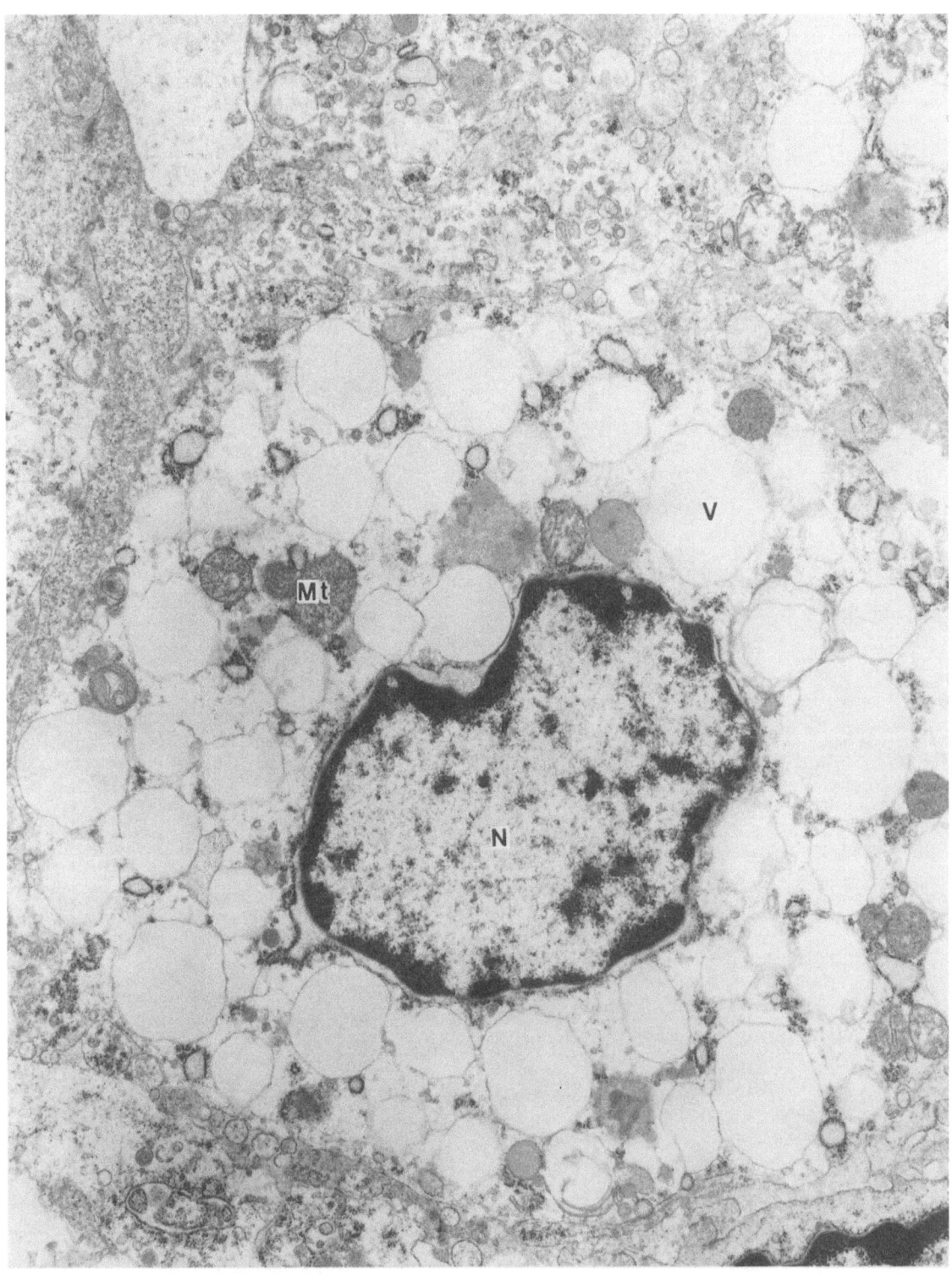

Fig. 2.5. *Pleomorphic xanthoastrocytoma* (the same case as in Fig. 2.1). A typical tumor cell has numerous lipid vacuoles (*V*) in the cytoplasm. *N* nucleus, *Mt* mitochondrion. × 10 000

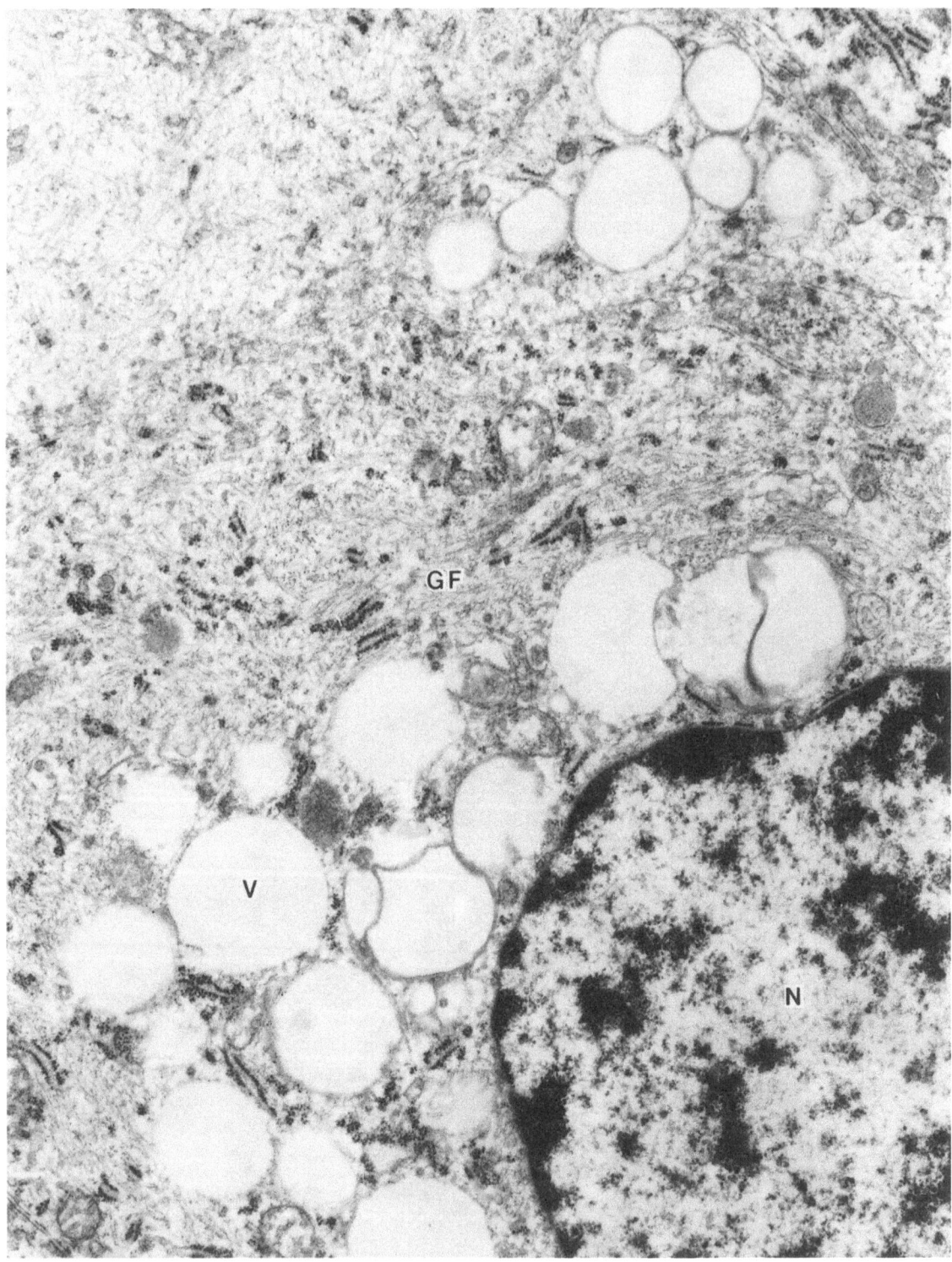

Fig. 2.6. *Pleomorphic xanthoastrocytoma* (the same case as in Fig. 2.1). The tumor cell with many lipid vacuoles (*V*) reveals prominent glial filaments (*GF*). *N* nucleus. × 20 000

3. Subependymal Giant Cell Astrocytoma

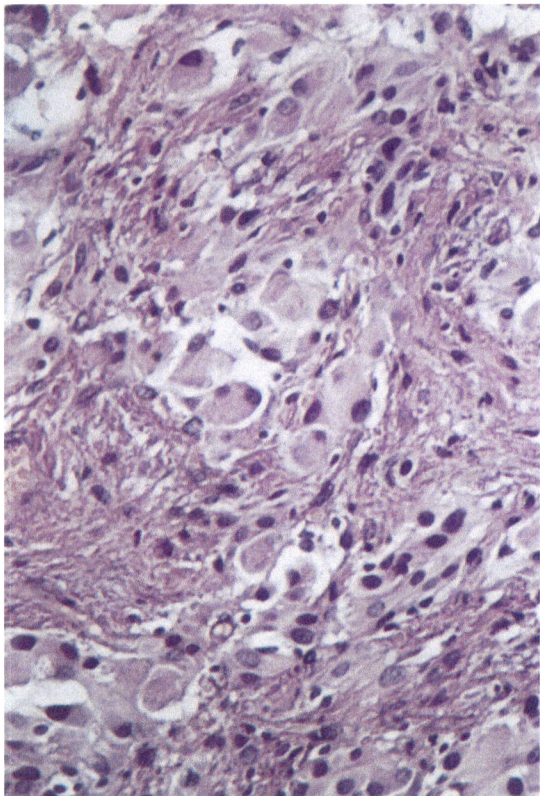

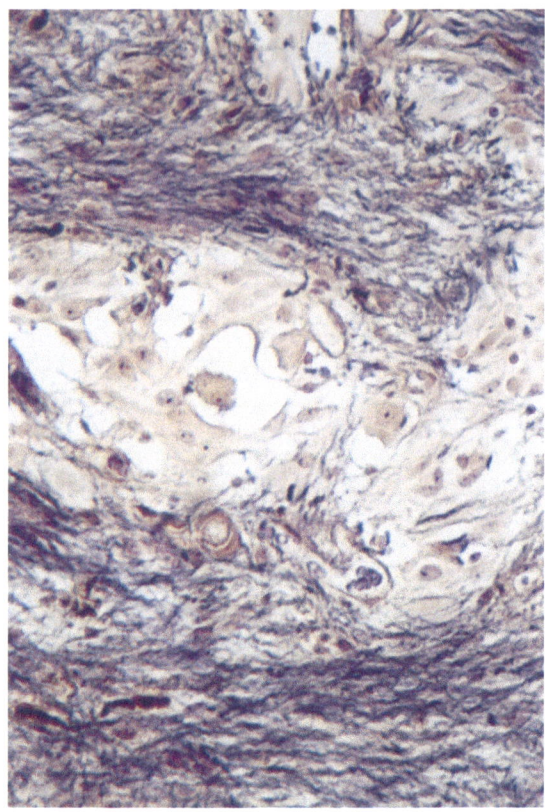

Fig. 3.1. *Subependymal giant cell astrocytoma* arose intraventricularly in a 15-year-old girl with tuberous sclerosis. The tumor consists of bizarre giant cells and elongated small cells. H and E, × 180

Fig. 3.2. *Subependymal giant cell astrocytoma* (the same case as in Fig. 3.1). The giant cells are surrounded by elongated small cells with fibrillary processes. Phosphotungstic acid hematoxylin, × 180

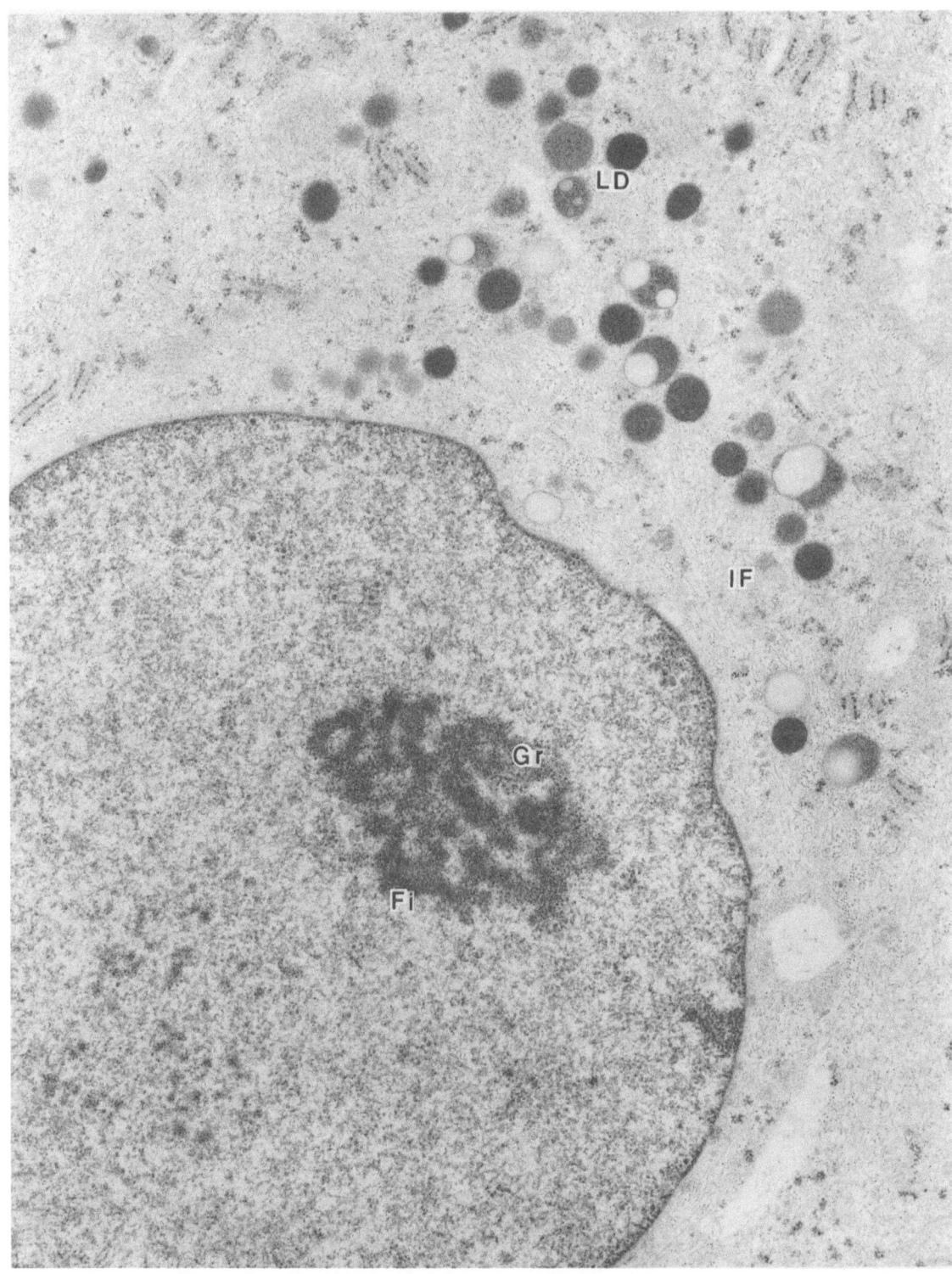

Fig. 3.3. *Subependymal giant cell astrocytoma* (the same case as in Fig. 3.1). The giant cell has a regular round nucleus with reticular nucleolonema in which light granular (*Gr*) and dense filamentous (*Fi*) components can be discerned. Intermediate filaments (*IF*) and lipid droplets (*LD*) are seen in the cytoplasm. × 13 000

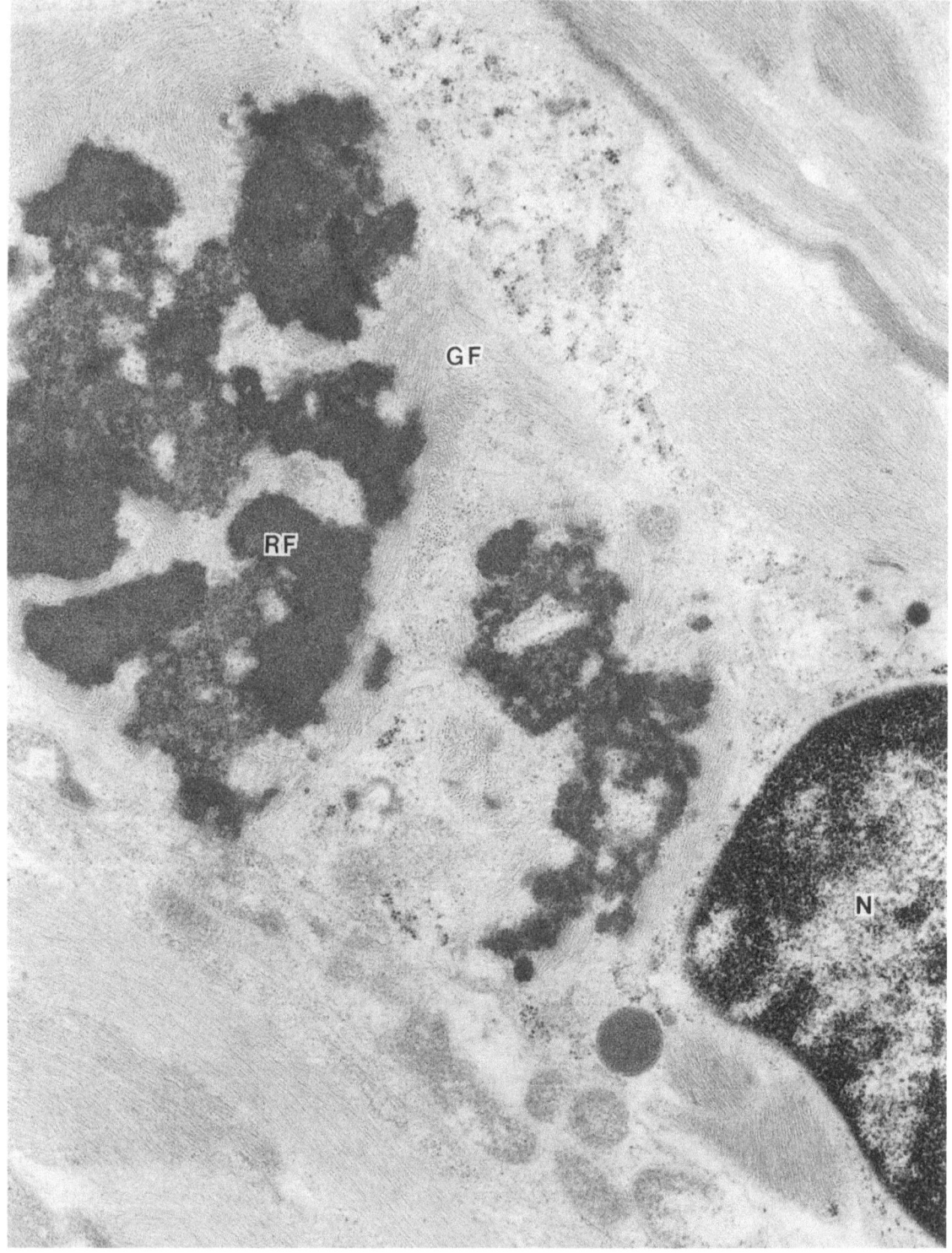

Fig. 3.4. *Subependymal giant cell astrocytoma* (the same case as in Fig. 3.1). The small cell contains Rosenthal fibers (*RF*) associated with abundant glial filaments (*GF*). *N* nucleus. × 25000

4. Anaplastic Astrocytoma

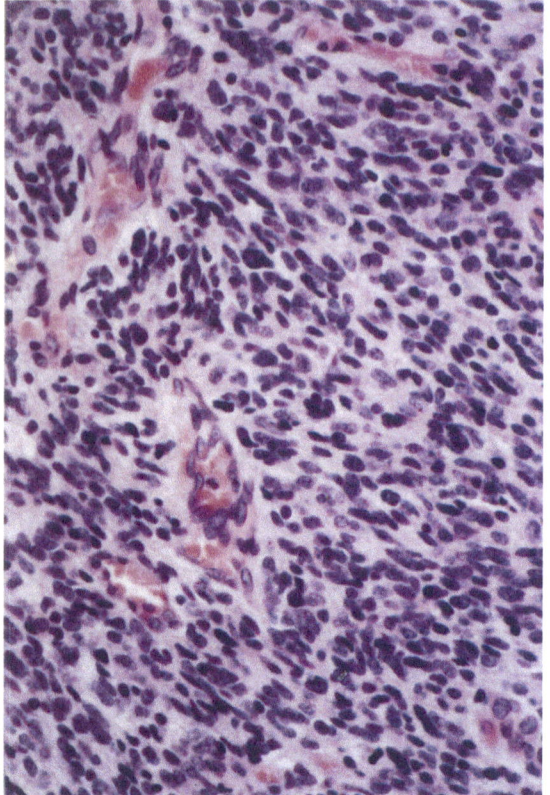

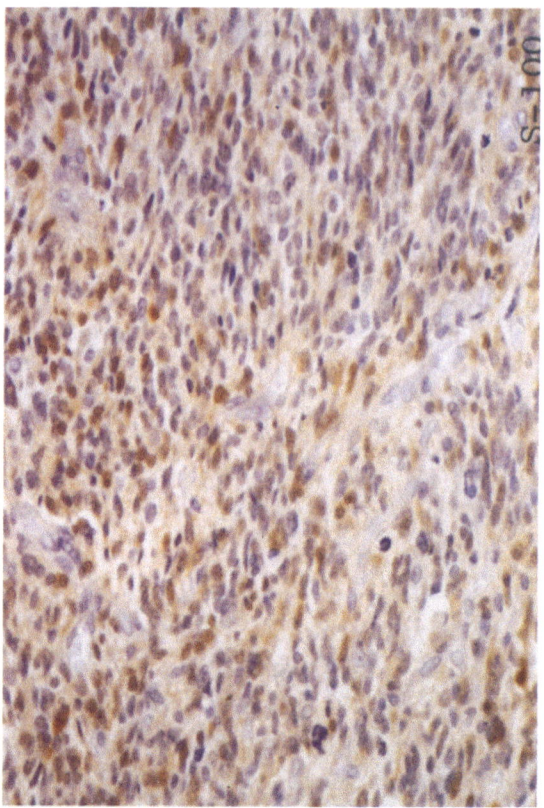

Fig. 4.1. *Anaplastic astrocytoma* of the right parietal lobe in a 52-year-old man. The tumor shows increased cellularity, moderate anaplasia as evident in hyperchromatism, prominent small blood vessels, and no necrosis. H and E, × 180

Fig. 4.2. *Anaplastic astrocytoma* (the same case as in Fig. 4.1). A brown reaction product, indicating positive staining for S-100 protein, is seen in both the cytoplasm and nuclei of most tumor cells, though it is relatively less intense than that of the fibrillary astrocytoma (cf. Fig. 1.2b). Indirect immunoperoxidase method counterstained with hematoxylin, × 180

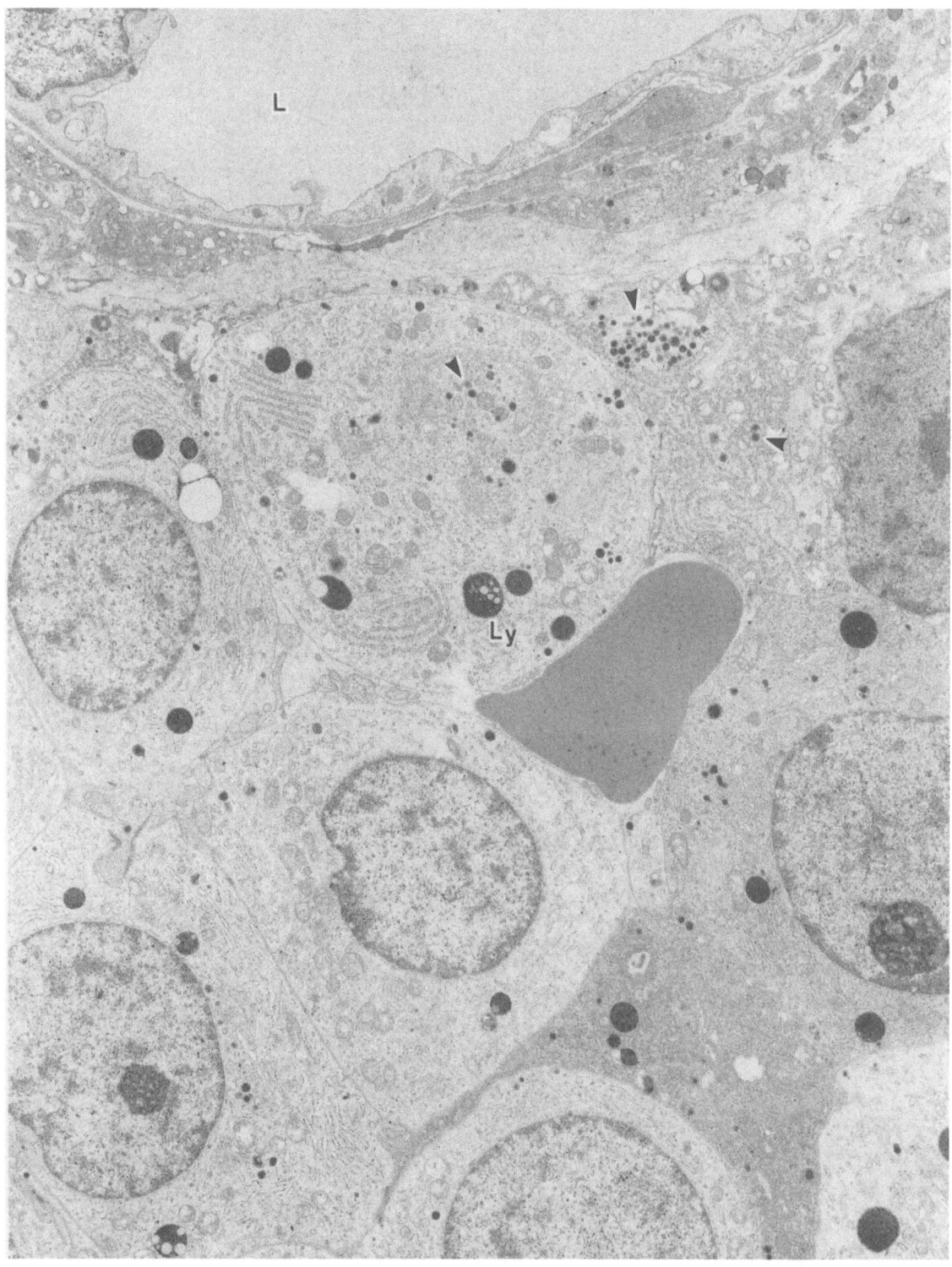

Fig. 4.3. *Anaplastic astrocytoma* (the same case as in Fig. 4.1). At a lower magnification, the tumor cells resemble each other in terms of relatively well-developed organelles, including lysosomes (*Ly*) and small electron-dense granules (*arrowheads*). *L* capillary lumen. × 6500

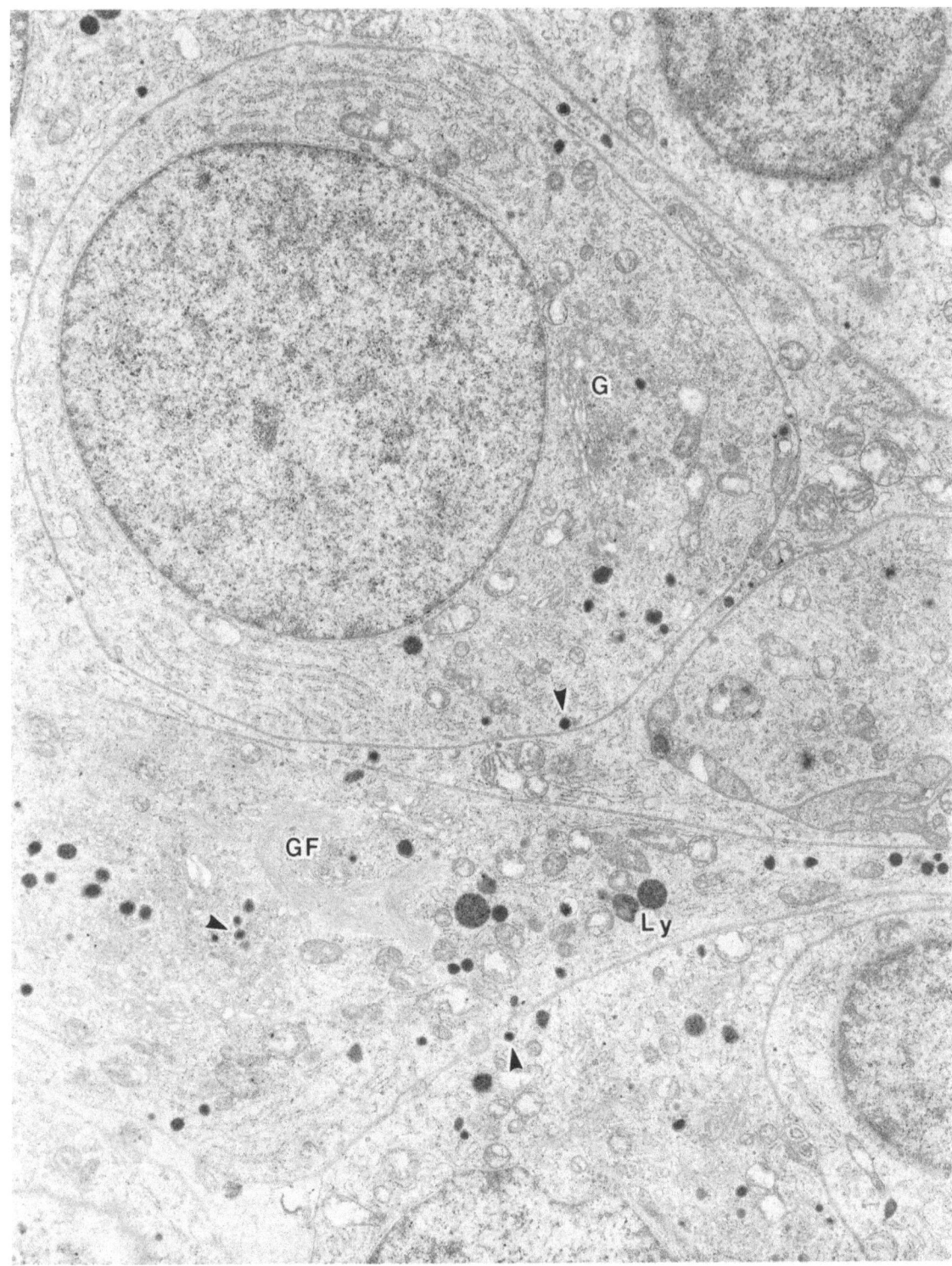

Fig. 4.4. *Anaplastic astrocytoma* (the same case as in Fig. 4.1). The tumor cells with round nuclei have fairly well-developed organelles and unusual small electron-dense granules (*arrowheads*) in addition to lysosomes (*Ly*) and occasional glial filaments (*GF*). There is no intercellular junctional apparatus. *G* Golgi apparatus. × 8500

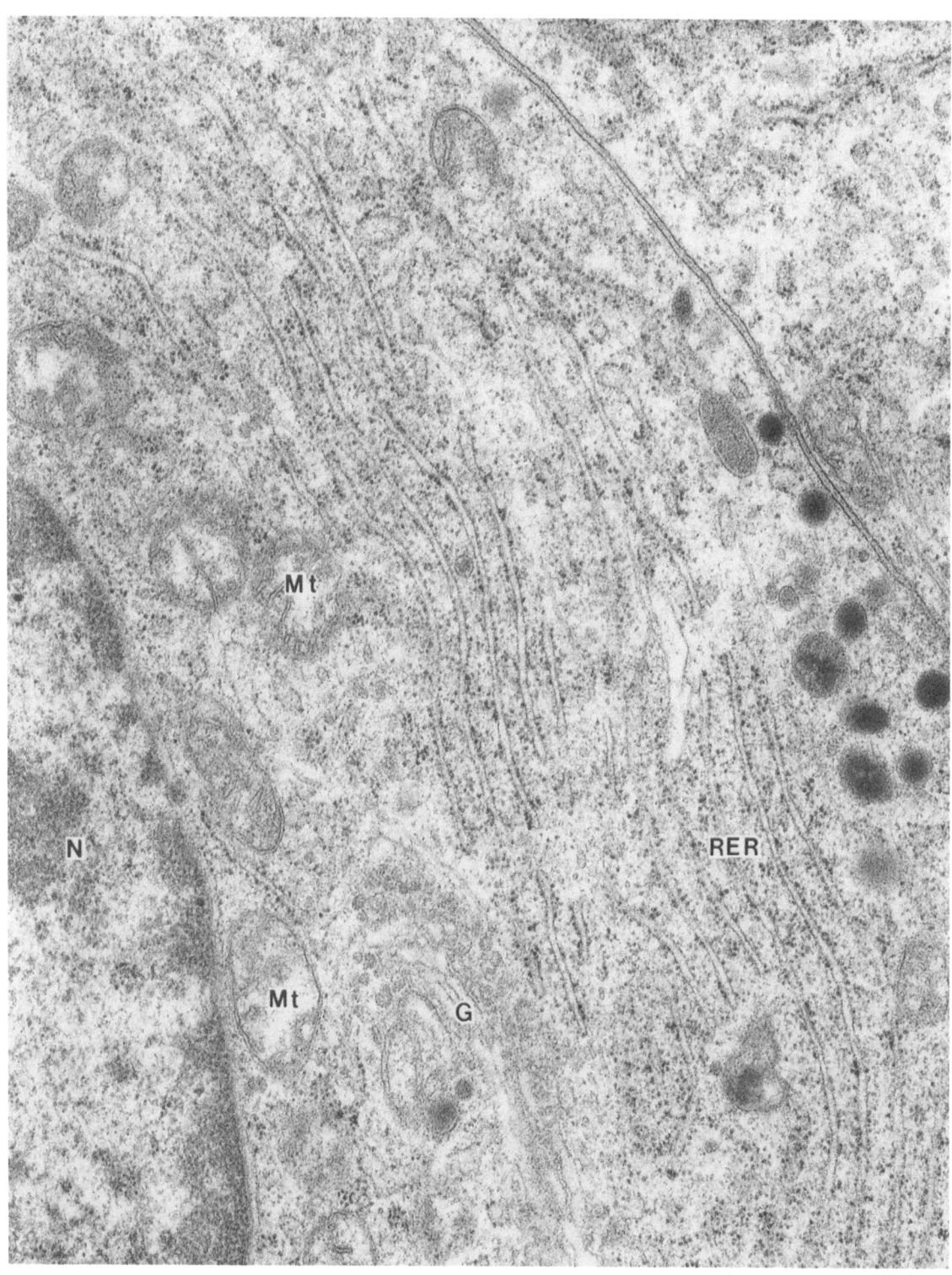

Fig. 4.5. *Anaplastic astrocytoma* (the same case as in Fig. 4.1). There are relatively well-developed organelles, including rough endoplasmic reticulum (*RER*), mitochondria (*Mt*), Golgi apparatus (*G*), and unusual electron-dense granules. *N* nucleus. × 34 000

5. Oligodendroglioma

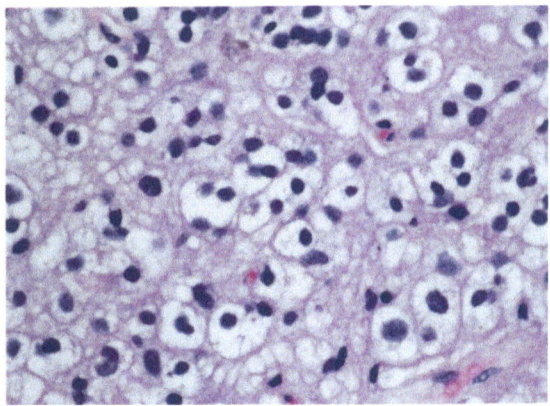

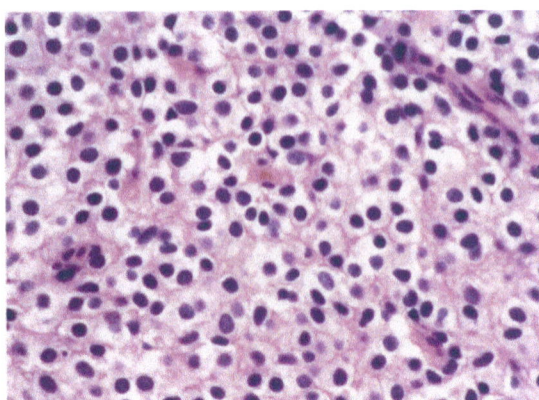

Fig. 5.1. *Oligodendroglioma* of the right frontal lobe in a 52-year-old woman. The tumor cells are characterized by prominent perinuclear cytoplasmic halos and slight nuclear pleomorphism. H and E, × 160

Fig. 5.2. *Oligodendroglioma* of the right frontal lobe in a 30-year-old man. The tumor is composed of densely packed cells with perinuclear cytoplasmic halos. H and E, × 160

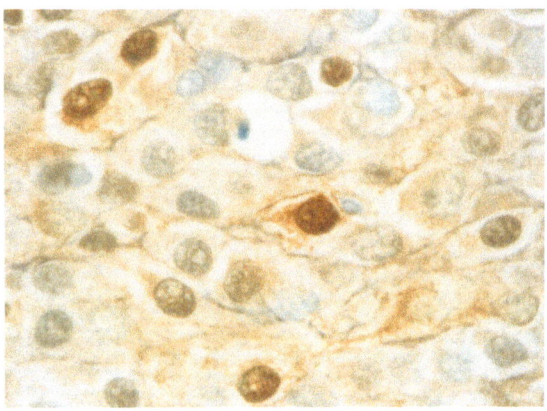

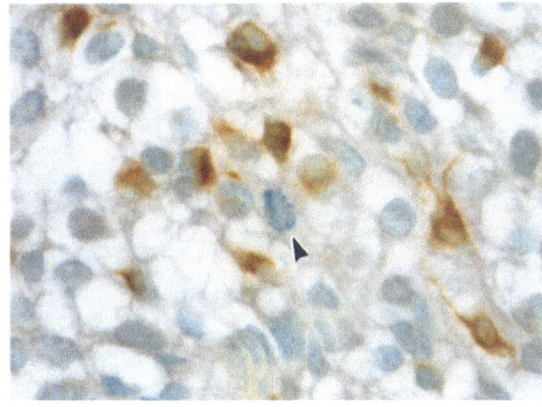

Fig. 5.3. *Oligodendroglioma* (the same case as in Fig. 5.2). A positive reaction for S-100 protein is observed both in the nuclei and cytoplasm of some cells. Peroxidase antiperoxidase method counterstained with methyl green, × 320

Fig. 5.4. *Oligodendroglioma* (the same case as in Fig. 5.2). Glial fibrillary acidic protein (GFAP) is localized in the cytoplasm of some cells. The *arrowhead* indicates a cell in mitosis. Peroxidase antiperoxidase method counterstained with methyl green, × 320

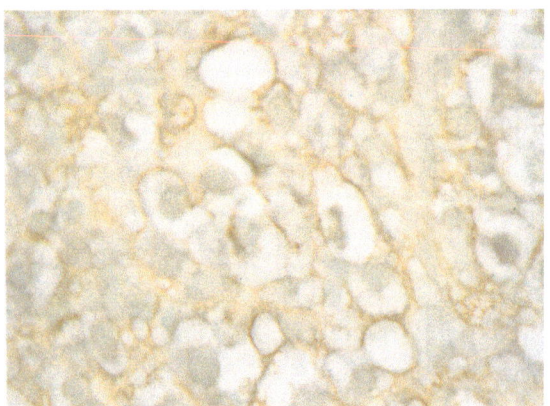

Fig. 5.5. *Oligodendroglioma* (the same case as in Fig. 5.2). A weak, but unequivocally positive staining is revealed on the cell surfaces following reaction with anti-Leu 7 mouse monoclonal antibody. Peroxidase antiperoxidase method counterstained with methyl green, × 320

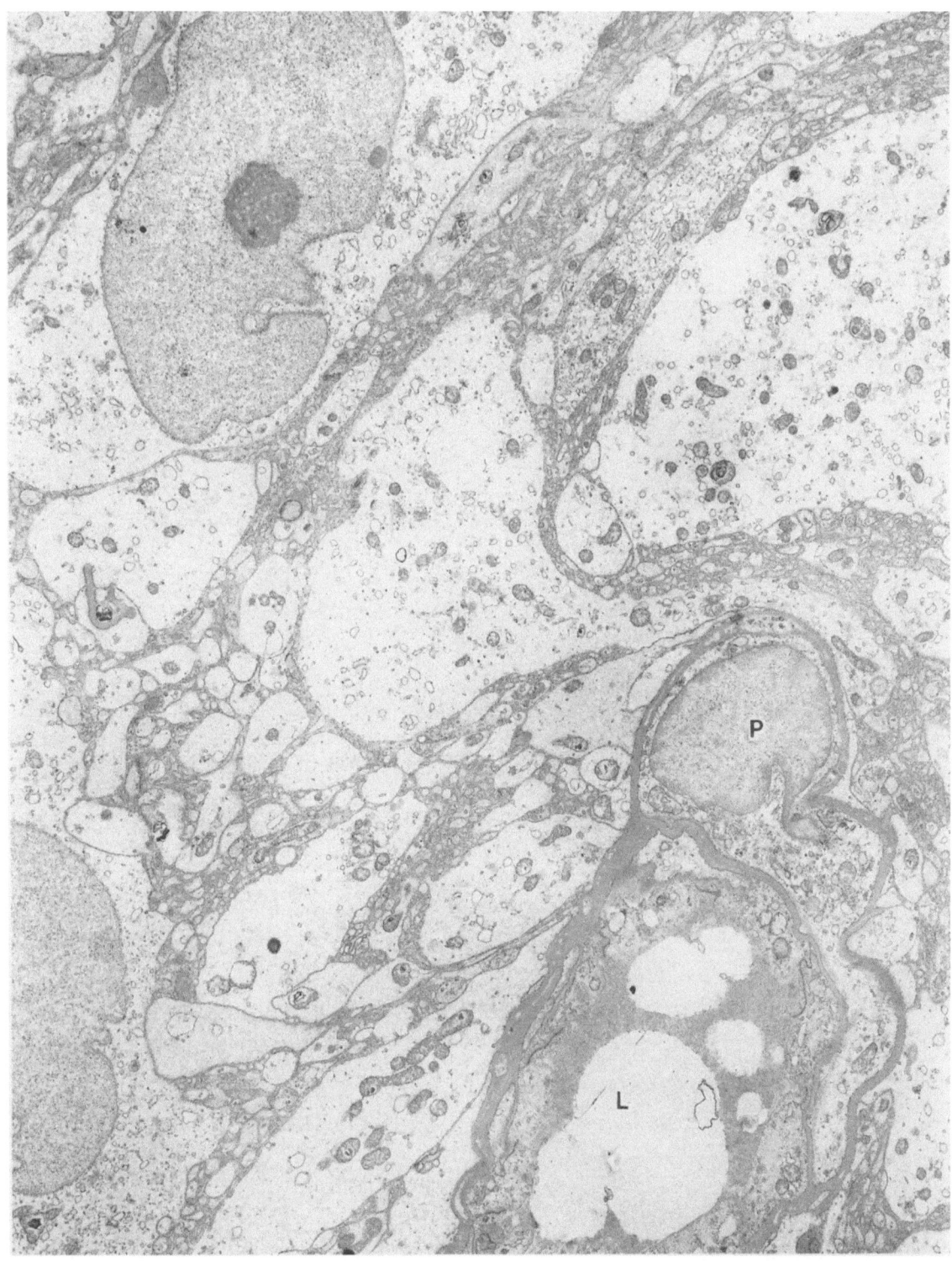

Fig. 5.6. *Oligodendroglioma* (the same case as in Fig. 5.1). The watery appearance of the well-defined cytoplasm of formalin-fixed tumor cells coincides with the perinuclear cytoplasmic halos seen under the light microscope. *L* capillary lumen, *P* pericyte. × 5800

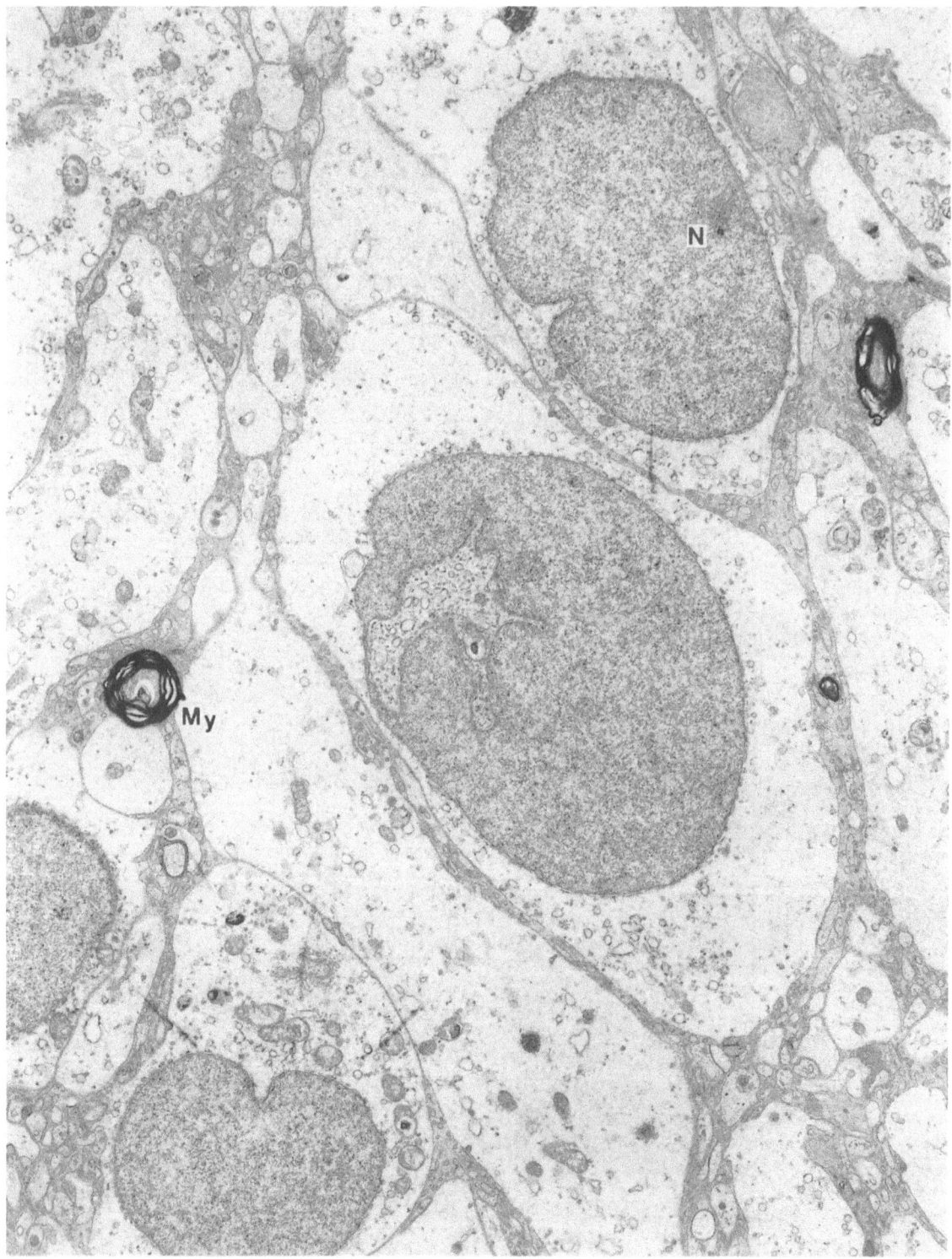

Fig. 5.7. *Oligodendroglioma* (the same case as in Fig. 5.1). Irregular nuclear shapes and aberrant myelin (*My*) are sometimes observed. *N* nucleus. Fixed with formalin, × 7700

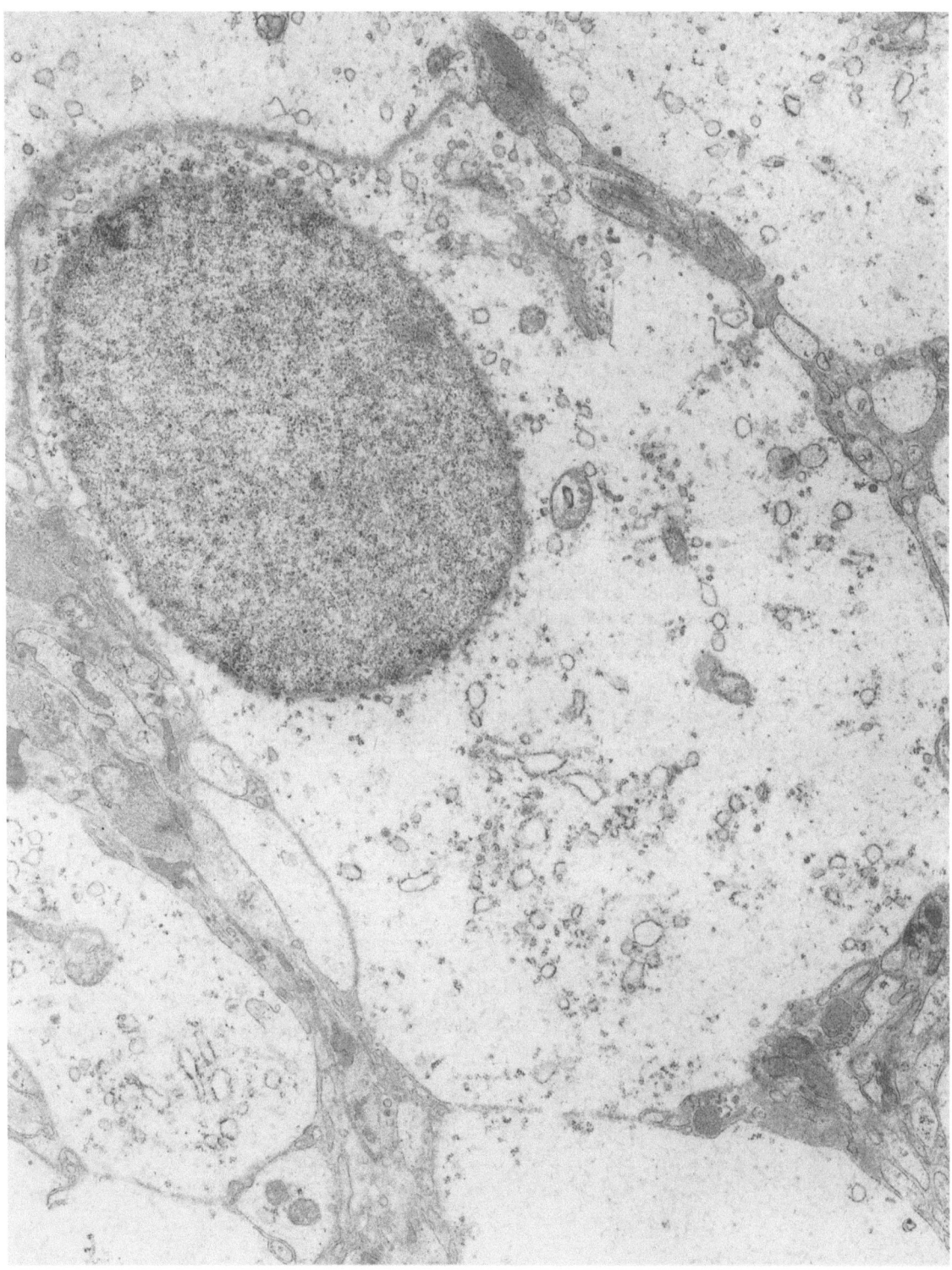

Fig. 5.8. *Oligodendroglioma* (the same case as in Fig. 5.1). Higher magnification of a typical tumor cell discloses the lack of organelles and intercellular junctions. Fixed with formalin, × 13 000

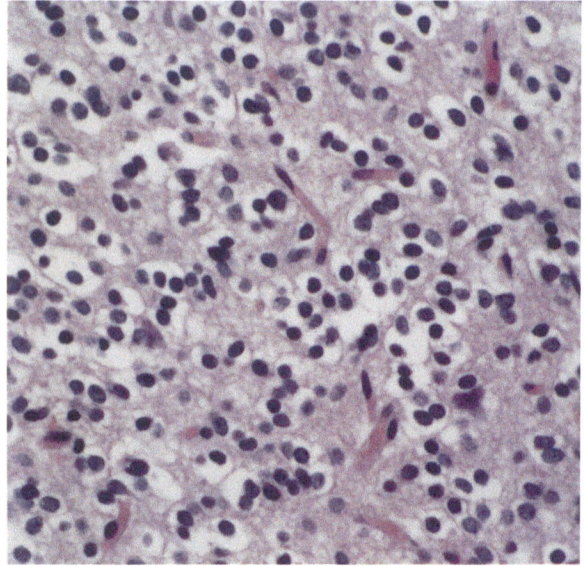

a

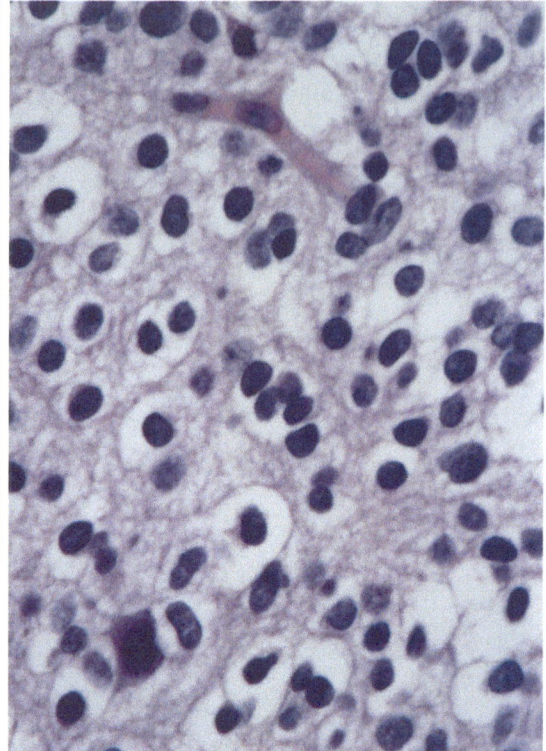

b

Fig. 5.9a, b. *Oligodendroglioma* of the right temporal lobe in a 54-year-old man. The tumor cells have round nuclei, which are surrounded by clear cytoplasm enclosed with well-defined membranes. Some thin-walled blood vessels are also visible. H and E; **a** × 180, **b** × 360

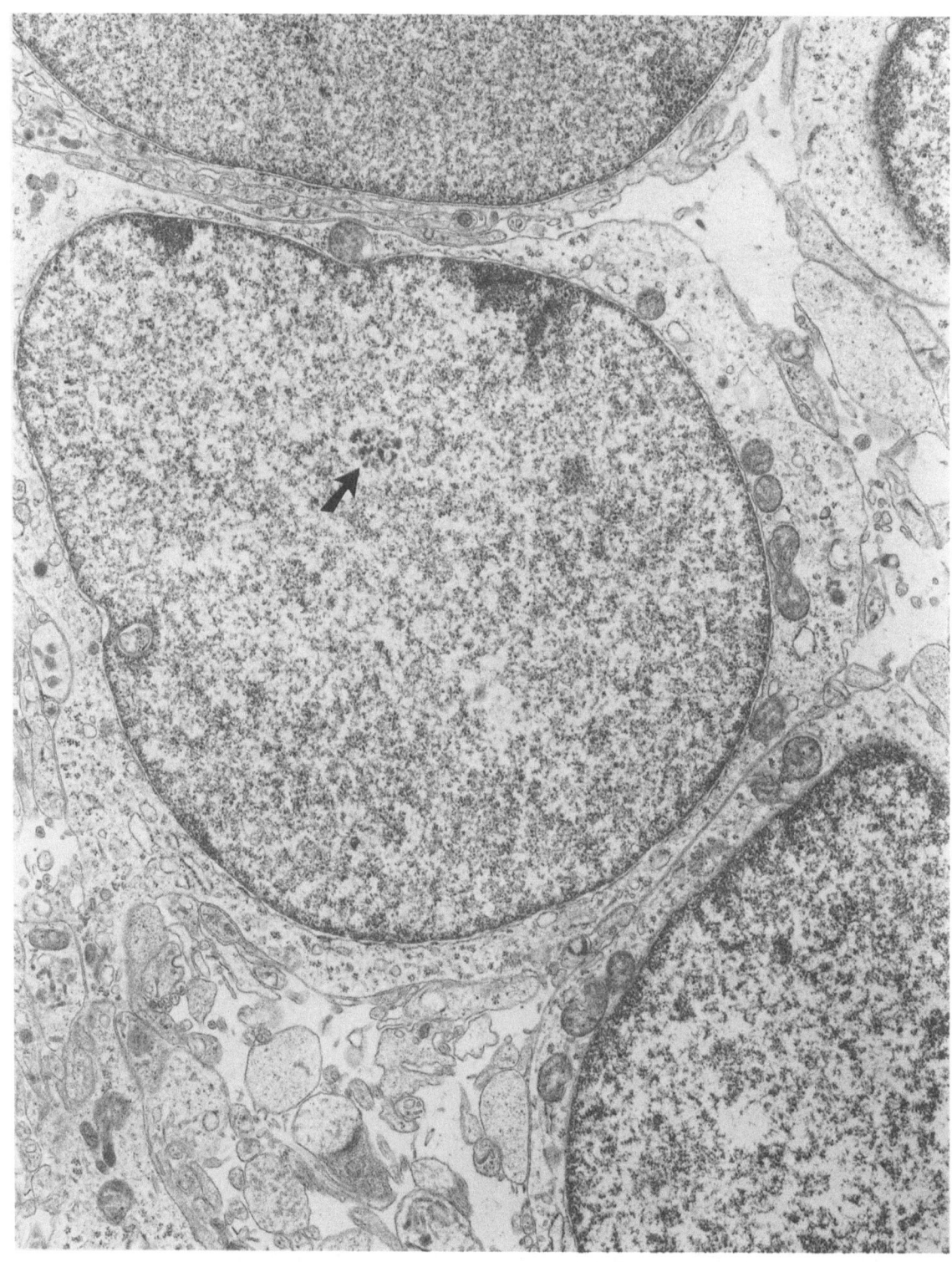

Fig. 5.10. *Oligodendroglioma* (the same case as in Fig. 5.9). The tumor cells reveal relatively well-preserved narrow cytoplasm, regular nuclei with scattered euchromatin, and an occasional nuclear body (*arrow*). × 14 000

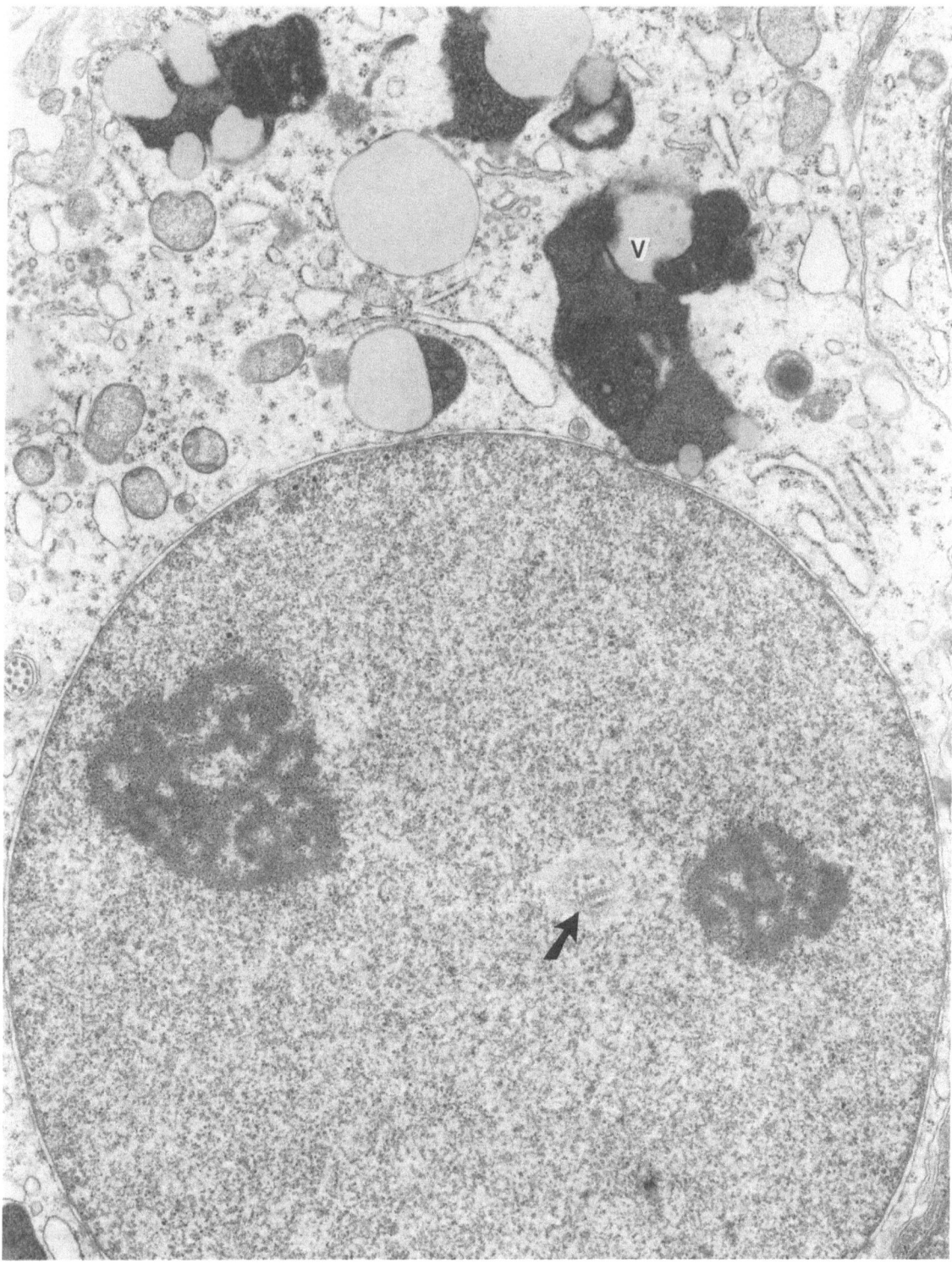

Fig. 5.11. *Oligodendroglioma* (the same case as in Fig. 5.9). A typical tumor cell has a round nucleus with nucleoli and relatively well-preserved cytoplasm with autophagic vacuoles (*V*). The *arrow* indicates a nuclear body. × 20 000

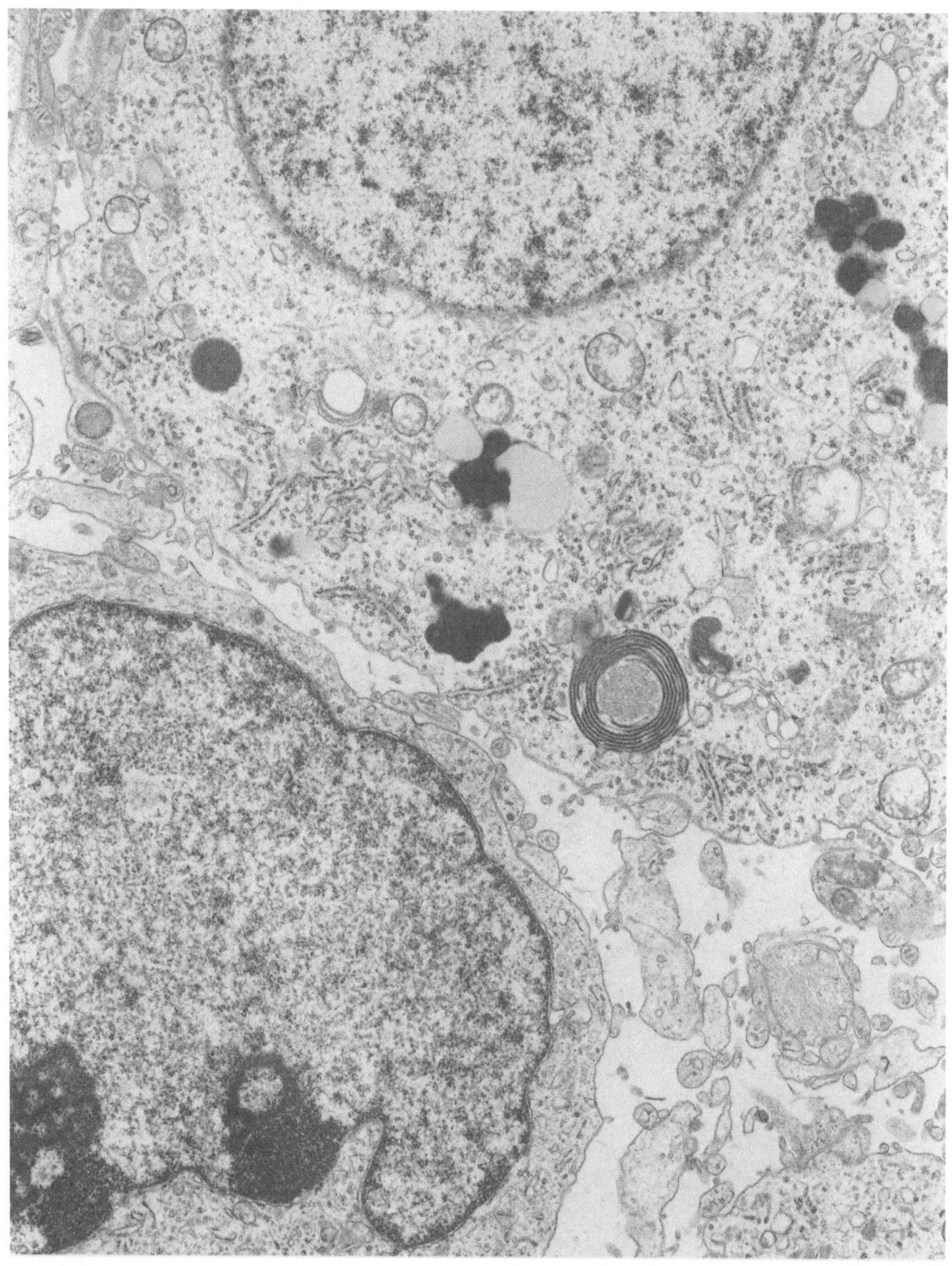

Fig. 5.12. *Oligodendroglioma* (the same case as in Fig. 5.9). A laminated membranous structure as well as autophagic vacuoles are seen in the cytoplasm of a tumor cell. × 13 000

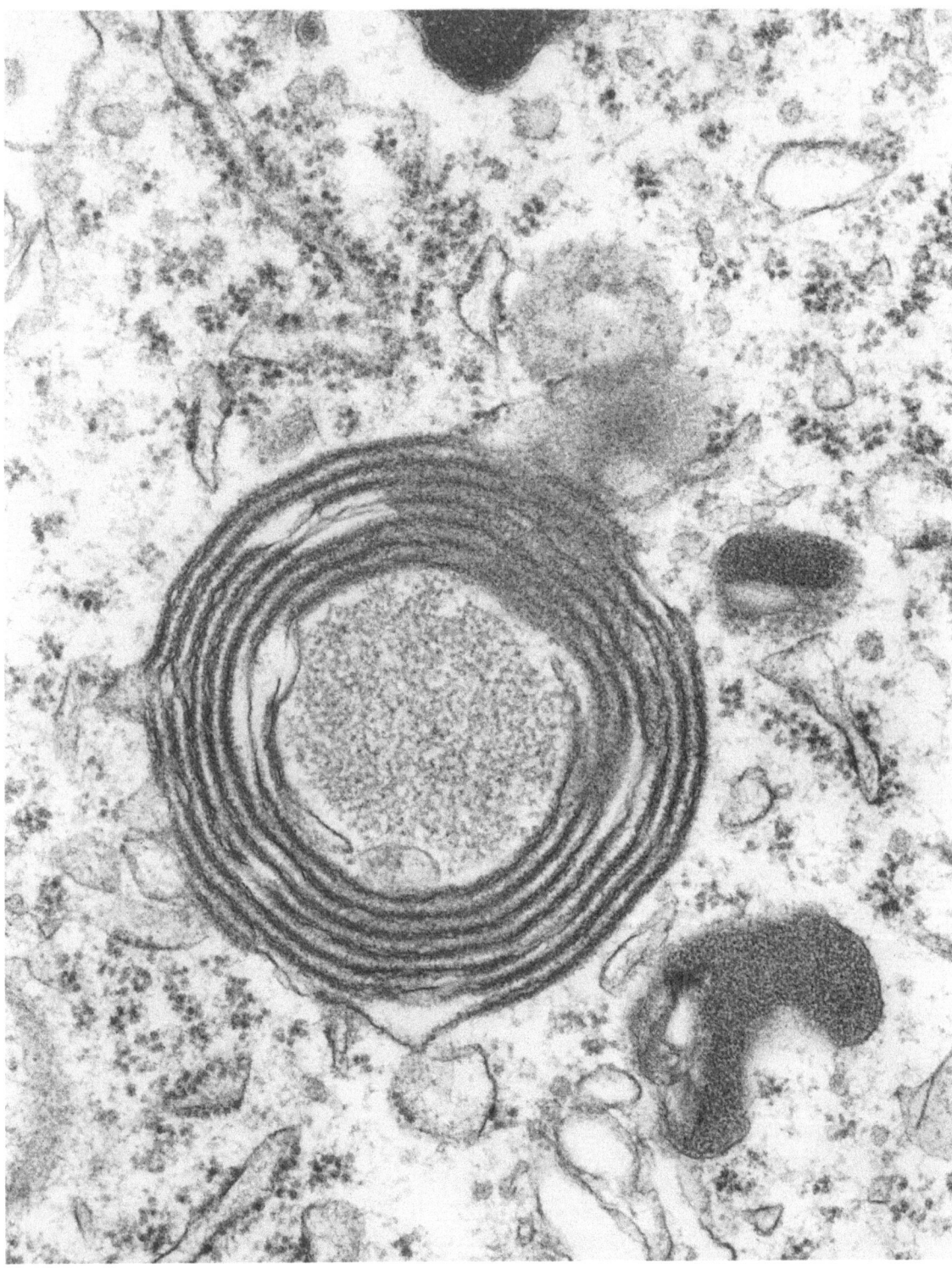

Fig. 5.13. *Oligodendroglioma* (the same case as in Fig. 5.9). Higher magnification shows the details of a laminated membranous structure surrounding the amorphous substance. × 76000

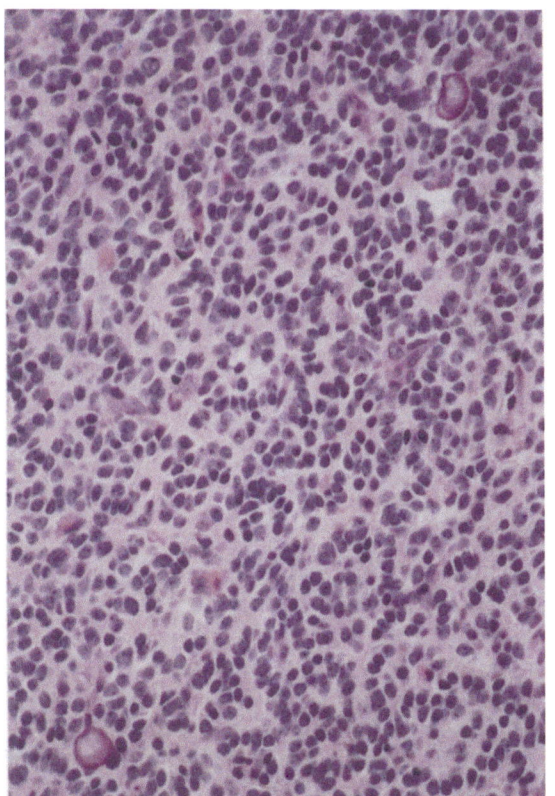

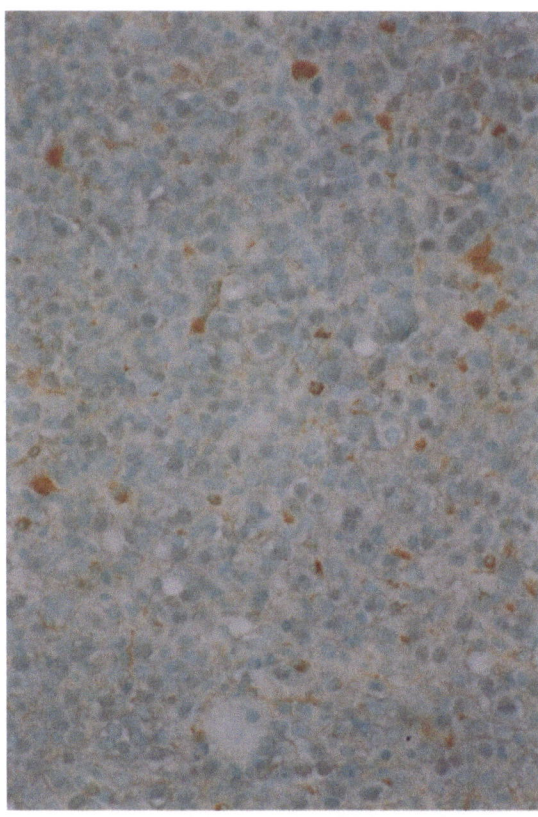

Fig. 5.14. *Oligodendroglioma* of the left frontal lobe in a 42-year-old woman. The tumor consists of cells with round to oval nuclei. A perinuclear halo is not evident in this area. Note some calcospherites. H and E, × 180

Fig. 5.15. *Oligodendroglioma* (the same case as in Fig. 5.14). A few cells show positive staining for GFAP. Peroxidase antiperoxidase method counterstained with methyl green, × 180

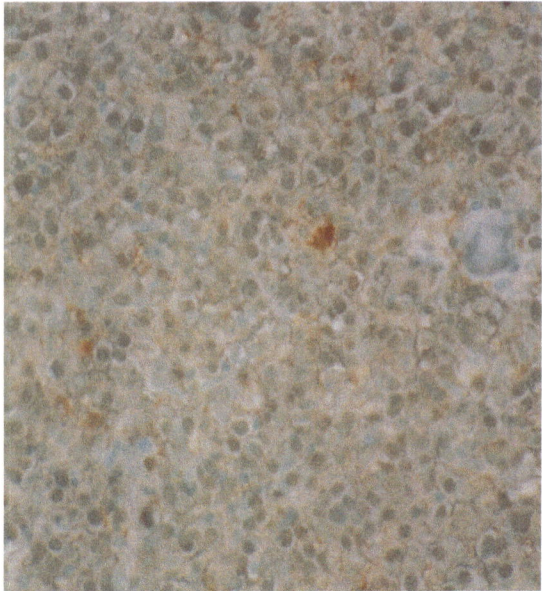

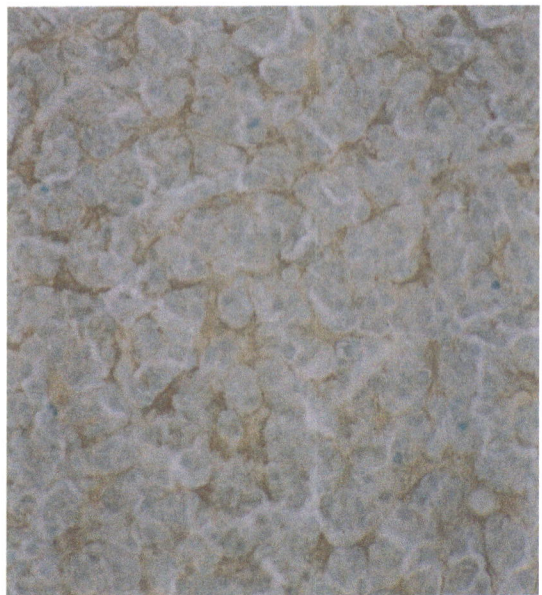

Fig. 5.16. *Oligodendroglioma* (the same case as in Fig. 5.14). A weak, but unequivocally positive reaction for S-100 protein is discernible in both the cytoplasm and nuclei of most tumor cells. Peroxidase antiperoxidase method counterstained with methyl green, × 180

Fig. 5.17. *Oligodendroglioma* (the same case as in Fig. 5.14). A faint, but unequivocally positive reaction is localized among the tumor cells after incubation with anti-Leu 7 mouse monoclonal antibody. Peroxidase antiperoxidase method counterstained with methyl green, × 180

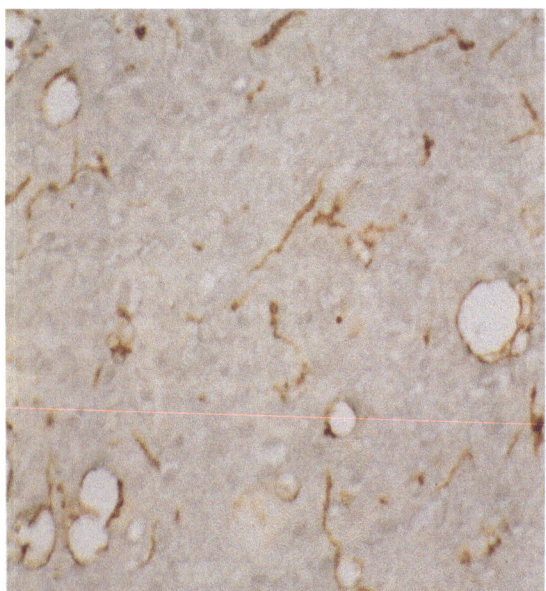

Fig. 5.18. *Oligodendroglioma* (the same case as in Fig. 5.14). Sporadic positive staining for myelin basic protein (*MBP*) is observed throughout the section. Peroxidase antiperoxidase method counterstained with methyl green, × 180

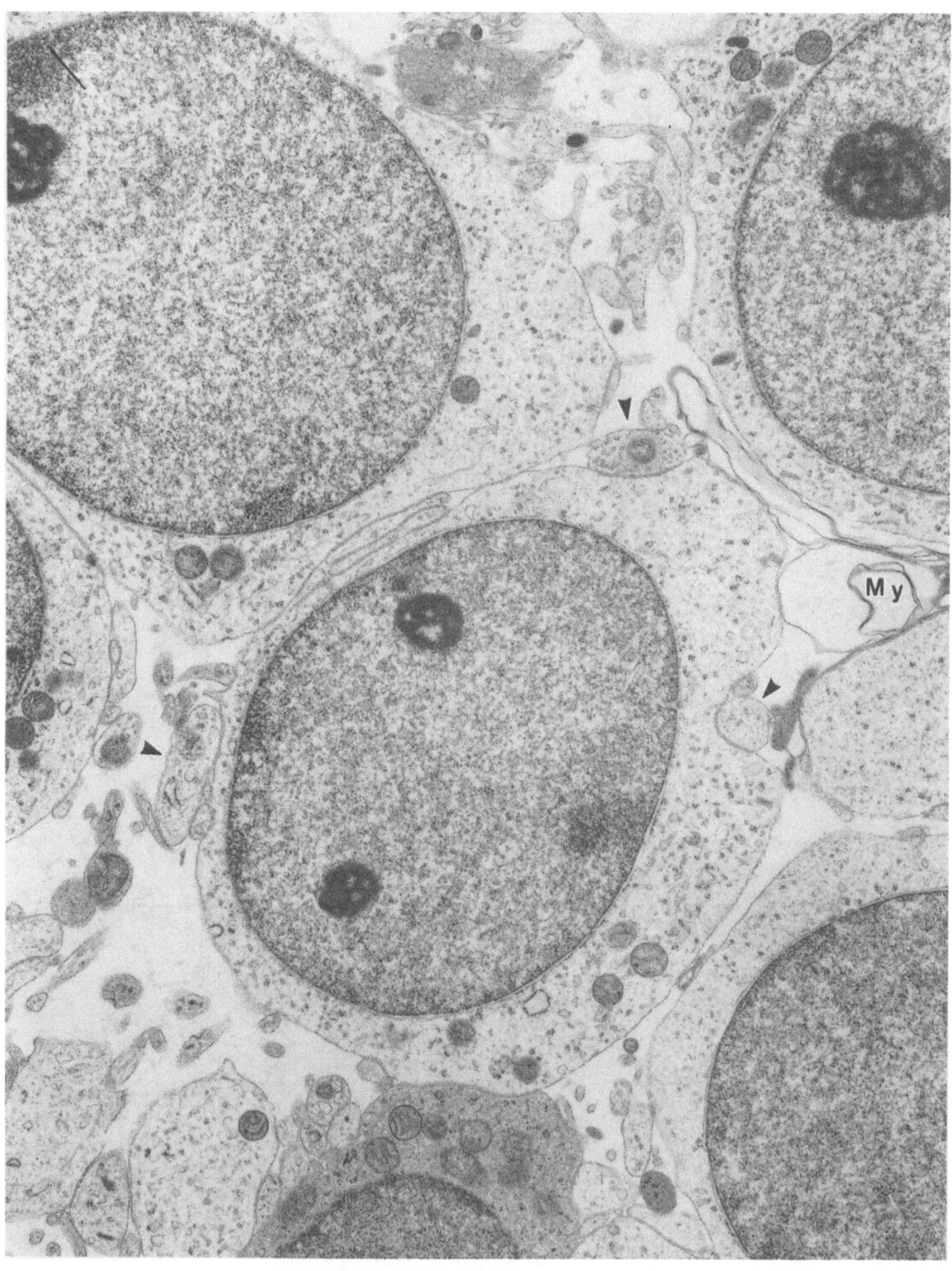

Fig. 5.19. *Oligodendroglioma* (the same case as in Fig. 5.14). The tumor cells have round nuclei with prominent nucleoli and clear cytoplasm with scanty organelles. Transversely sectioned cytoplasmic processes (*arrowheads*) and aberrant myelin (*My*) are discernible. × 12 700

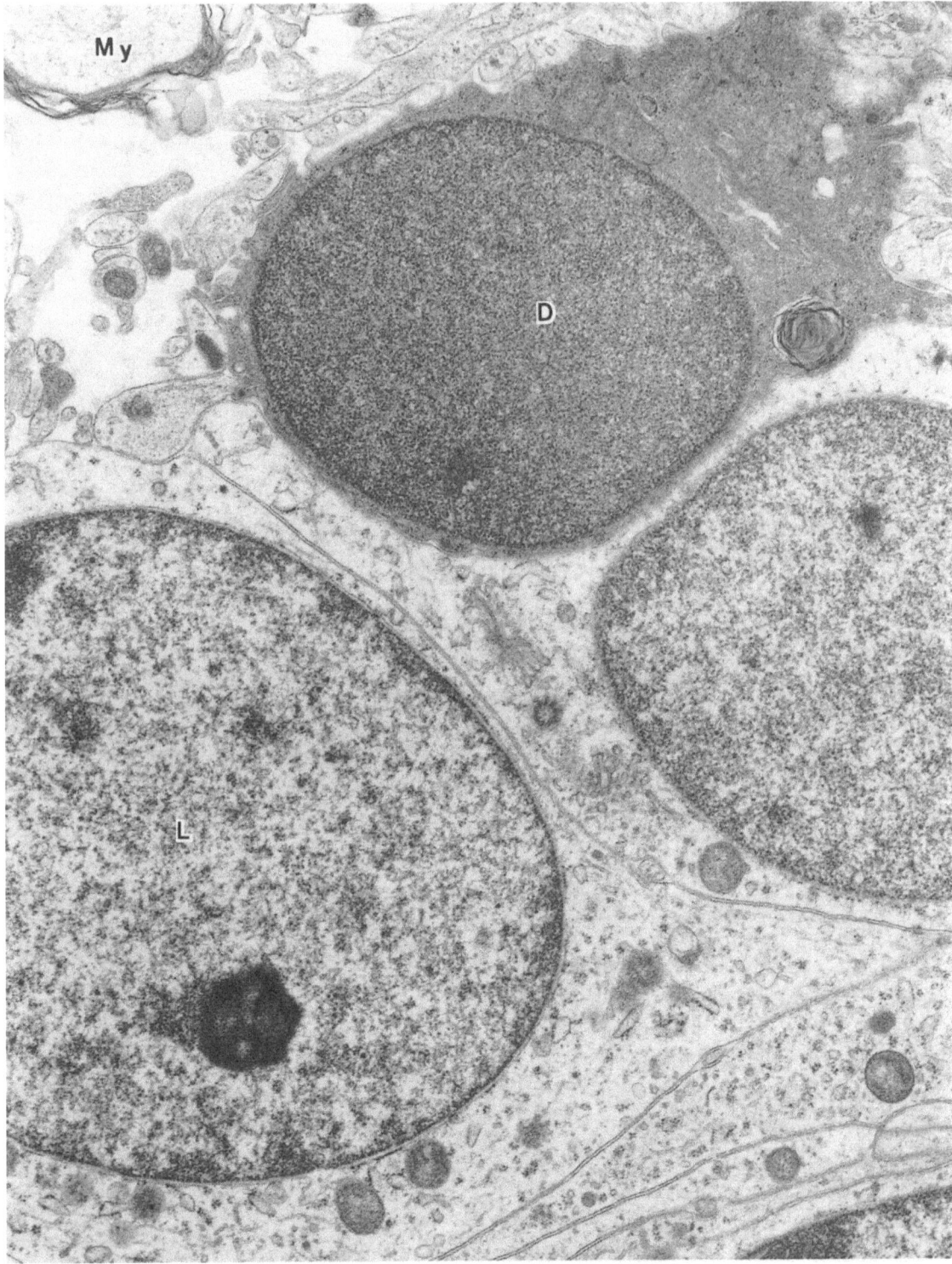

Fig. 5.20. *Oligodendroglioma* (the same case as in Fig. 5.14). A dark tumor cell (*D*) is commonly found among light tumor cells (*L*). No intercellular junctional apparatus is seen. *My* aberrant myelin. × 16 000

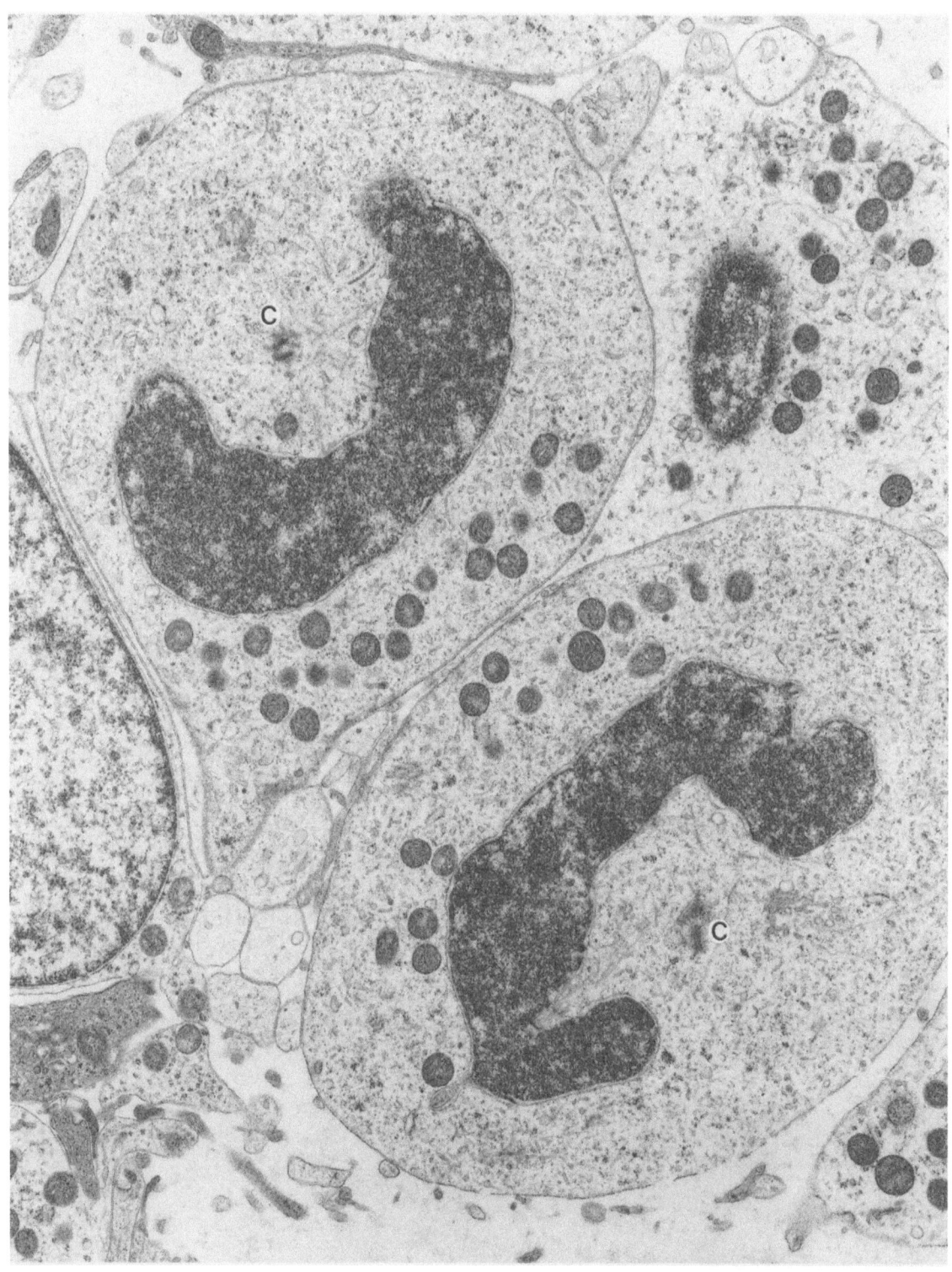

Fig. 5.21. *Oligodendroglioma* (the same case as in Fig. 5.14). Two daughter cells are completed shortly after cytokinesis. *C* centriole. × 14 000

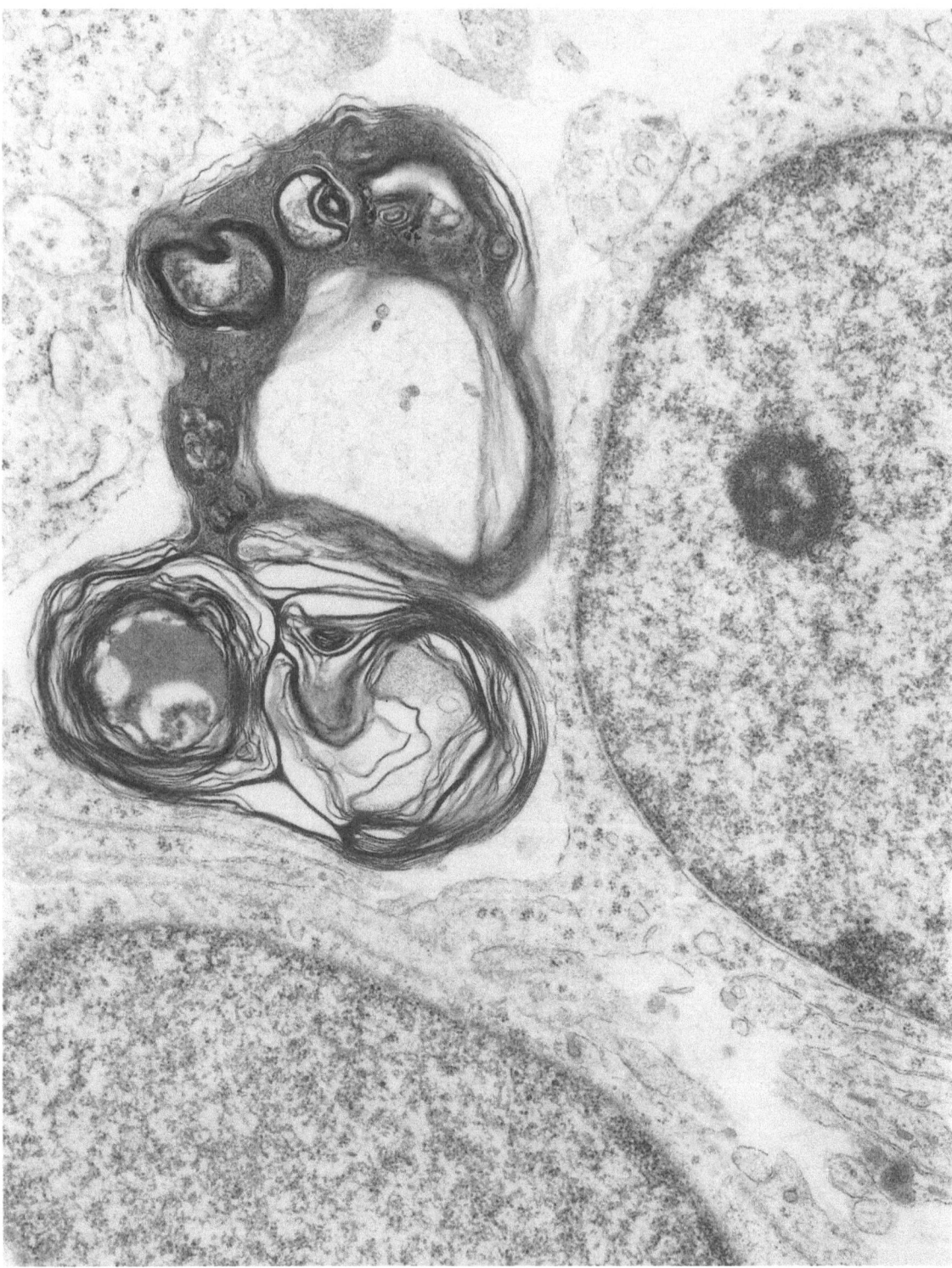

Fig. 5.22. *Oligodendroglioma* (the same case as in Fig. 5.14). Strange configurations of myelin surround the amorphous substance instead of the axon. × 24 600

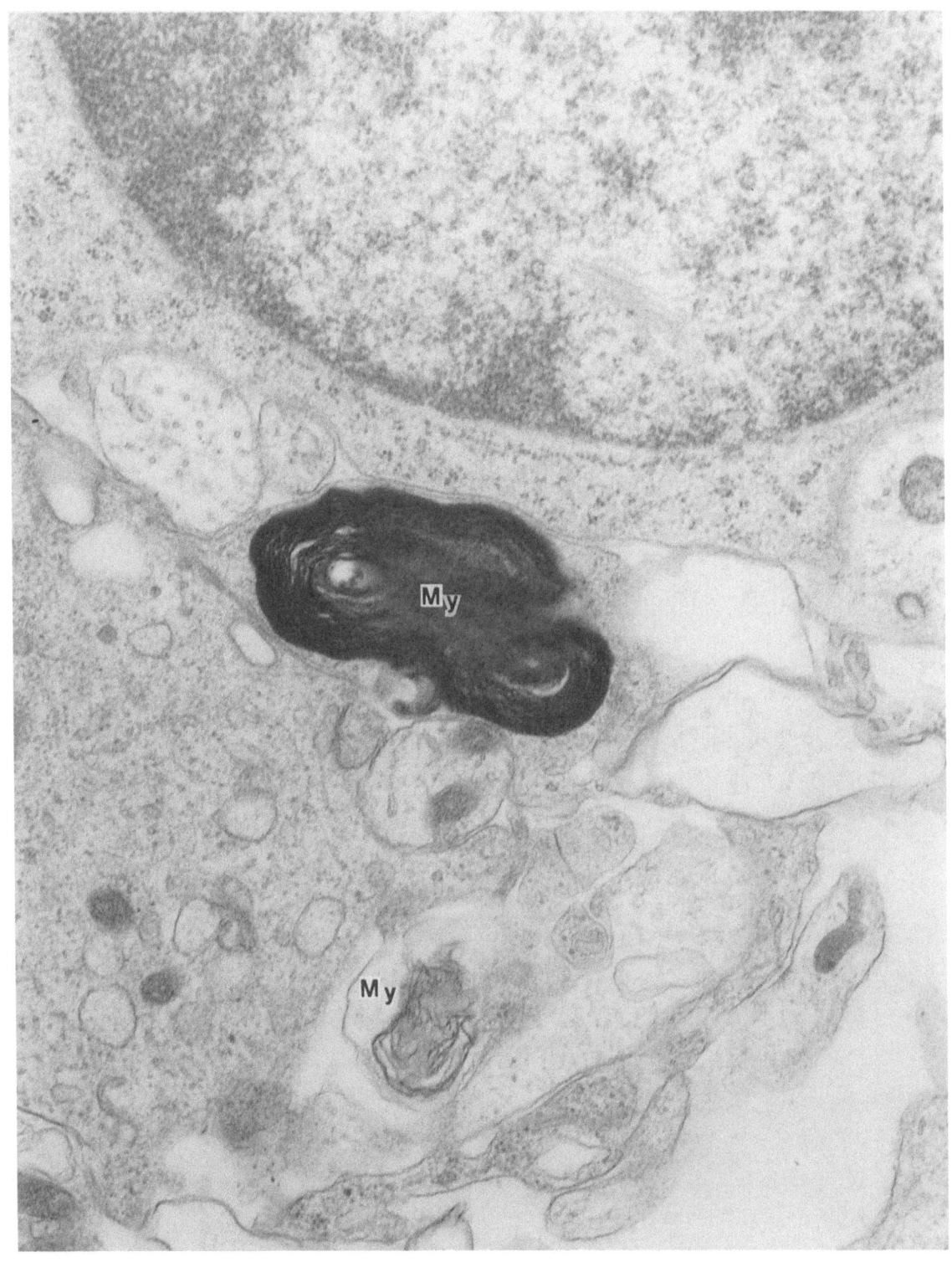

Fig. 5.23. *Oligodendroglioma* (the same case as in Fig. 5.14). Aberrant myelin (*My*) indicates a close correlation between this tumor and oligodendrocytes. × 38 500

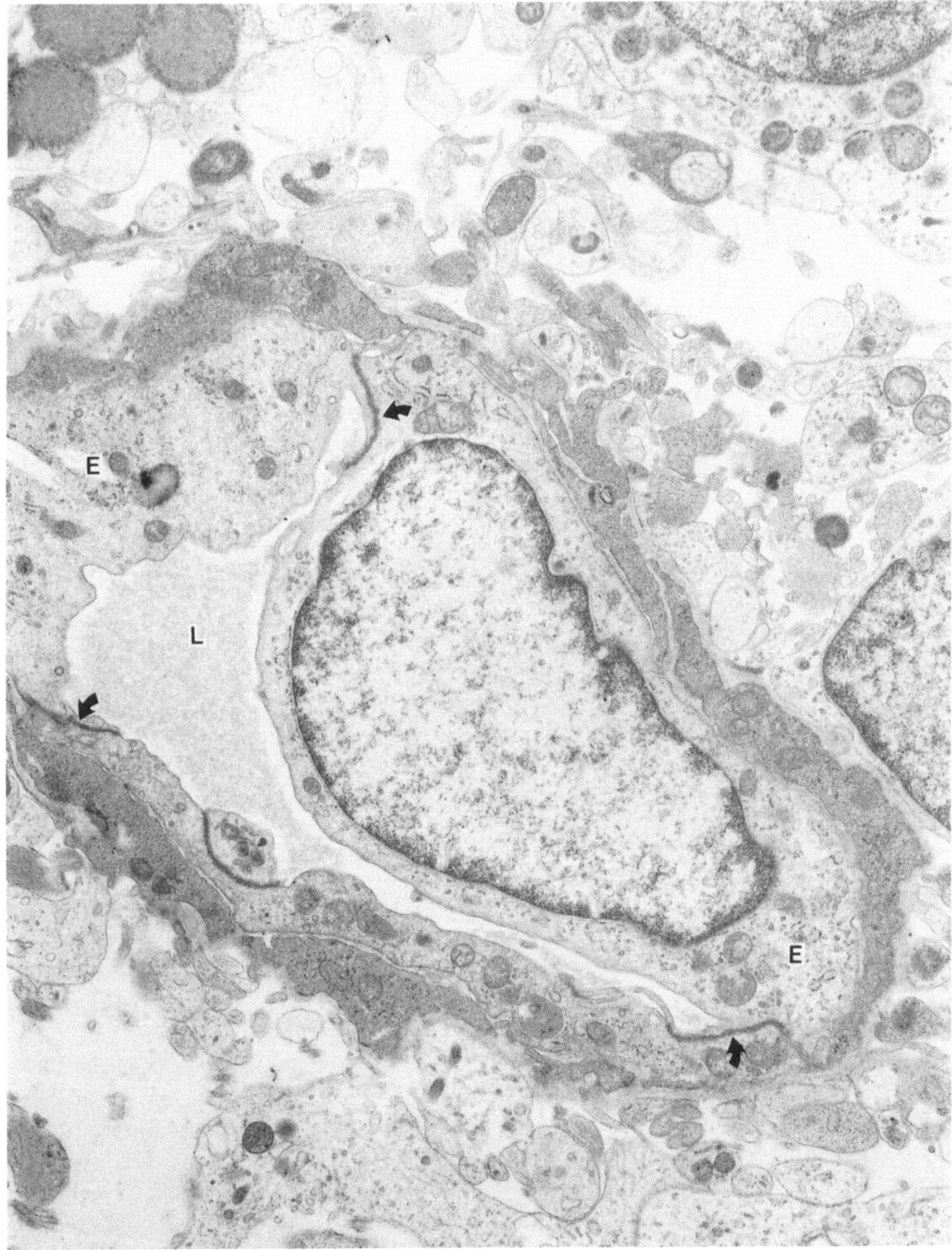

Fig. 5.24. A capillary in *oligodendroglioma* (the same case as in Fig. 5.14). Tight junctions (*arrows*) are seen between endothelial cells (*E*). *L* capillary lumen. × 12 700

6. Ependymoma

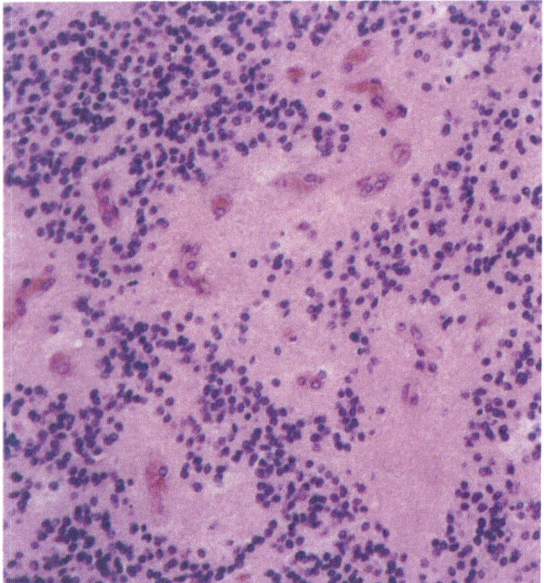

Fig. 6.1. *Ependymoma* of the fourth ventricle in a 5-year-old girl. The tumor consists of polygonal cells with very granular round nuclei, forming zones of high nuclear density and anuclear perivascular sleeves. H and E, × 90

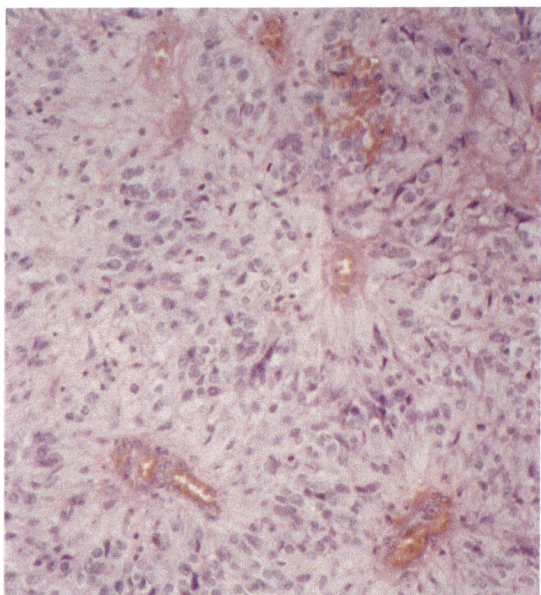

Fig. 6.2. *Ependymoma* of the left lateral ventricle in a 40-year-old man. The tumor is characterized by perivascular arrangement of the cells with long cytoplasmic processes attaching to the wall of blood vessels (pseudorosettes). H and E, × 180

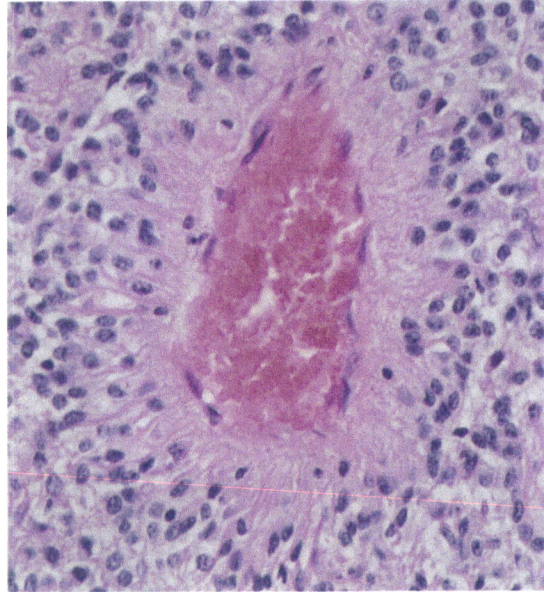

Fig. 6.3. *Ependymoma* (the same case as in Fig. 6.2). Delicately fibrillated cells form a radial pattern around a blood vessel. H and E, × 360

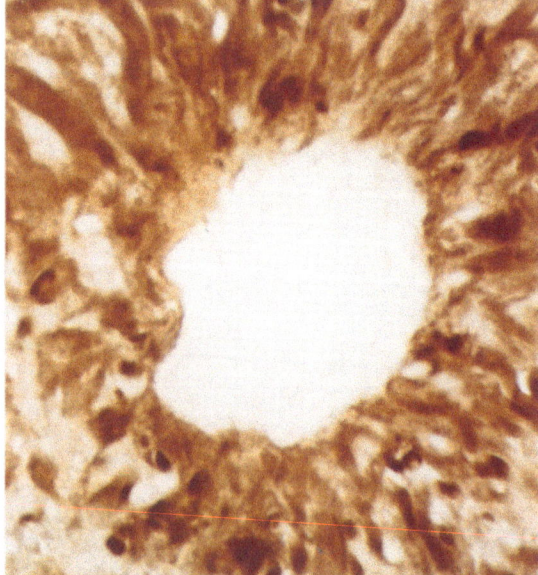

Fig. 6.4. *Ependymoma* (the same case as in Fig. 6.2). The fibrillated cells forming pseudorosettes are intensely positive for S-100 protein, Indirect immunoperoxidase method without counterstain, × 360

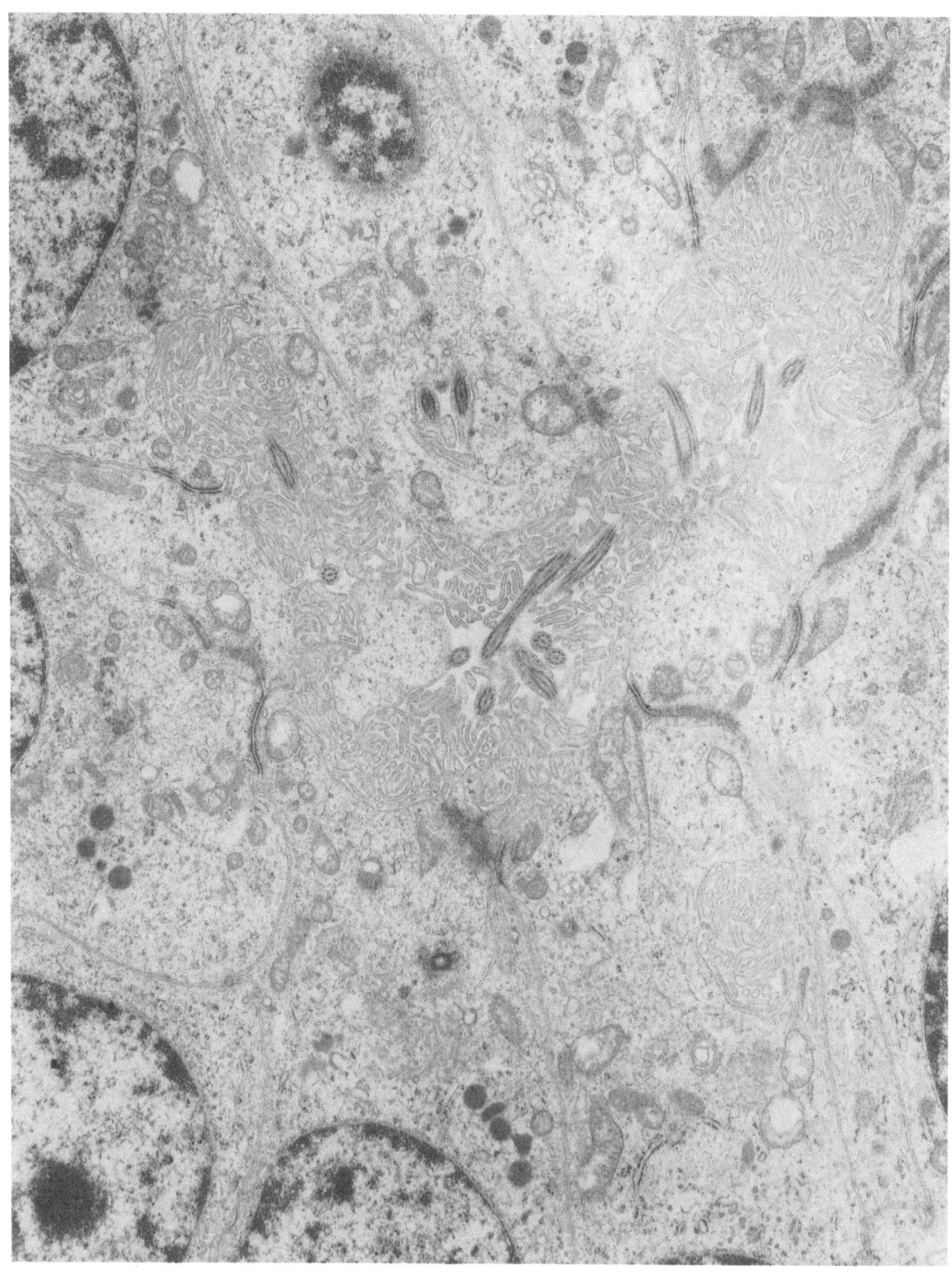

Fig. 6.5. *Ependymoma* (the same case as in Fig. 6.1). Many cilia and microvilli fill the lumen of an ependymal rosette. Intercellular junctional appratus are prominent near the luminal surfaces of tumor cells. × 10 000

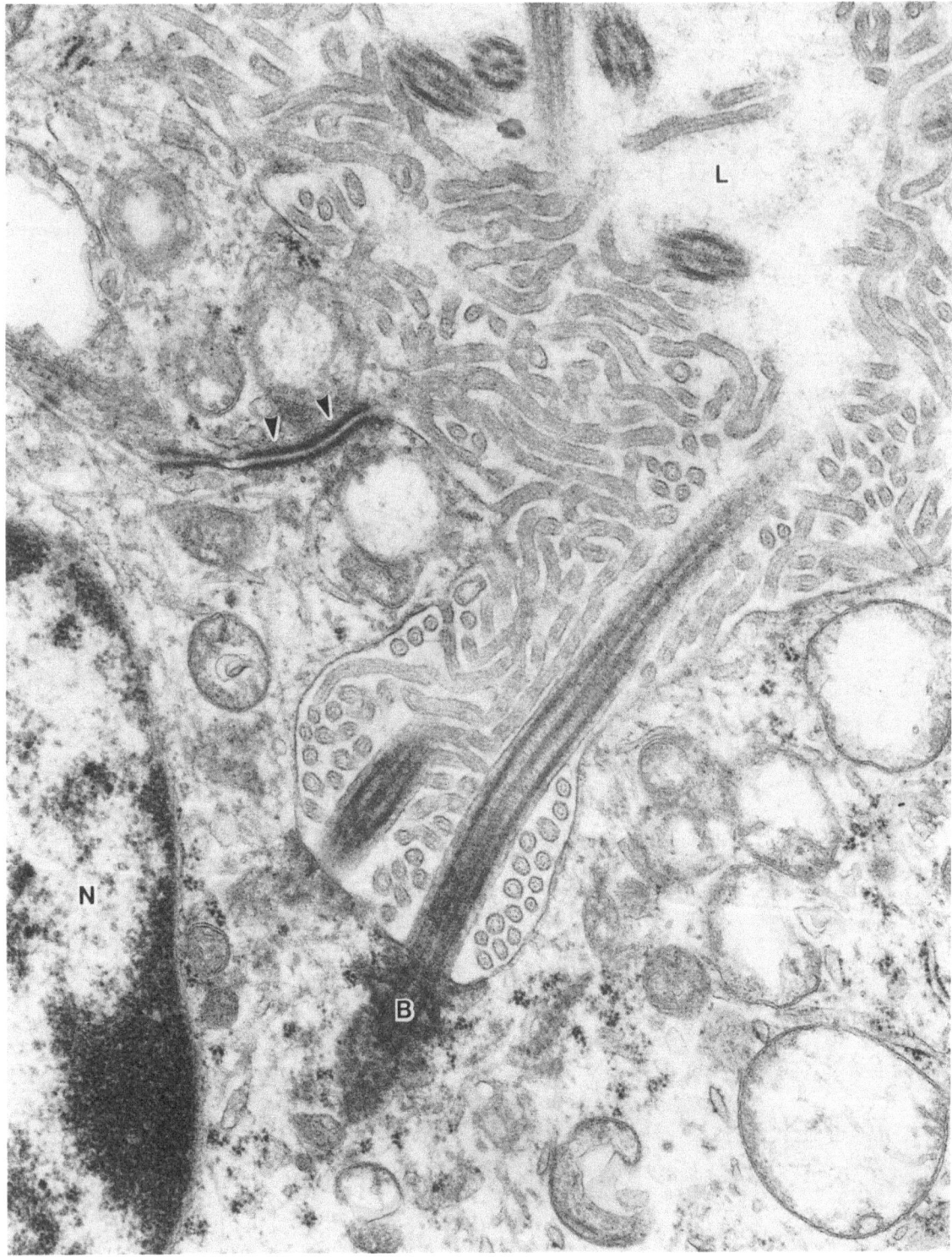

Fig. 6.6. *Ependymoma* (the same case as in Fig. 6.1). Higher magnification reveals details of the junctional apparatus (*arrowheads*), cilia, and microvilli in the lumen (*L*) of an ependymal rosette. *B* basal body of cilium, *N* nucleus. × 38 400

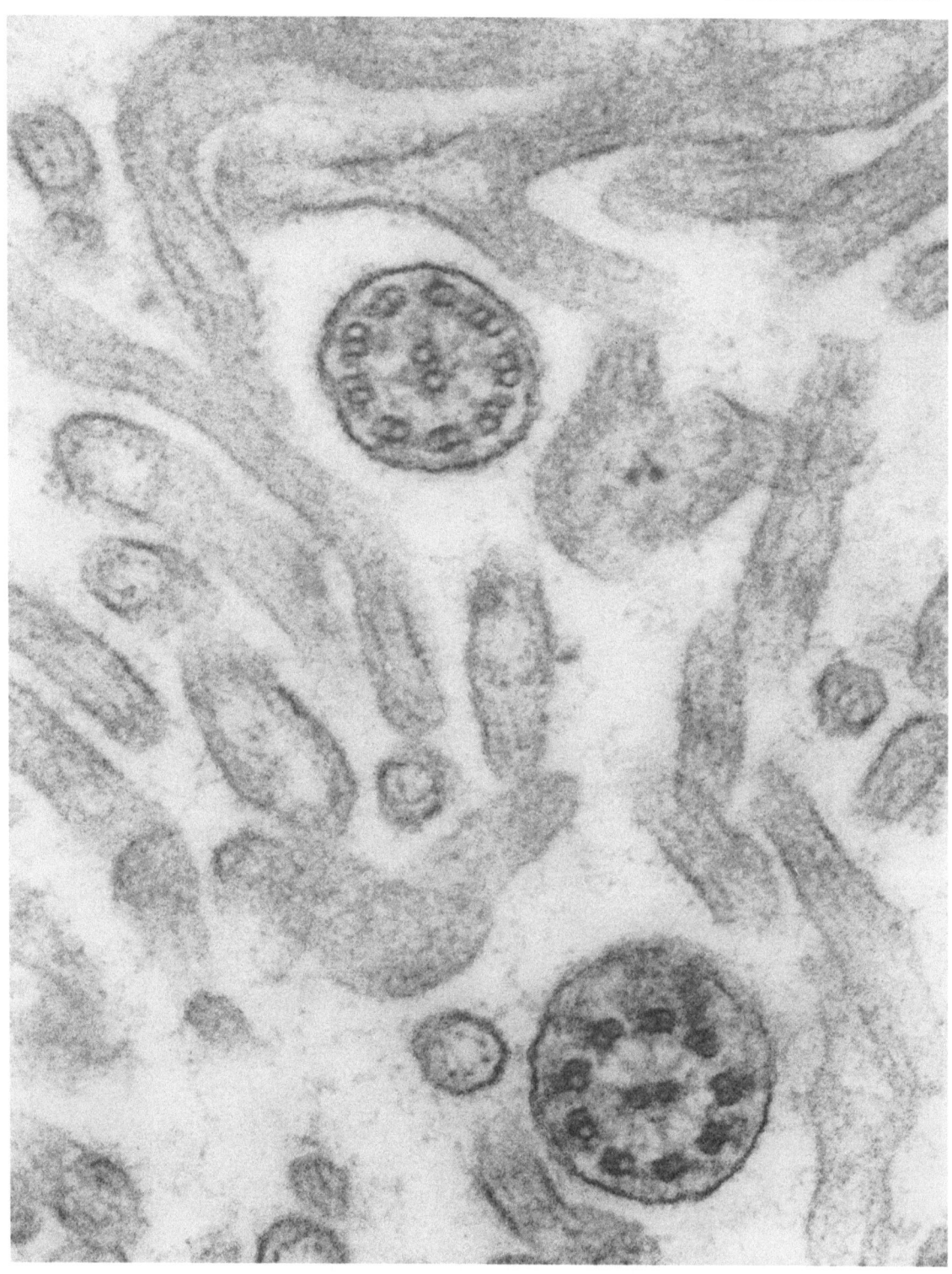

Fig. 6.7. *Ependymoma* (the same case as in Fig. 6.1). Cross sections of cilia show "9 + 2" arrangement of microtubules. × 159 000

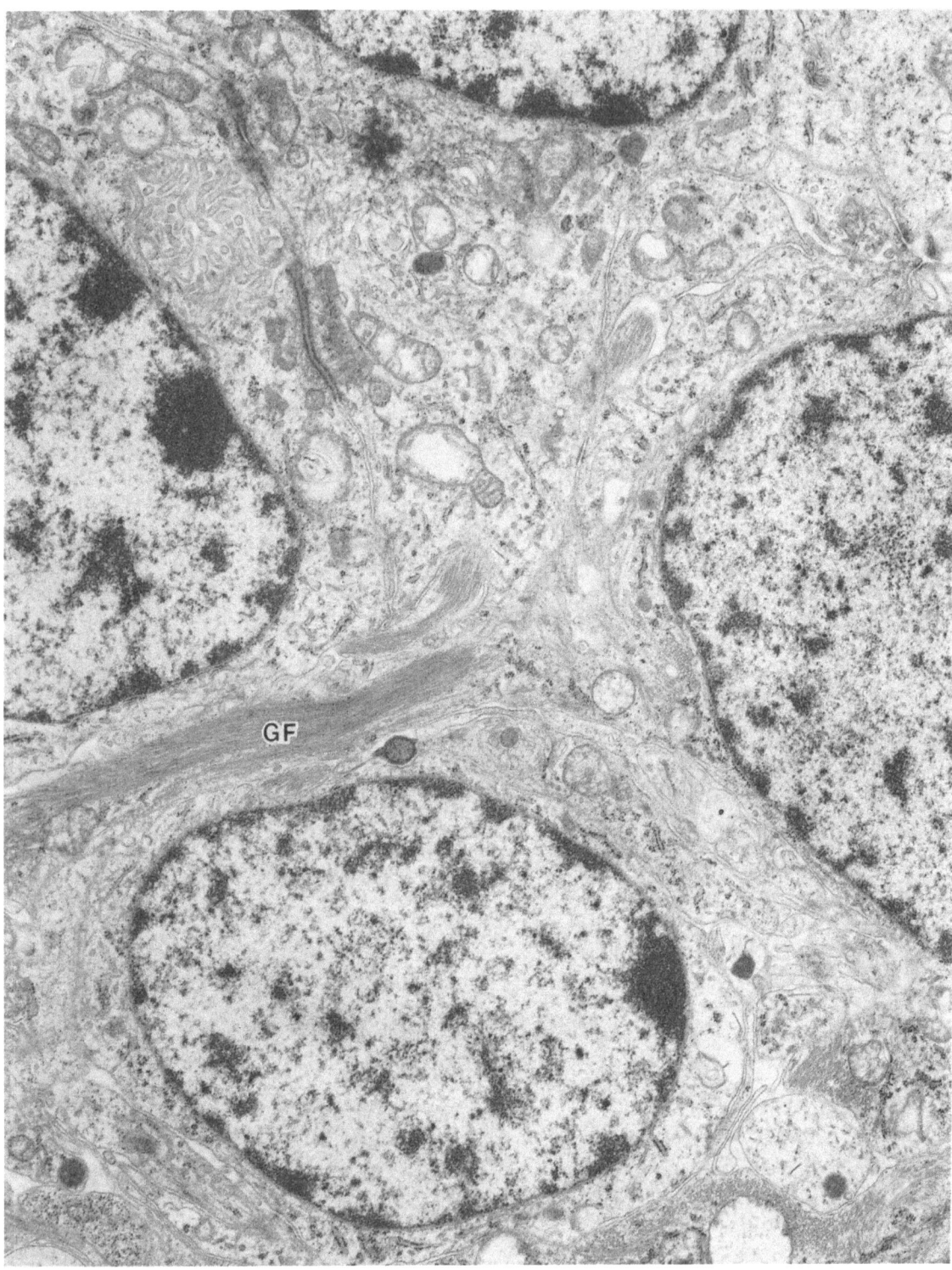

Fig. 6.8. *Ependymoma* (the same case as in Fig. 6.1). There are occasional long cell processes filled with bundles of glial filaments (*GF*). × 14100

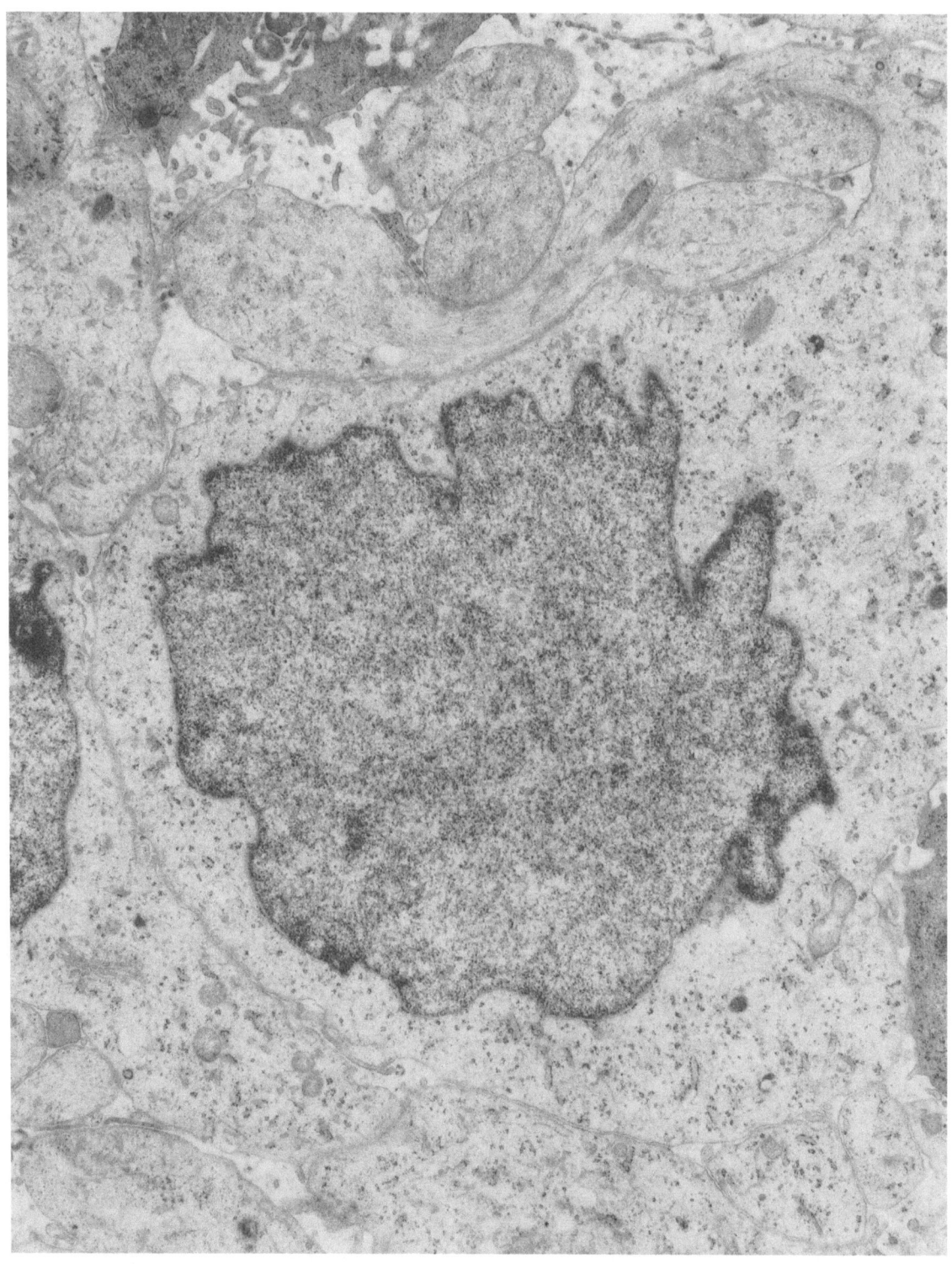

Fig. 6.9. *Ependymoma* (the same case as in Fig. 6.1). The tumor cell has an irregular nucleus and a long cell process containing glial filaments. × 24000

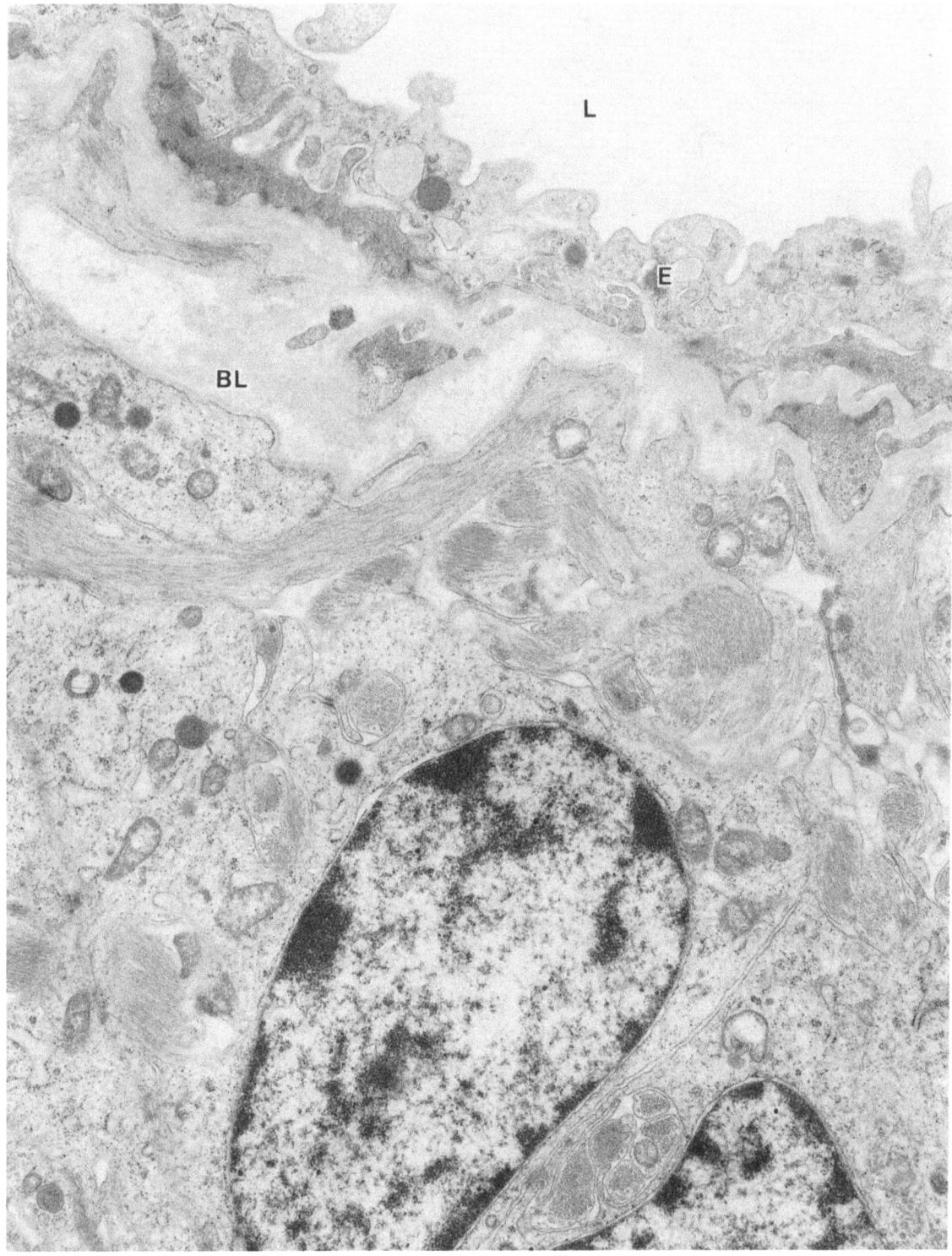

Fig. 6.10. *Ependymoma* (the same case as in Fig. 6.1). Many cell processes with or without glial filaments attach to the prominent basal lamina (*BL*). *L* capillary lumen, *E* endothelial cell. × 14 100

7. Choroid Plexus Papilloma

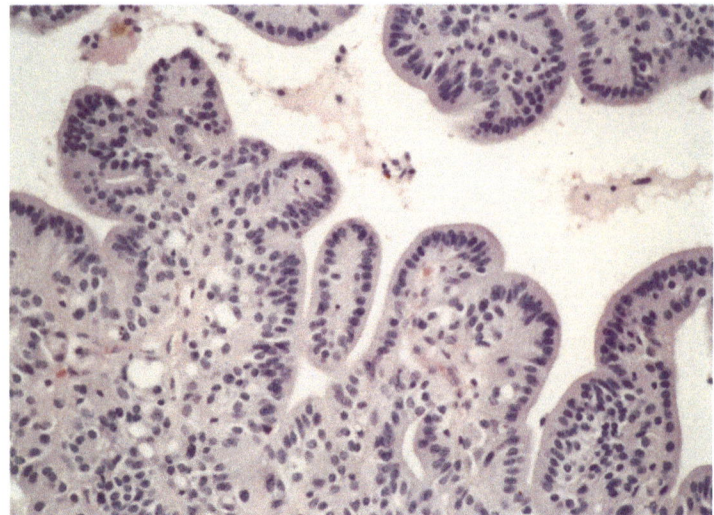

Fig. 7.1. *Choroid plexus papilloma* of the left lateral ventricle in a 34-year-old man. The tumor is characterized by a papillary structure, which is composed of columnar cells; however, as observed in this case, partial disorganization or crowding of the columnar cells is usually found. H and E, × 160

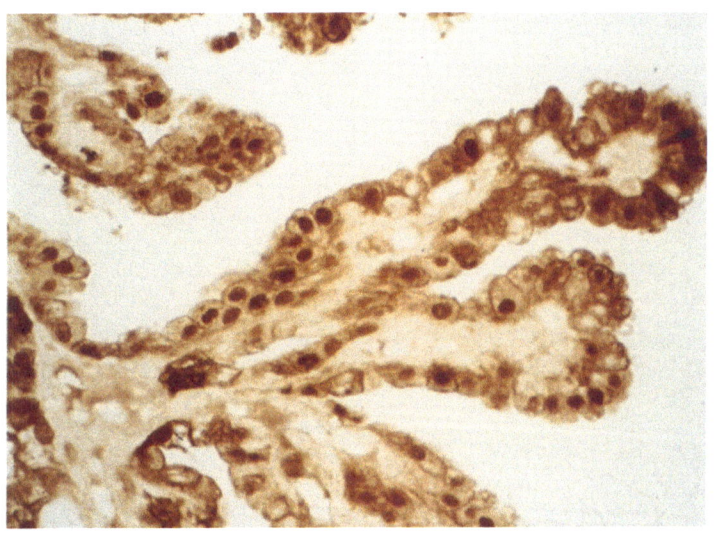

Fig. 7.2. *Choroid plexus papilloma* of the left lateral ventricle in a 37-year-old man. Intensely positive staining for S-100 protein is seen in many nuclei of the columnar cells. Indirect immunoperoxidase method without counterstain, × 160

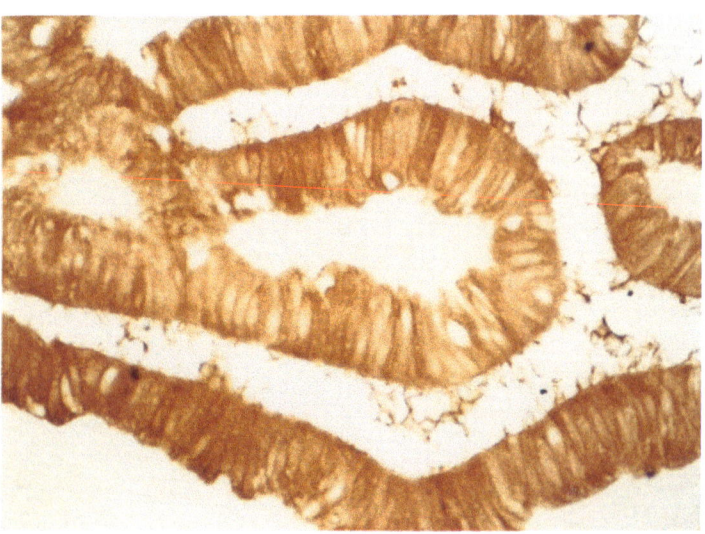

Fig. 7.3. *Choroid plexus papilloma* of the right lateral ventricle in a 5-month-old male infant. The tumor consists of higher columnar cells and shows a positive reaction for S-100 protein in the cytoplasm but not in the nuclei. Indirect immunoperoxidase method without counterstain, × 160

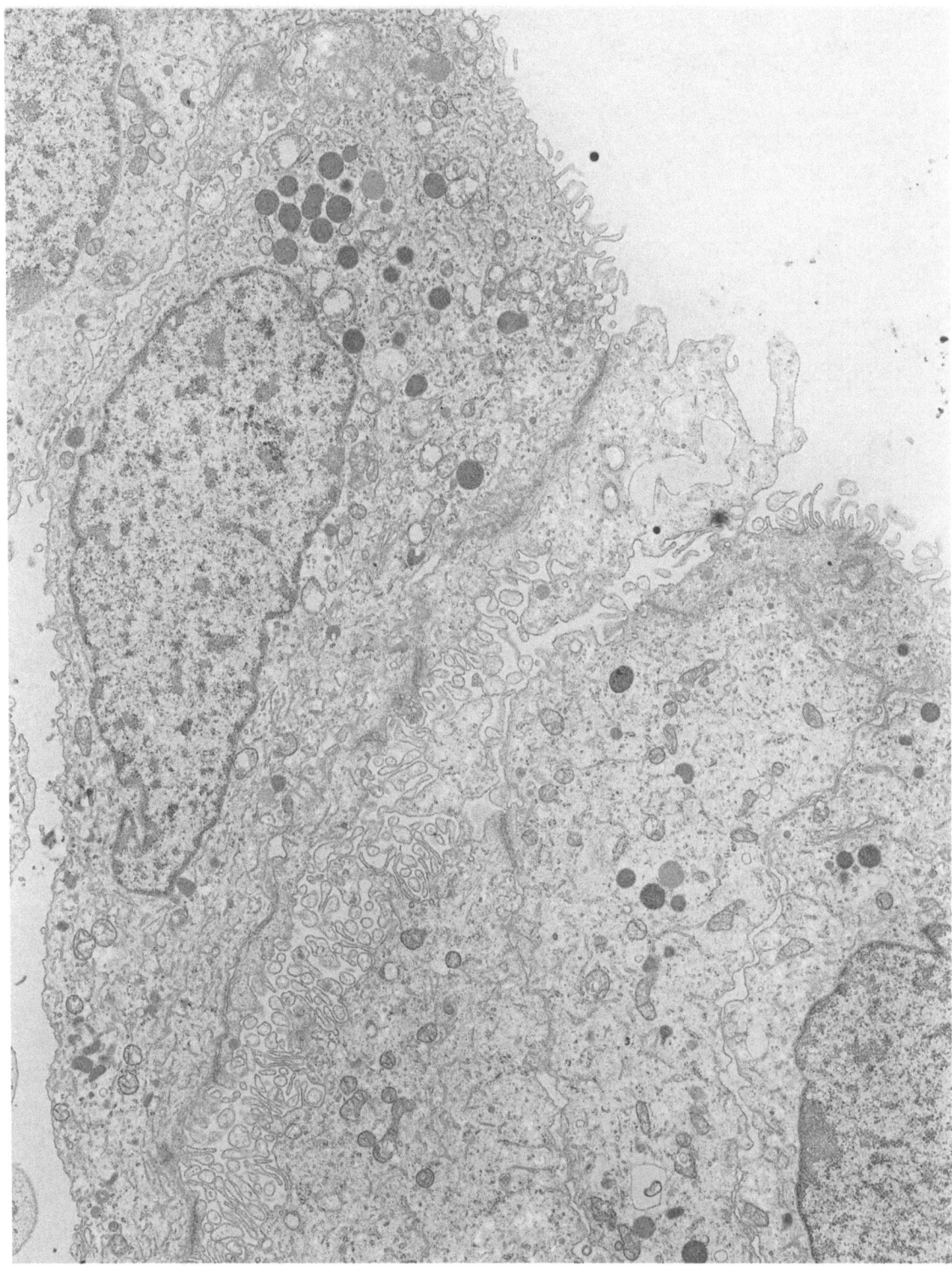

Fig. 7.4. *Choroid plexus papilloma* (the same case as in Fig. 7.1). Typical columnar tumor cells have numerous microvilli and intercellular junctional apparatus but no cilia. Electron-dense lysosomal granules are prominent in this case. × 7500

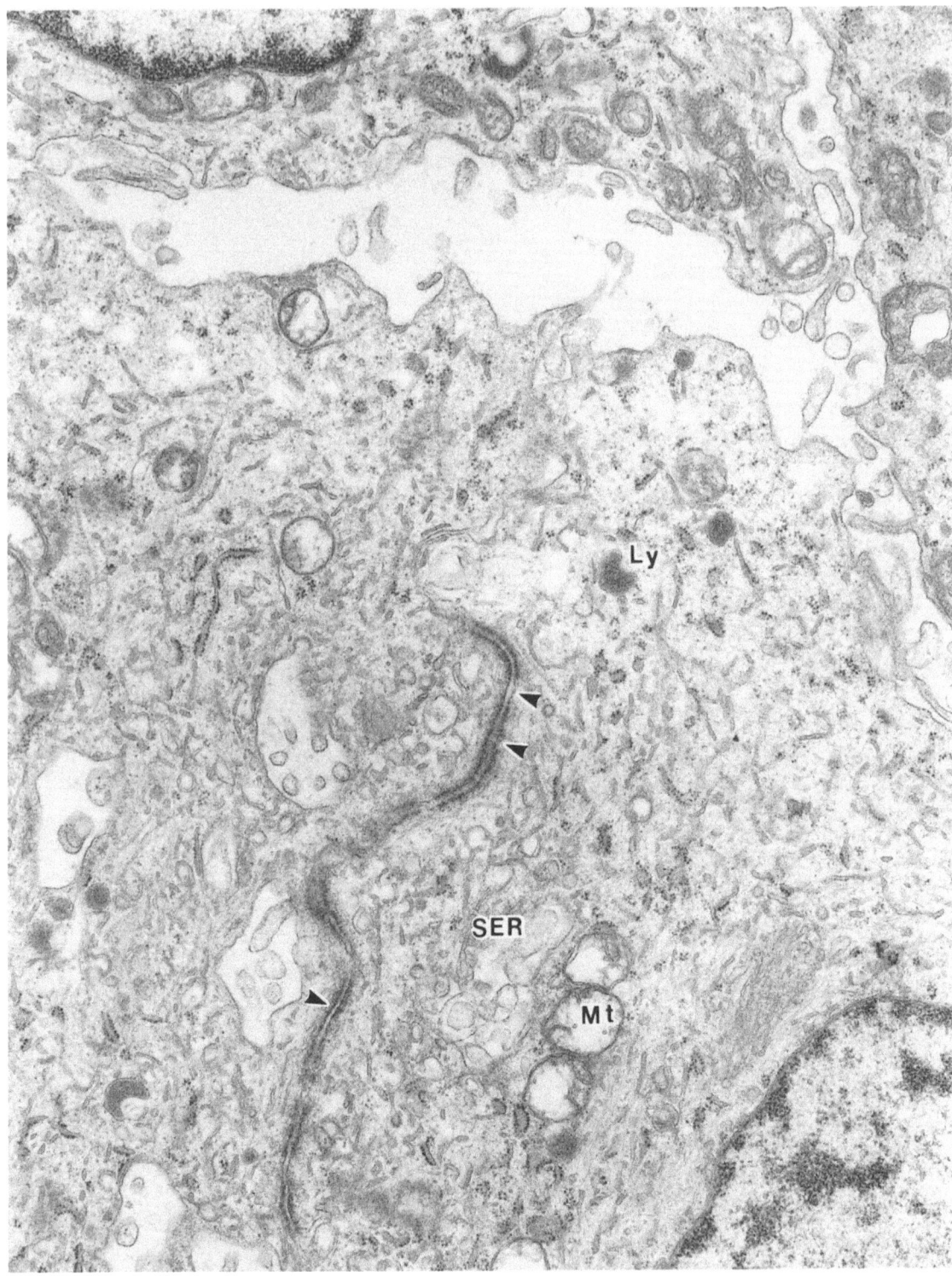

Fig. 7.5. *Choroid plexus papilloma* (the same case as in Fig. 7.1). Higher magnification reveals details of the intercellular junctional apparatus (*arrowheads*) and well-developed organelles, including smooth endoplasmic reticulum (*SER*), mitochondria (*Mt*), and lysosomal granules (*Ly*). × 21 000

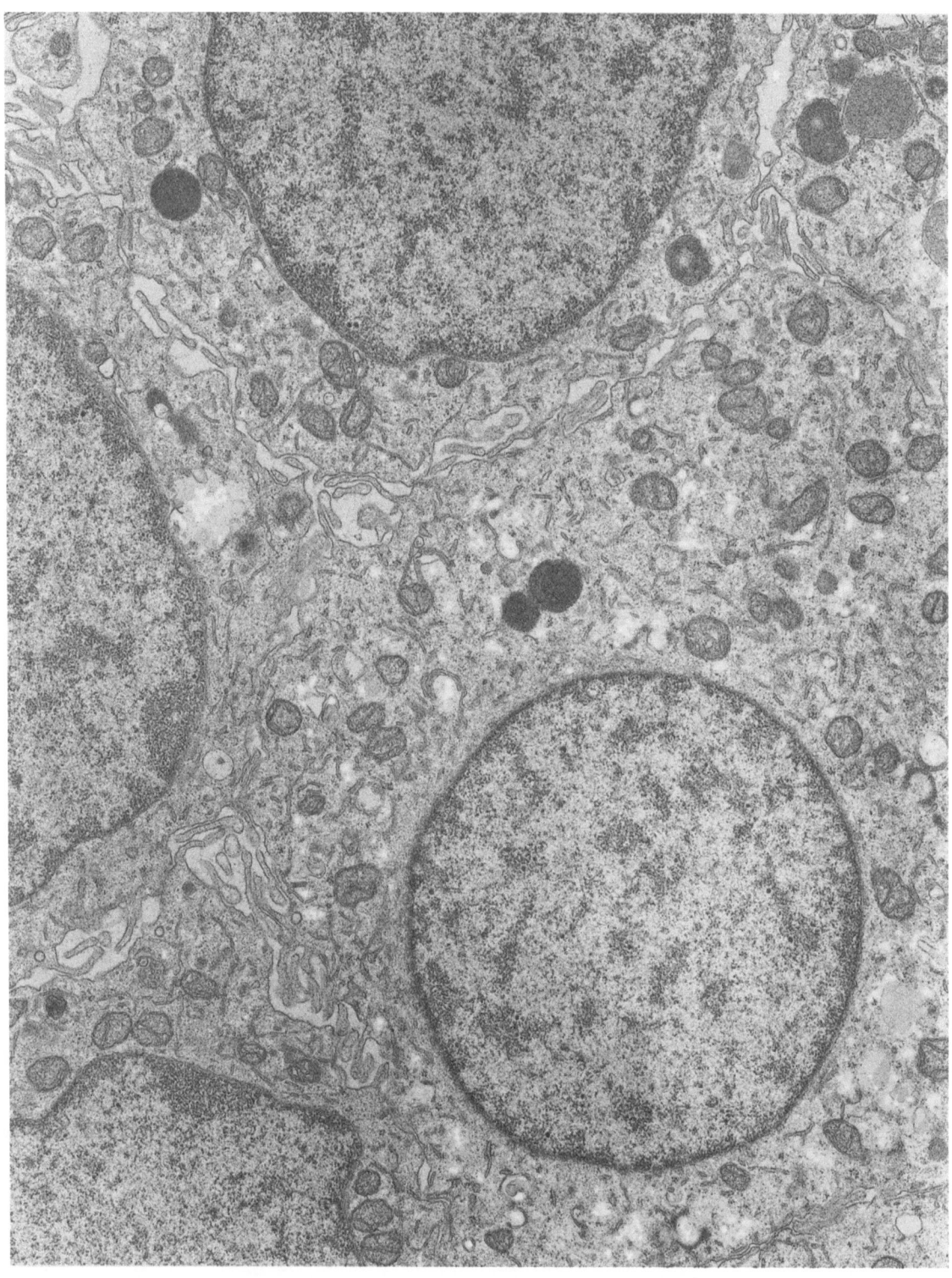

Fig. 7.6. *Choroid plexus papilloma* (the same case as in Fig. 7.1). The tumor cells with regular round nuclei are rich in organelles. × 14 700

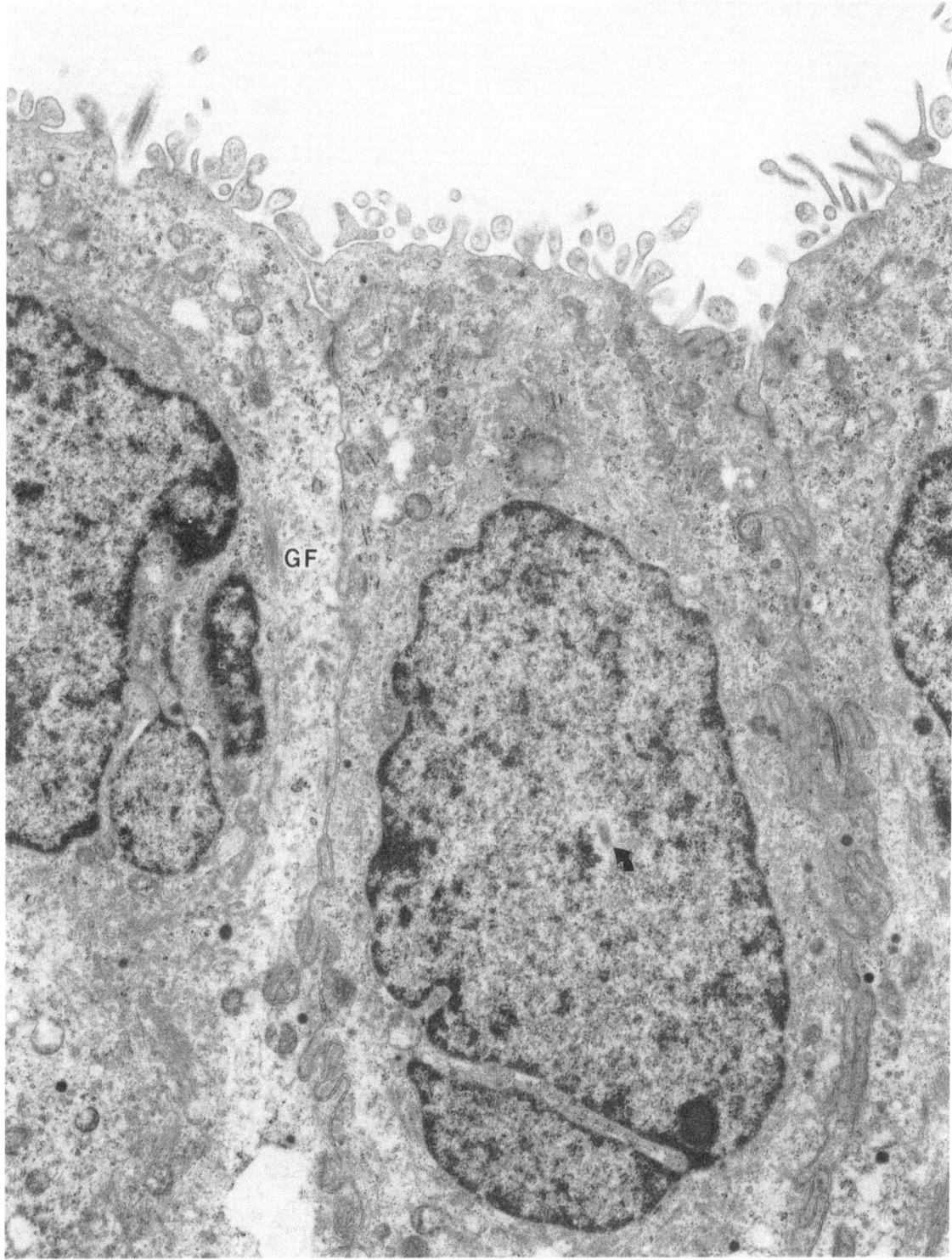

Fig. 7.7. *Choroid plexus papilloma* (the same case as in Fig. 7.2). The columnar cells show blunt microvilli and indented nuclei. Some tumor cells have 7- to 9-nm glial filaments (*GF*). The *arrow* indicates a filamentous intranuclear inclusion. × 14 700

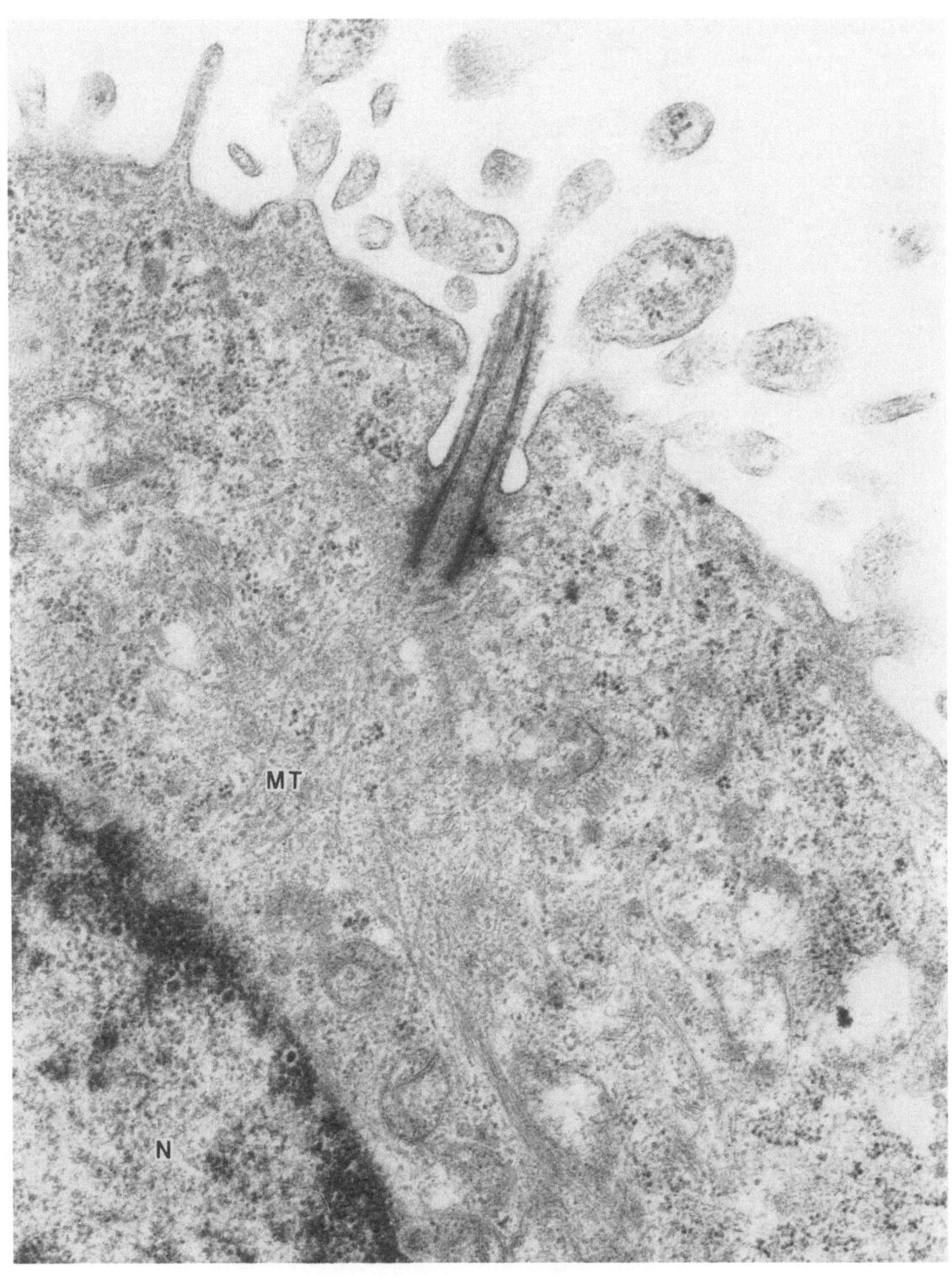

Fig. 7.8. *Choroid plexus papilloma* (the same case as in Fig. 7.2). A rare cilium is seen on the apical surface of the columnar cell. *MT* microtubules, *N* nucleus. × 42 000

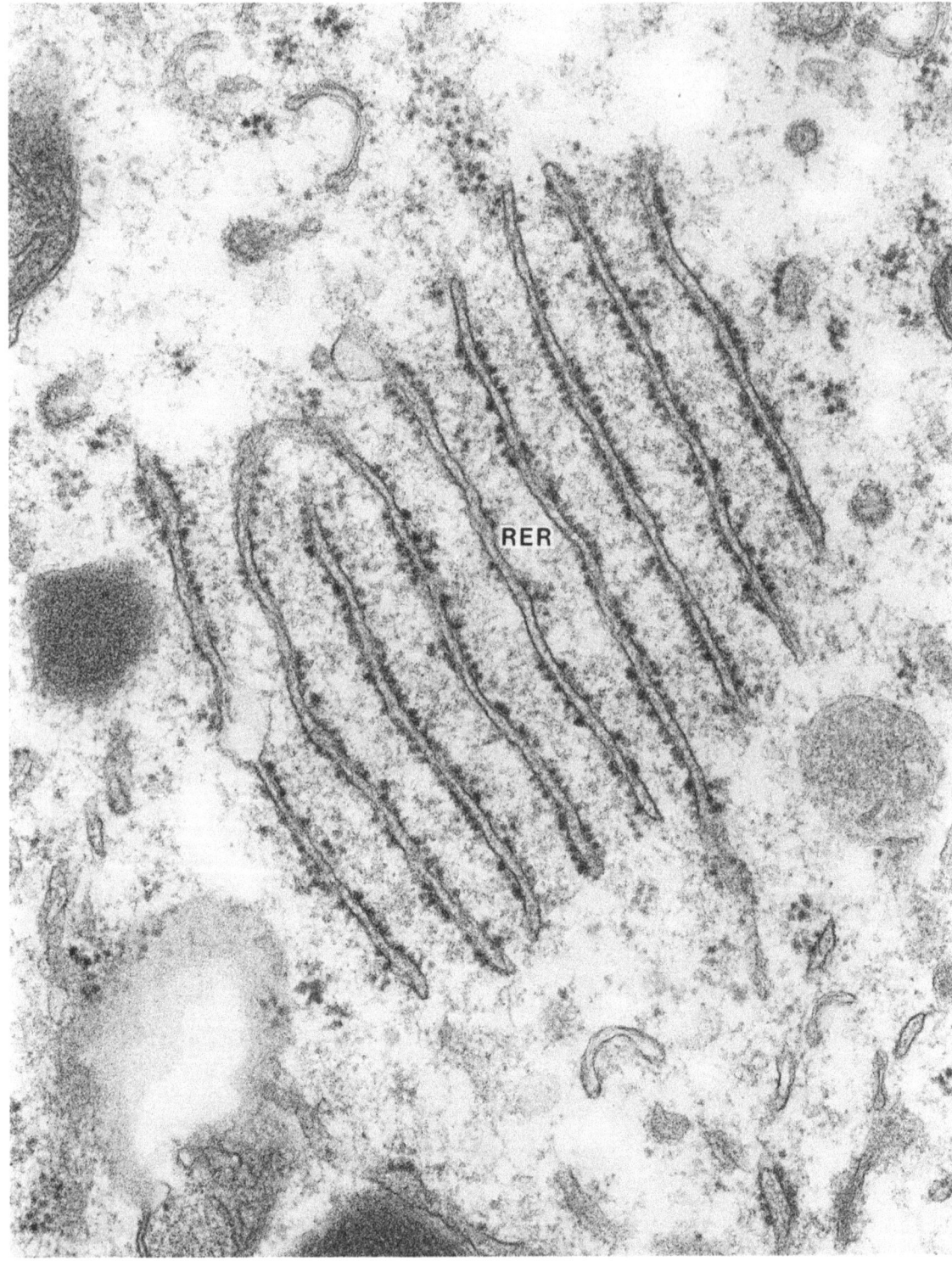

Fig. 7.9. *Choroid plexus papilloma* (the same case as in Fig. 7.2). Higher magnification shows details of the stacked rough endoplasmic reticulum (*RER*). × 70 000

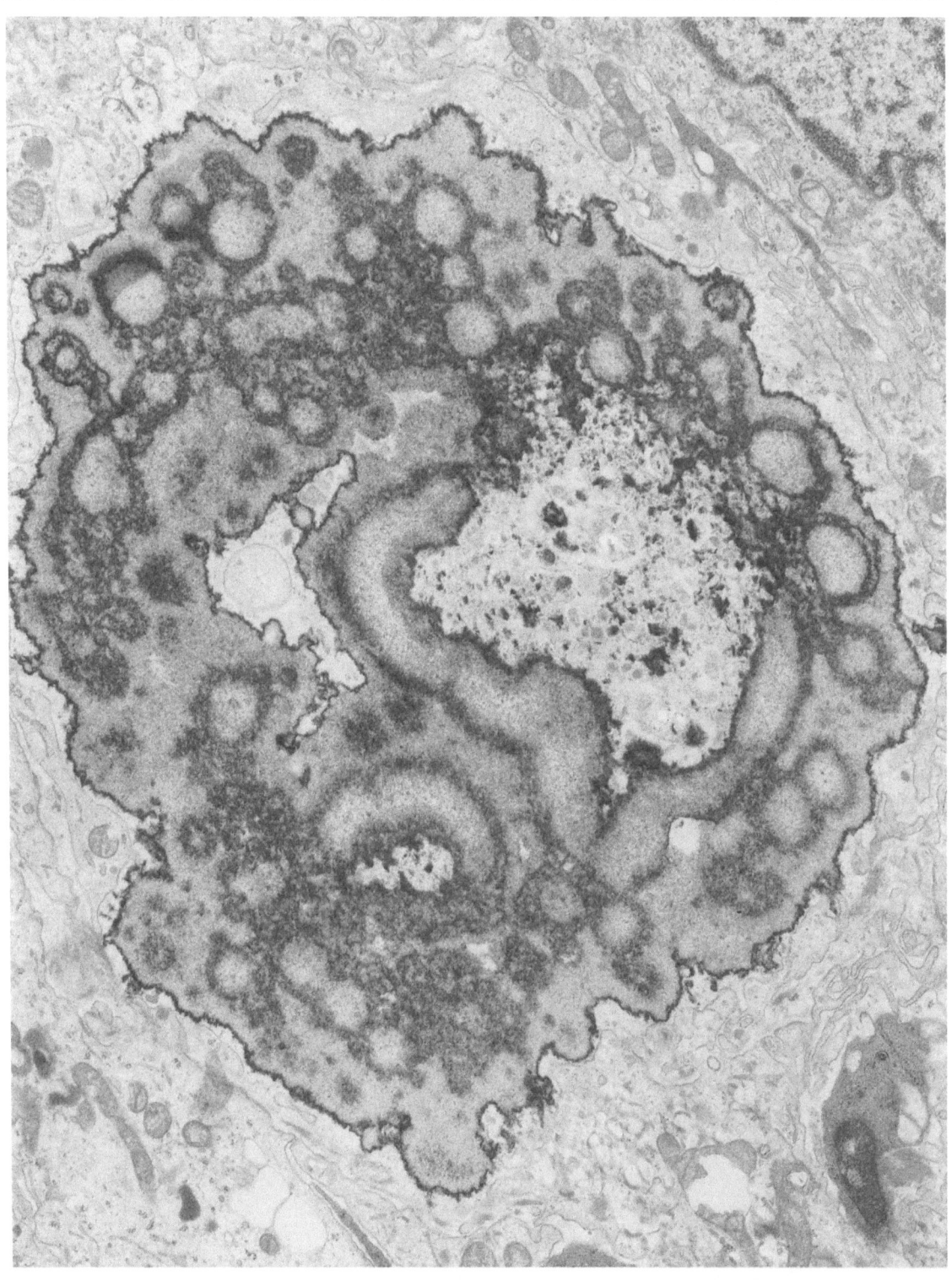

Fig. 7.10. *Choroid plexus papilloma* (the same case as in Fig. 7.2). Occasional intracytoplasmic calcification is seen as an irregularly shaped mass with a heterogeneous electron density. × 15 300

8. Glioblastoma

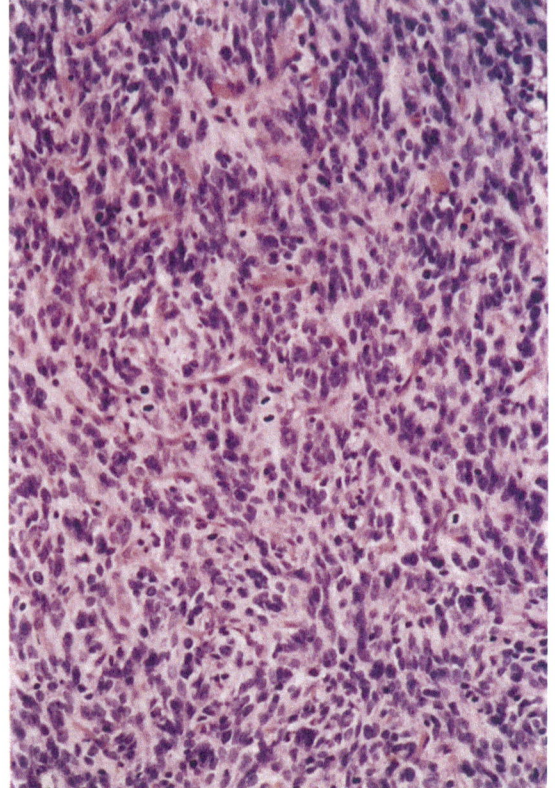

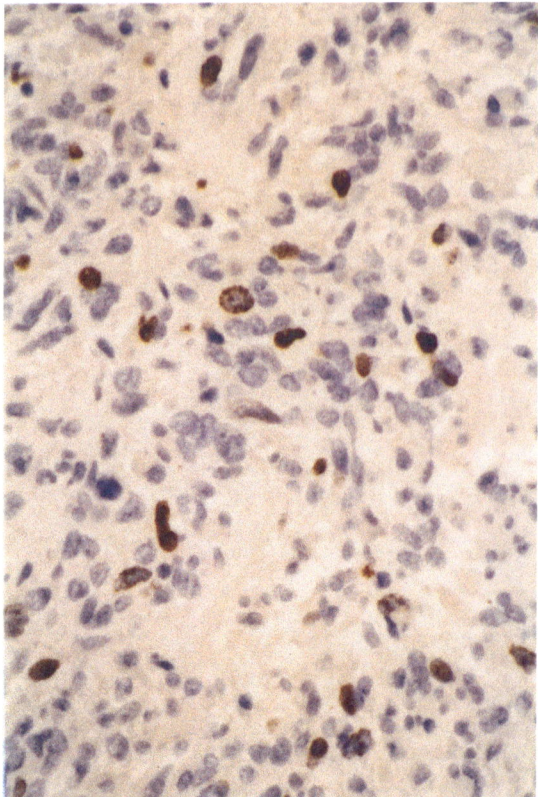

Fig. 8.1. *Glioblastoma* of the right frontal lobe in a 55-year-old man. This highly cellular tumor is characterized by numerous mitotic figures, hyperchromatism, and pleomorphism. The astrocytic lineage of the tumor cells is not evident. H and E, × 90

Fig. 8.2. *Glioblastoma* (the same case as in Fig. 8.1). Immunohistochemical examination reveals frequent nuclear uptake of bromodeoxyuridine, a thymidine analogue that is incoporated into nuclear DNA during the S (DNA synthesis) phase of the cell cycle. This result indicates the high proliferative potential of this tumor. Indirect immunoperoxidase method counterstained with hematoxylin, × 180

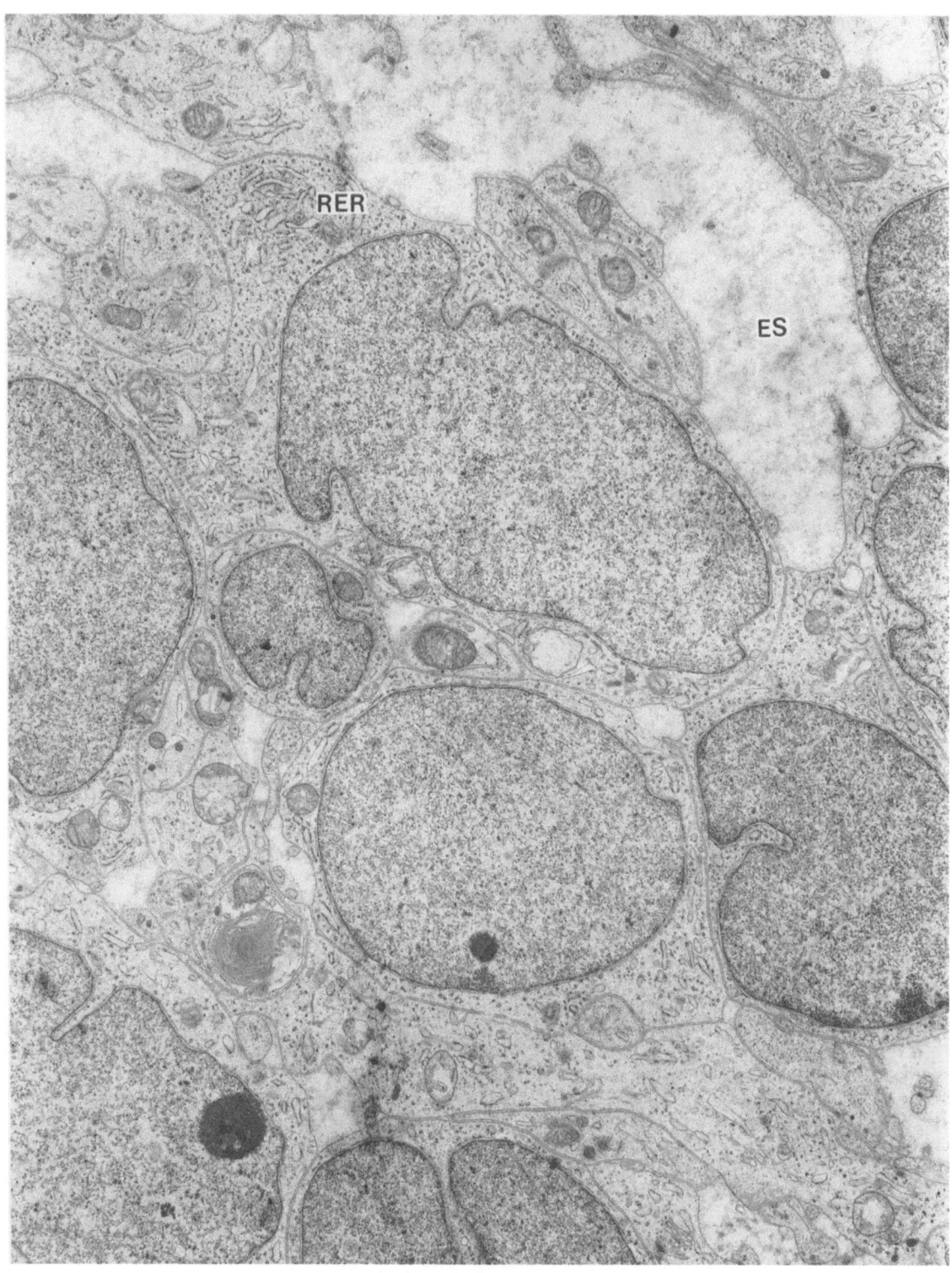

Fig. 8.3. *Glioblastoma* (the same case as in Fig. 8.1). The crowded tumor cells with irregularly shaped nuclei show relatively clear cytoplasm containing scattered free ribosome granules and rough endoplasmic reticulum (*RER*). This tumor is also characterized by the prominent extracellular space (*ES*) filled with electron-lucent proteinaceous fluid. × 8200

61

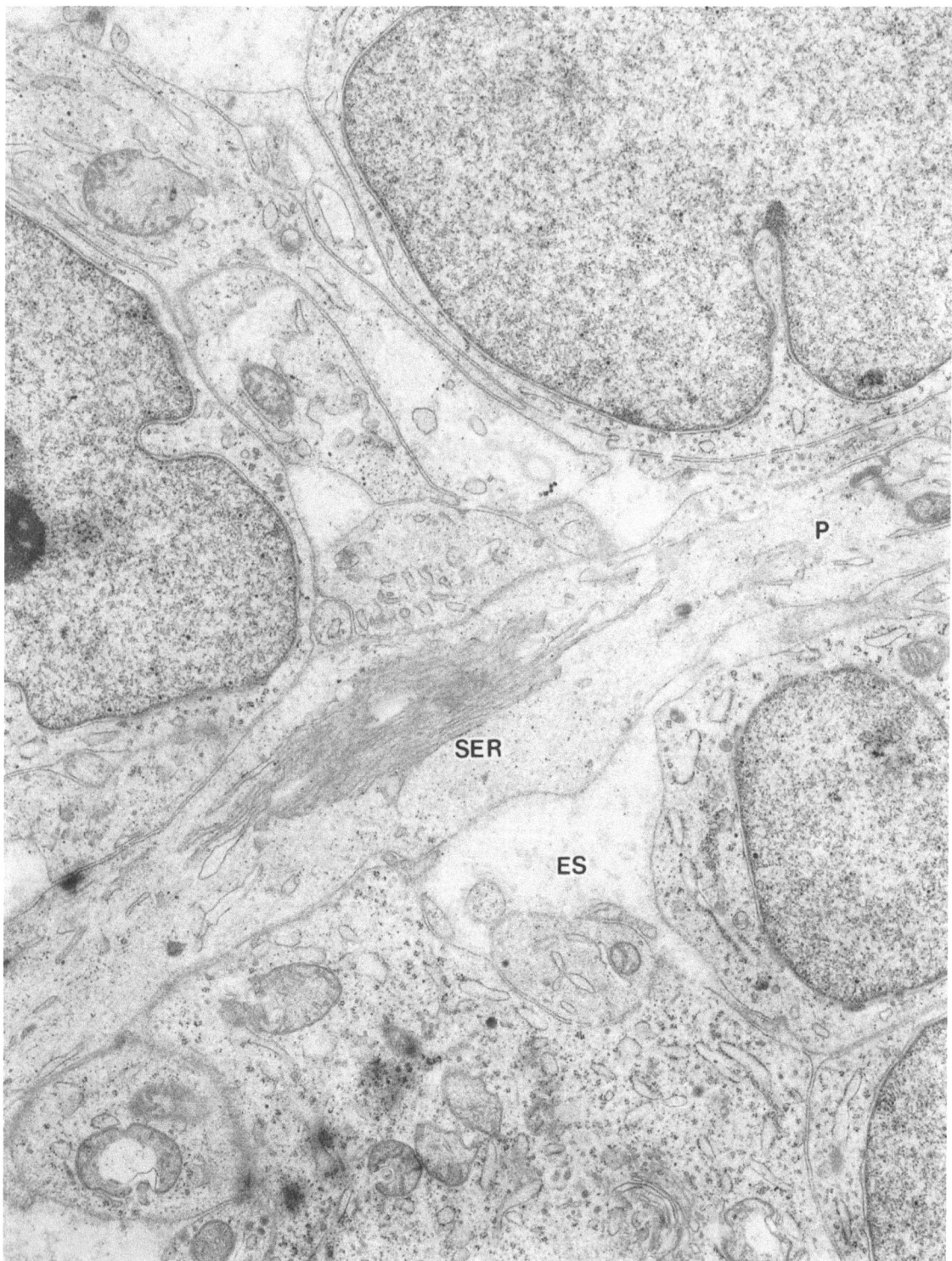

Fig. 8.4. *Glioblastoma* (the same case as in Fig. 8.1). A long cell process (*P*) in the center indicates the astrocyctic character of this tumor, though a bundle of glial filaments and intercellular junctional apparatus are not evident. *ES* extracellular space, *SER* smooth endoplasmic reticulum. × 13 600

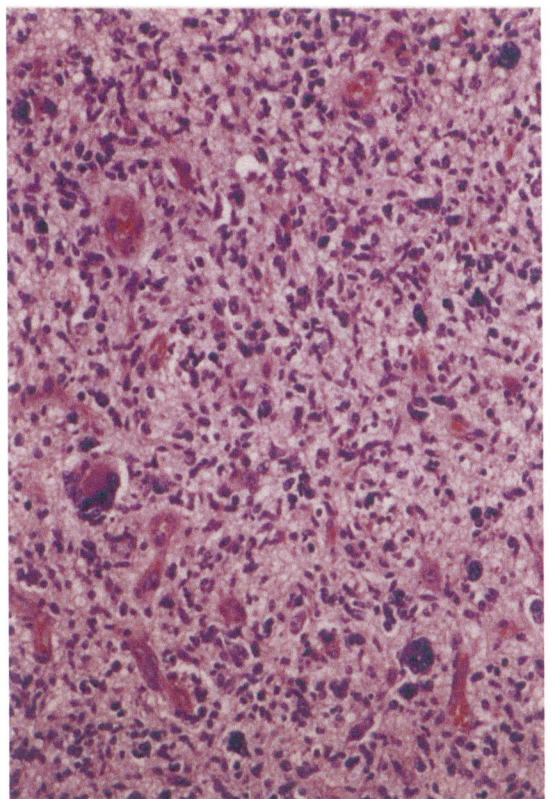 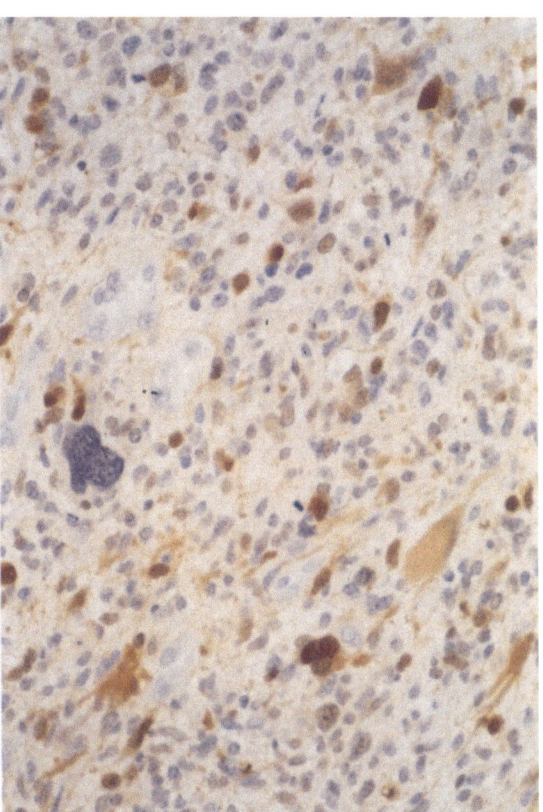

Fig. 8.5. *Glioblastoma* of the left occipital lobe in a 31-year-old man. The tumor is composed of pleomorphic glial cells with the patently astrocytic features of a translucent cytoplasm and process formation. Endothelial proliferation and nuclear gigantism are seen. H and E, × 90

Fig. 8.6. *Glioblastoma* (the same case as in Fig. 8.5). The intensity of the positive reaction for S-100 protein in both the cytoplasm and nuclei varies with individual cells. Indirect immunoperoxidase method counterstained with hematoxylin, × 180

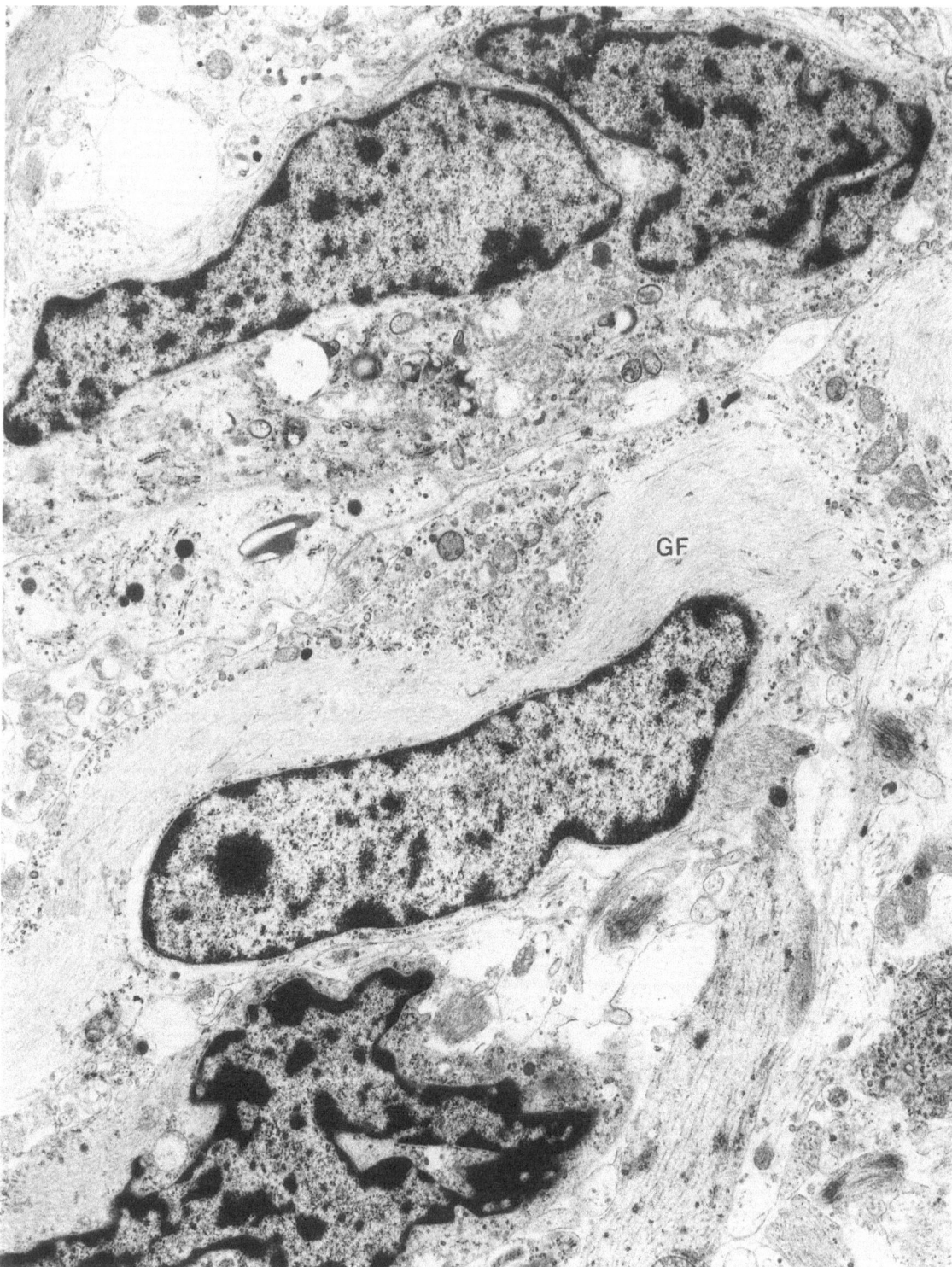

Fig. 8.7. *Glioblastoma* (the same case as in Fig. 8.5). The tumor cells show markedly irregular nuclei marginated with heterochromatin. In accordance with the astrocytic parentage of this glioblastoma, the tumor cells often bear abundant glial filaments (*GF*). × 11 300

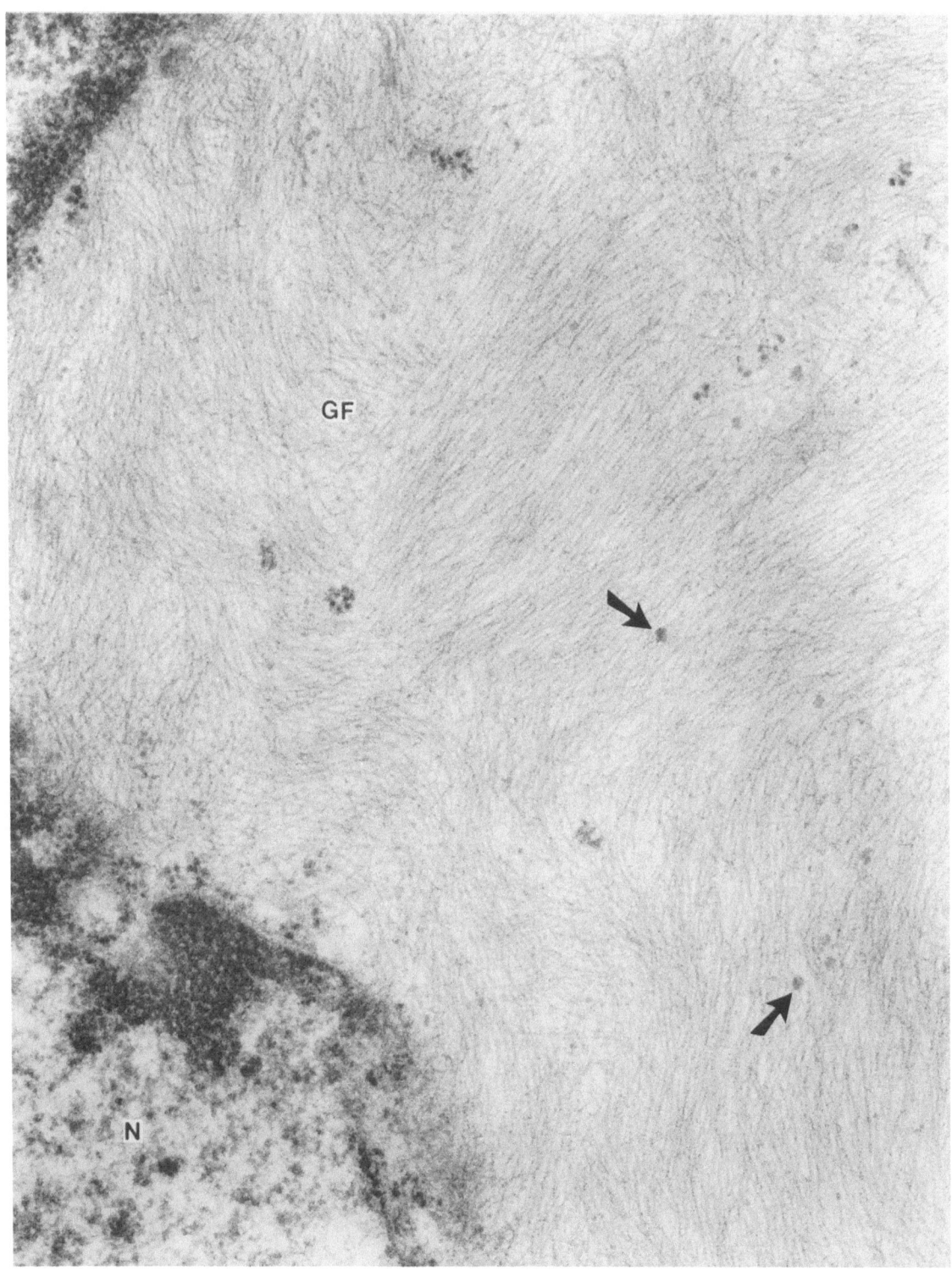

Fig. 8.8. Higher magnification of the intracytoplasmic glial filaments (*GF*) of a glioblastoma cell (the same case as in Fig. 8.5). The filaments are 6–9 nm in diameter. The electron-dense granules, approximately 30–40 nm in diameter, are monoparticulate glycogen (*arrows*). *N* nucleus. × 60 000

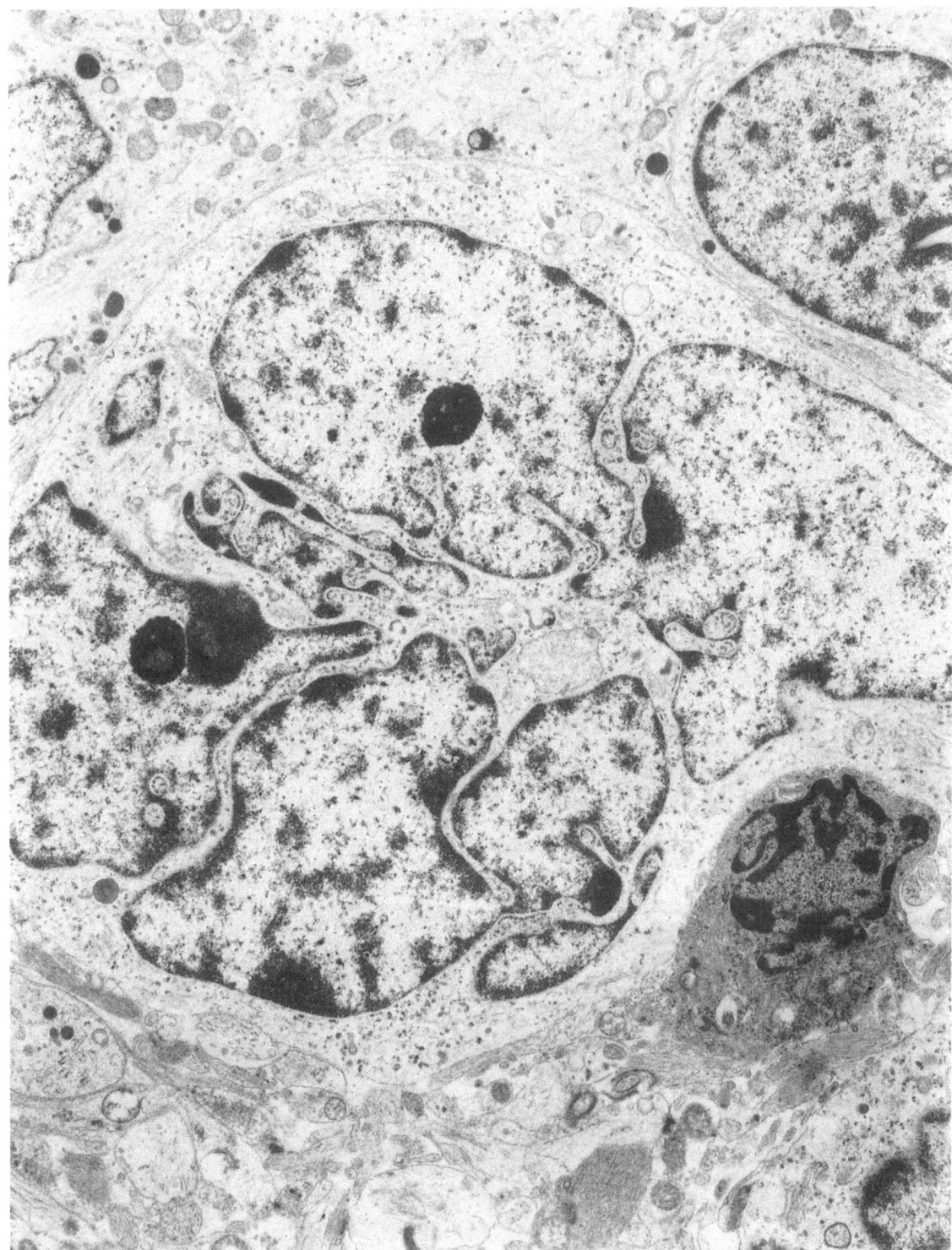

Fig. 8.9. A multinucleated giant cell is often present in a glioblastoma (the same case as in Fig. 8.5). × 11 300

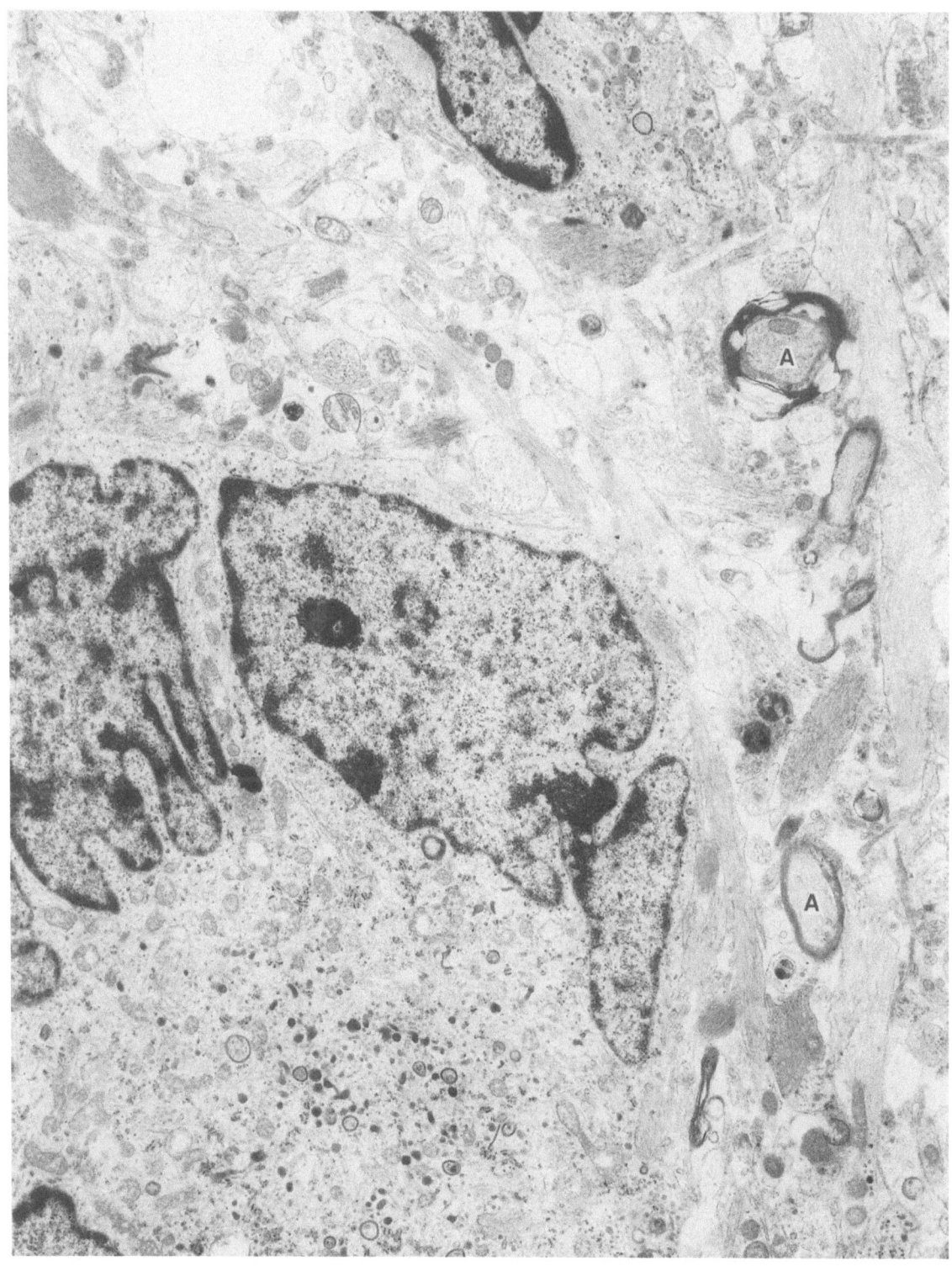

Fig. 8.10. *Glioblastoma* (the same case as in Fig. 8.5). A multinucleated giant cell is surrounded by astrocytic processes filled with glial filaments. Myelinated axons (*A*) entrapped in the tumor are also observed. × 9800

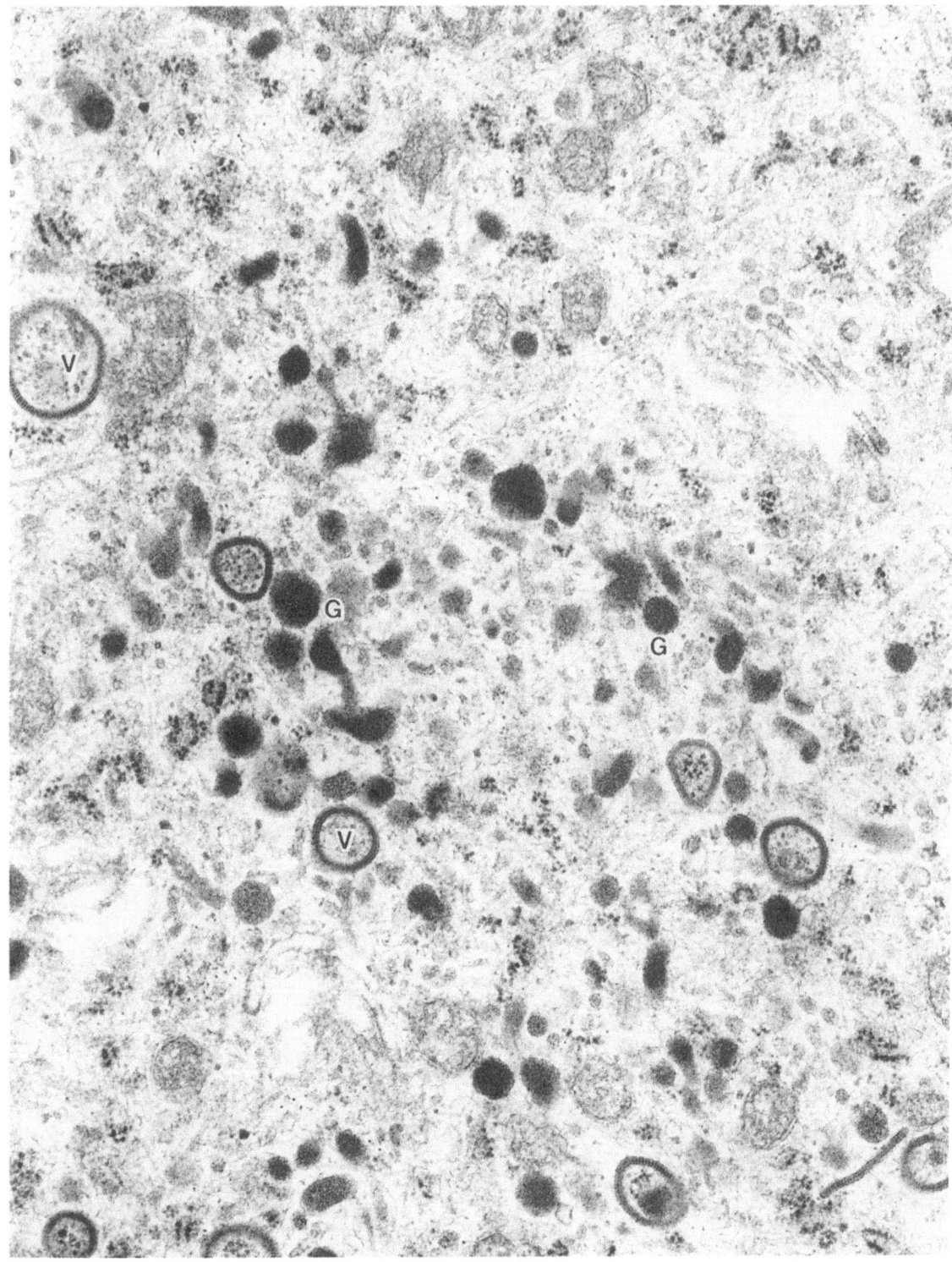

Fig. 8.11. Higher magnification of part of Fig. 8.10 reveals uniquely organized vesicles (*V*) and many uncharacterized dense granules (*G*) in the cytoplasm of a multinucleated giant cell. × 39 000

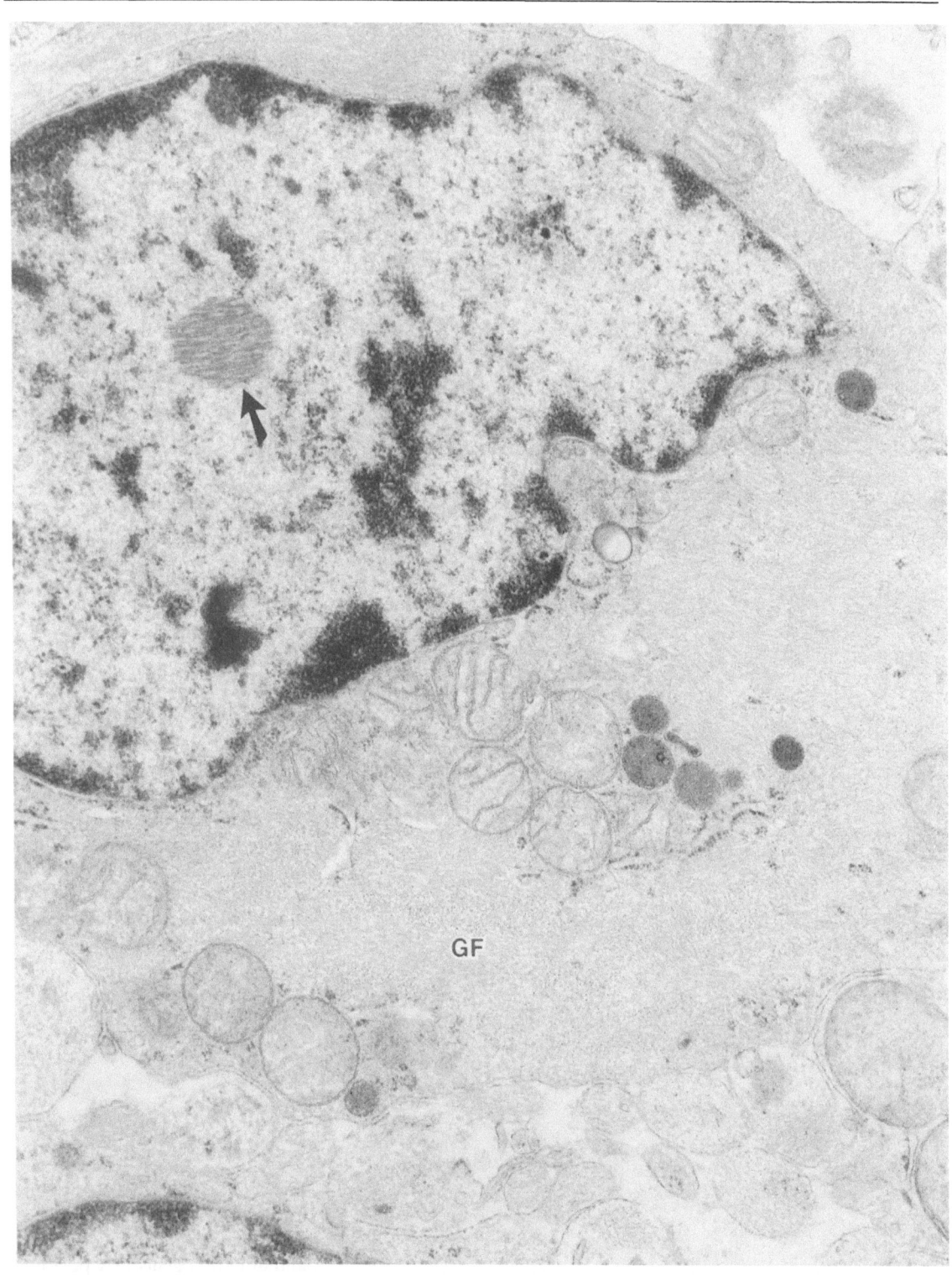

Fig. 8.12. A *glioblastoma* cell shows a filamentous intranuclear inclusion (*arrow*) and abundant intracyto-plasmic glial filaments (*GF*). × 25 400

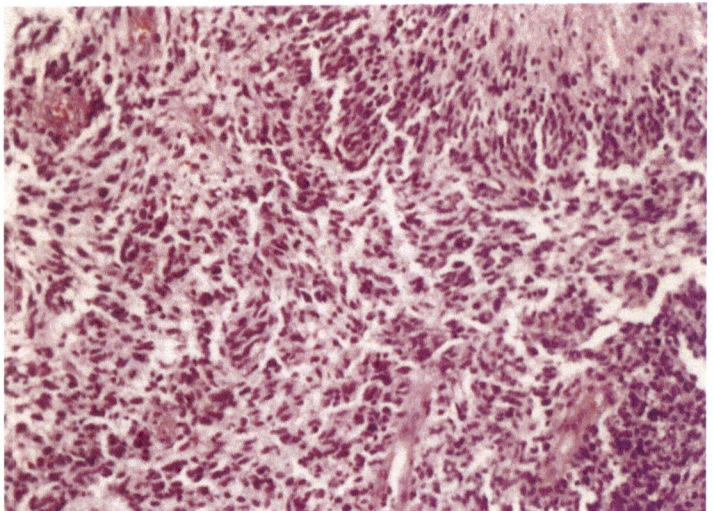

Fig. 8.13. *Glioblastoma* of the right frontal lobe in a 72-year-old man. The tumor is composed of small spindle-shaped cells and shows increased cellularity. H and E, × 80

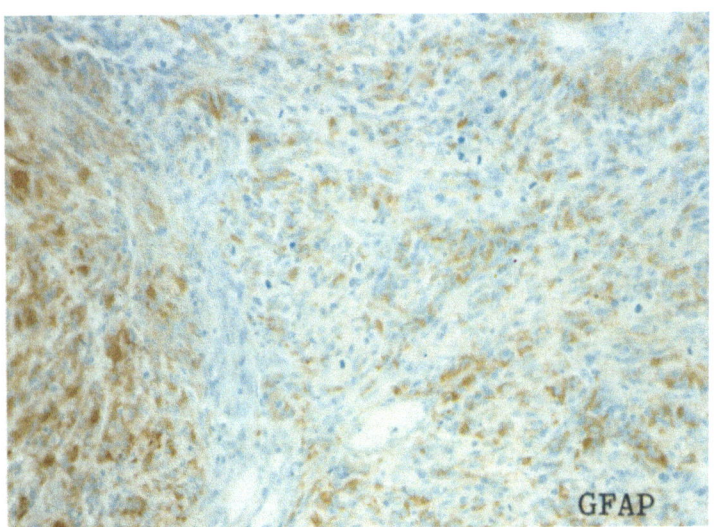

Fig. 8.14. *Glioblastoma* (the same case as in Fig. 8.13). Positive immunohistochemical staining for glial fibrillary acidic protein (GFAP) is not only weak but also heterogeneous in intensity among the tumor cells. Indirect immunoperoxidase method counterstained with methyl green, × 80

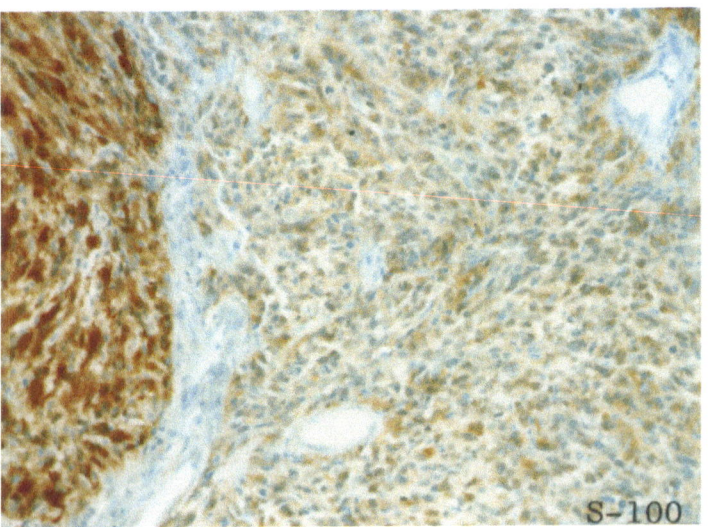

Fig. 8.15. *Glioblastoma* (the same case as in Fig. 8.13; similar area as in Fig. 8.14). A relatively weak and nonhomogeneously positive reaction for S-100 protein is evident among the tumor cells. Indirect immunoperoxidase method counterstained with methyl green, × 80

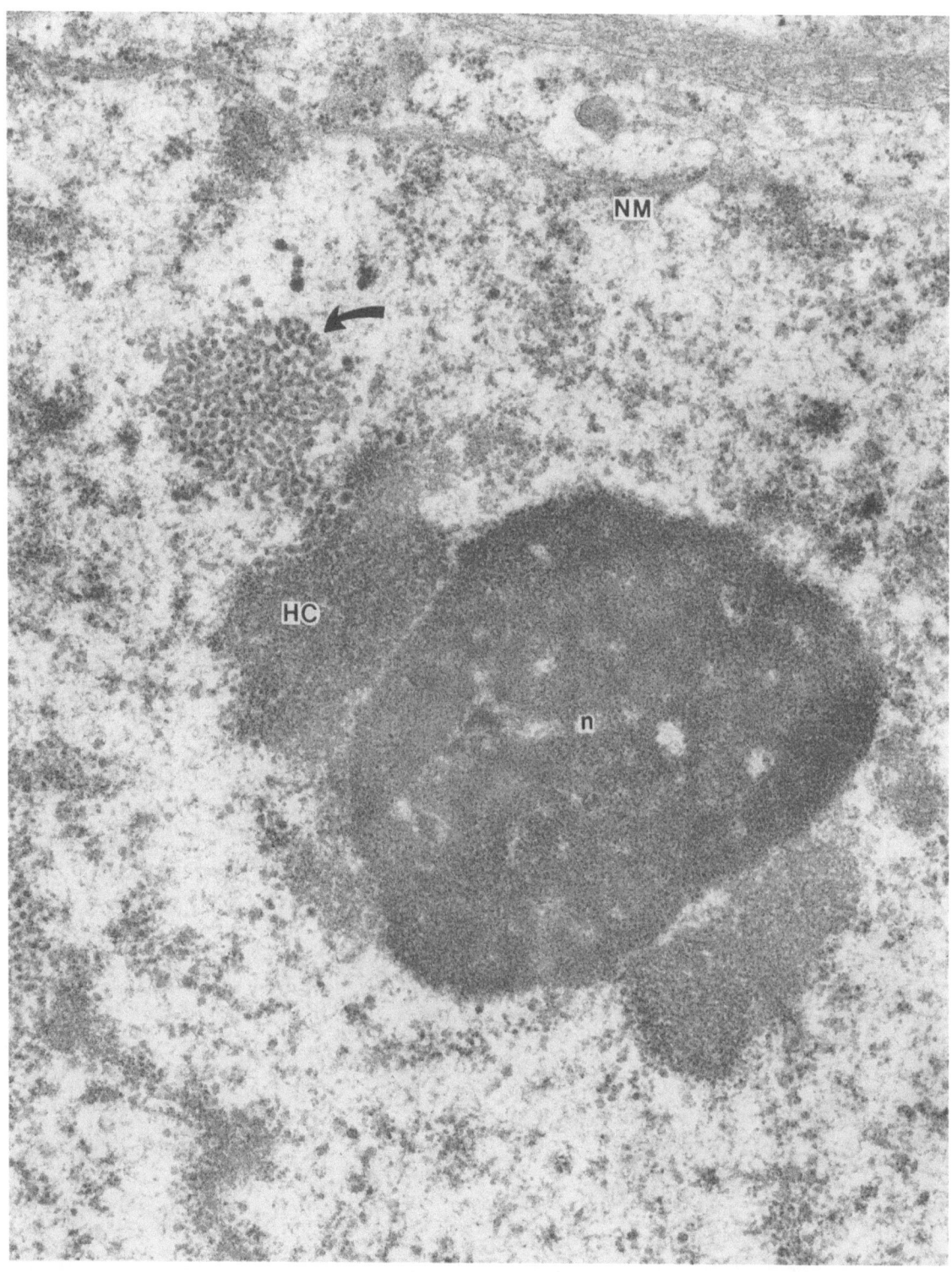

Fig. 8.16. *Glioblastoma* (the same case as in Fig. 8.13). Higher magnification shows an enlarged nucleolus (*n*) associated with heterochromatin (*HC*). Some perichromatin granules (30–40 nm in diameter) and clusters of interchromatin granules (*arrow*) are also discernible. *NM* nuclear membranes. × 34 300

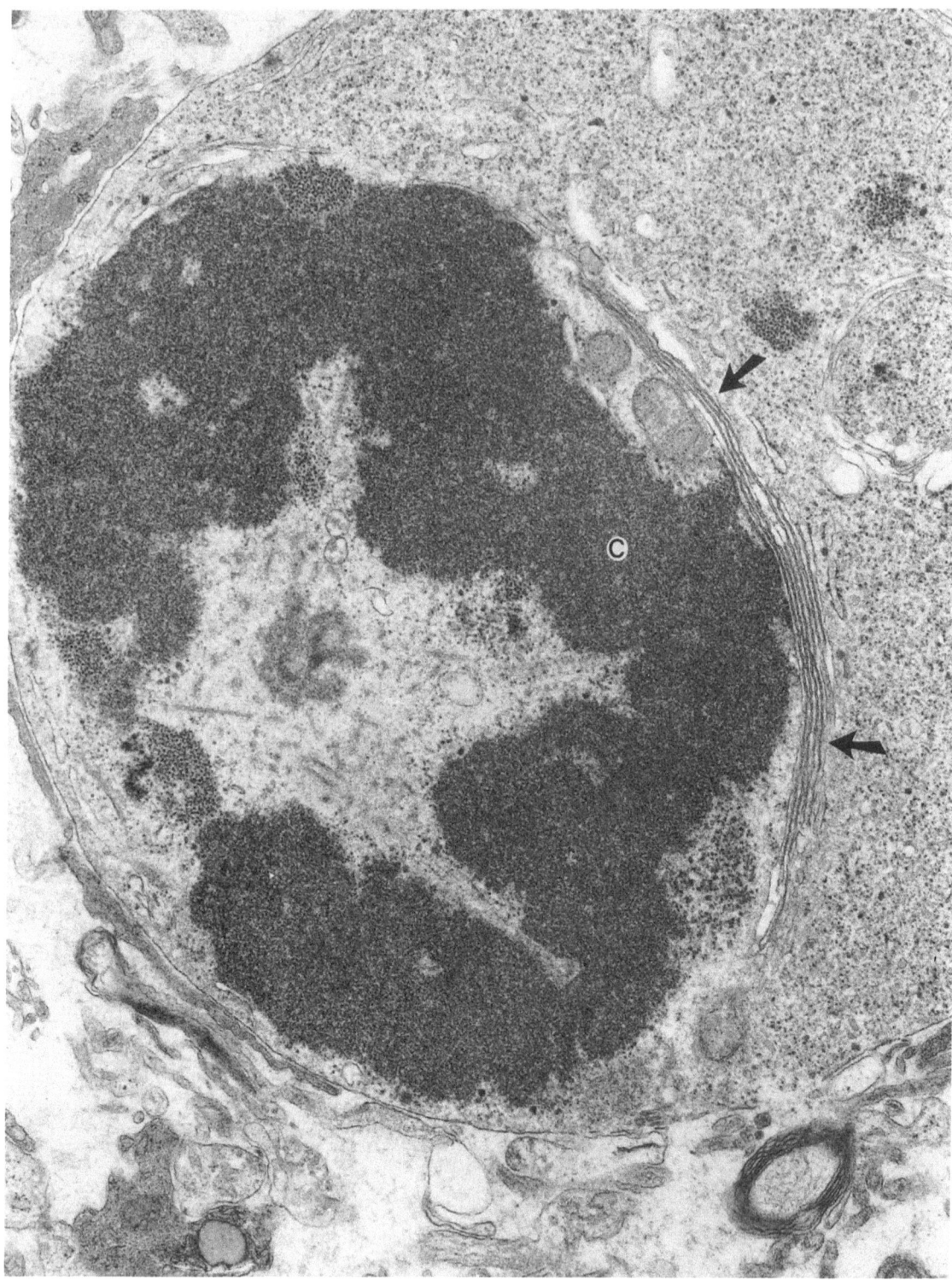

Fig. 8.17. *Glioblastoma* (the same case as in Fig. 8.13). A dividing tumor cell in telophase is reforming a new nuclear membranes (*arrows*) around the decondensing chromosome (*C*). × 24 000

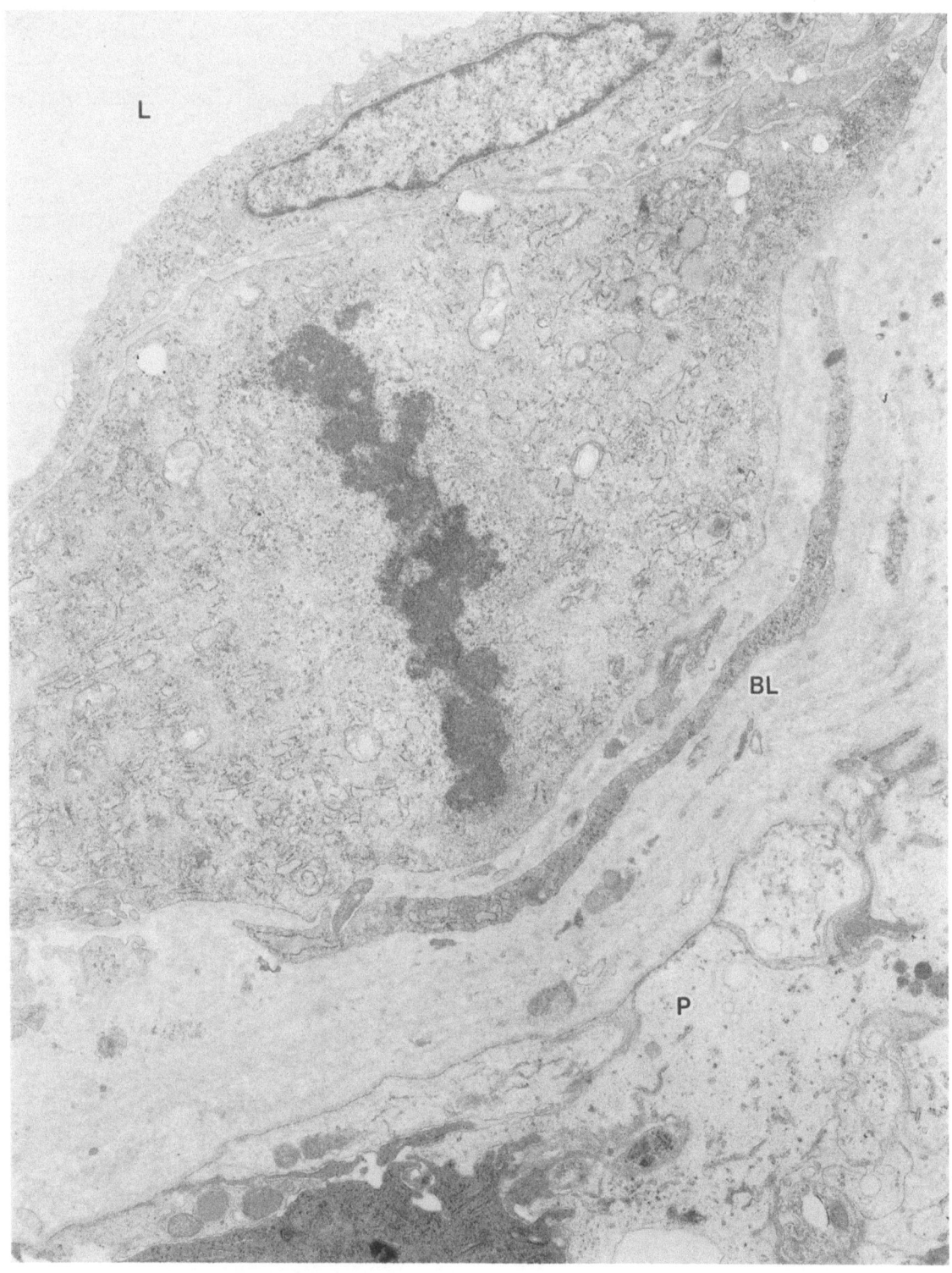

Fig. 8.18. A capillary endothelial cell in metaphase is found in a glioblastoma (the same case as in Fig. 8.13). Chromosomes are aligned at the metaphase plate. *L* capillary lumen, *BL* basal lamina, *P* astrocytic process of tumor cell. × 9500

9. Medulloblastoma

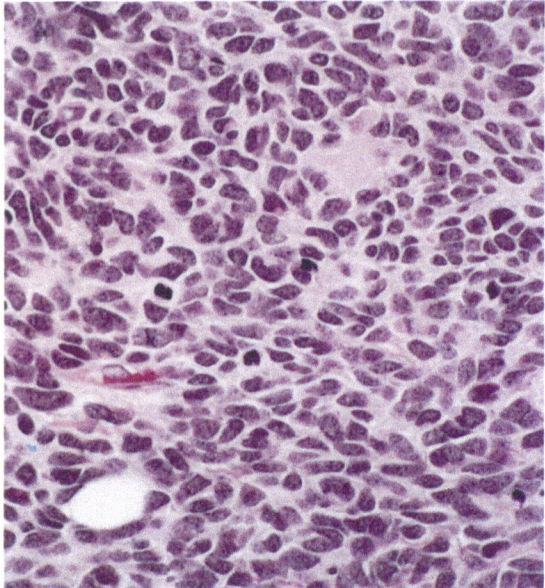

Fig. 9.1. *Medulloblastoma* of cerebellar vermis in a 7-year-old girl. The tumor is very cellular and consists of polygonal cells with sparse cytoplasm. Mitoses are common. H and E, × 300

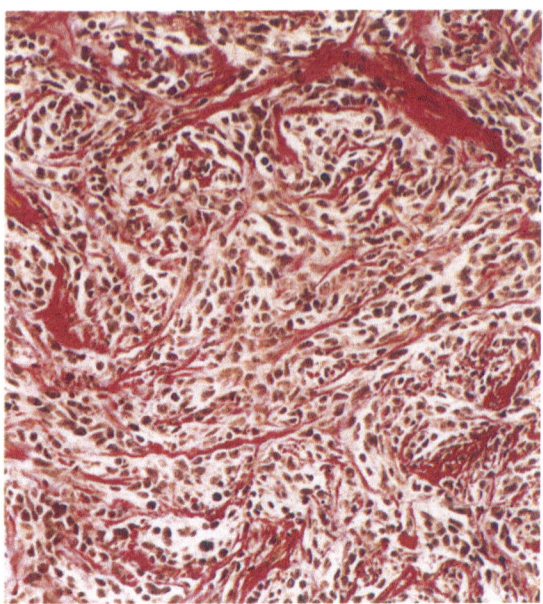

Fig. 9.2. *Medulloblastoma* (the same case as in Fig. 9.1). In parts of the tumor, sinuous linear trabeculae of tumor cells represent the "desmoplastic" type of medulloblastoma. Van Gieson, × 120

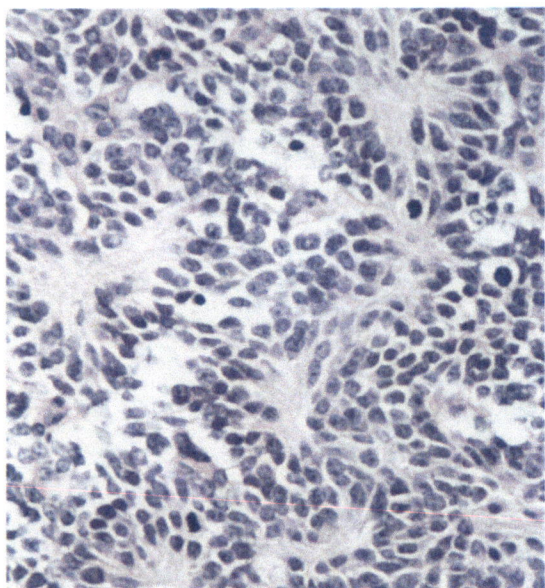

Fig. 9.3. *Medulloblastoma* of cerebellar vermis in an 8-year-old boy. Cellular rosettes and mitoses occur. H and E, × 240

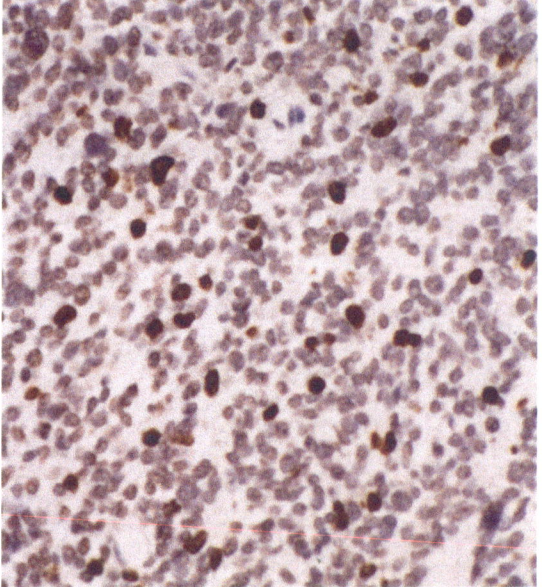

Fig. 9.4. *Medulloblastoma* of cerebellar vermis in an 11-year-old boy. Nuclear uptake of bromode-oxyuridine, a thymidine analogue, is immunohisto-chemically demonstrated in approximately 12% of the tumor cells, indicating the high proliferative potential of this tumor. Indirect immunoperoxidase method counterstained with hematoxylin, × 180

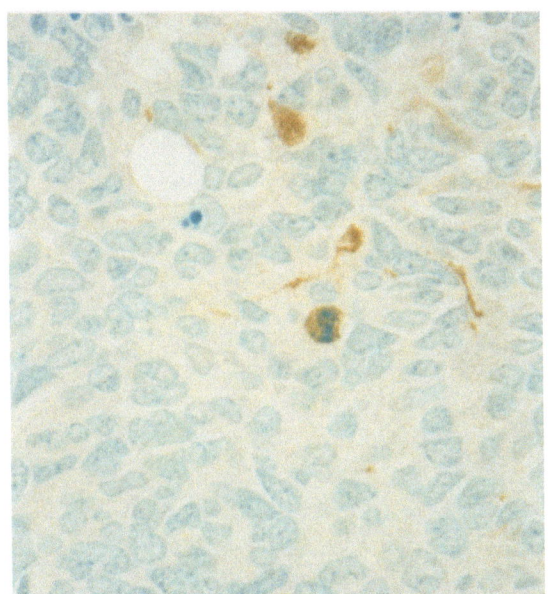 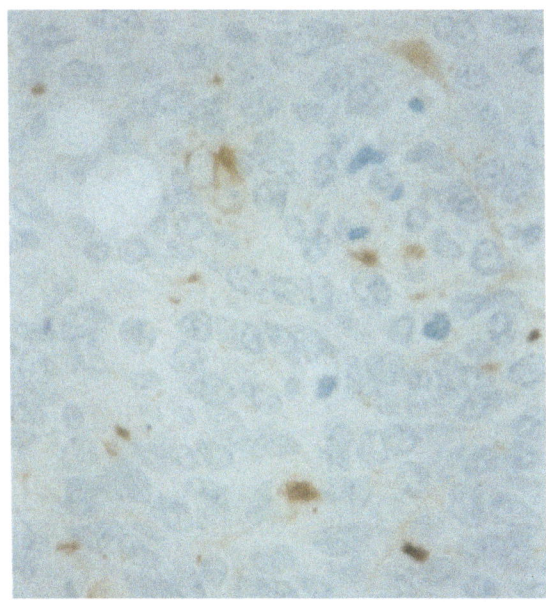

Fig. 9.5. *Medulloblastoma* (the same case as in Fig. 9.1). Some tumor cells reveal positive staining for S-100 protein. Indirect immunoperoxidase method counterstained with methyl green, × 360

Fig. 9.6. *Medulloblastoma* (the same case as in Fig. 9.1). Glial fibrillary acidic protein (GFAP)-positive cells are seen sporadically in the tumor. Indirect immunoperoxidase method counterstained with methyl green, × 360

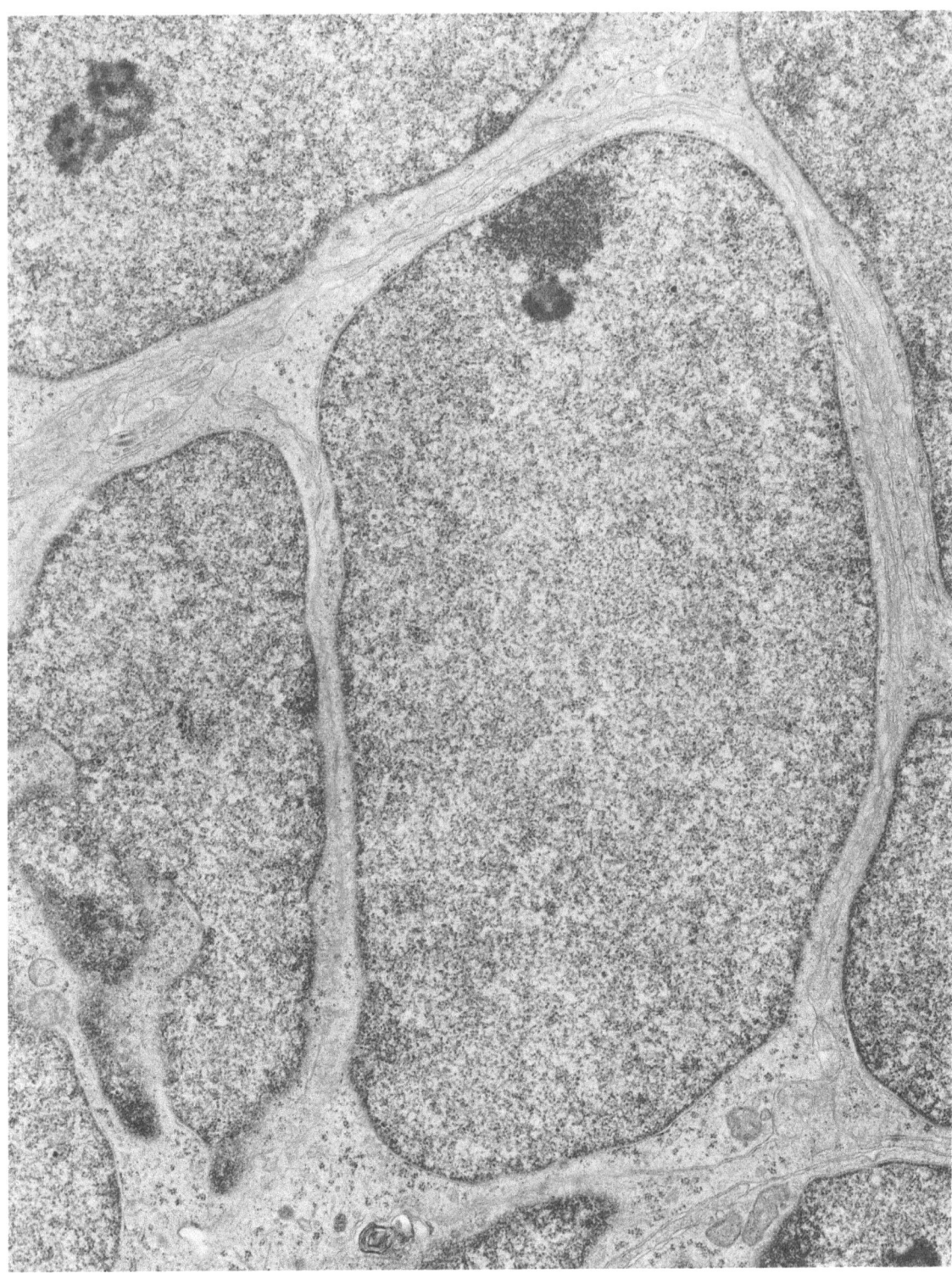

Fig. 9.7. *Medulloblastoma* (the same case as in Fig. 9.1). The tumor cells are very uniform. The cytoplasm is narrow with sparse organelles; the nucleus is dominant and contains euchromatin, indicating the primitive nature of the tumor. × 14900

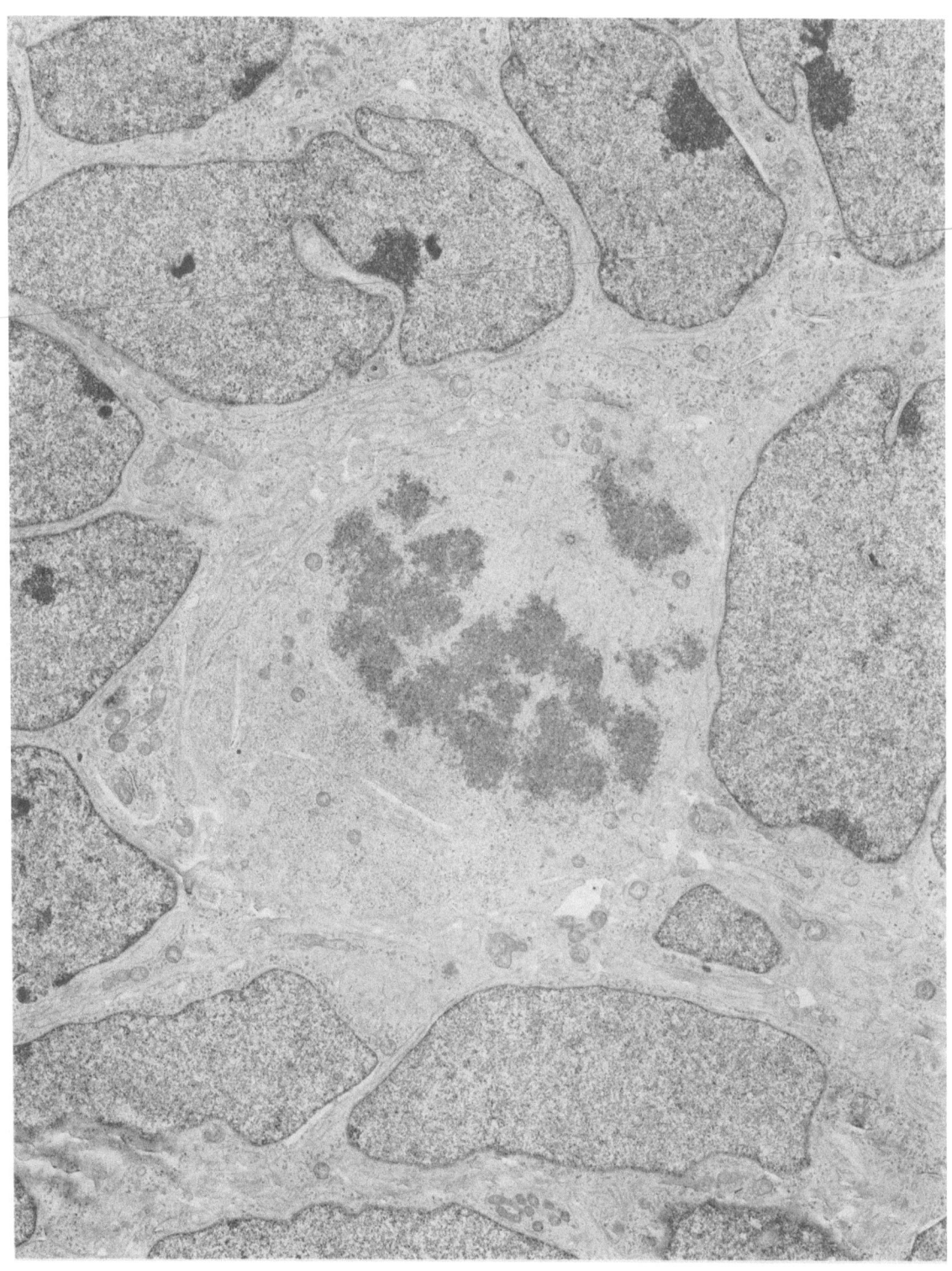

Fig. 9.8. *Medulloblastoma* (the same case as in Fig. 9.1). A mitotic nucleus is often found in the tumor. × 7700

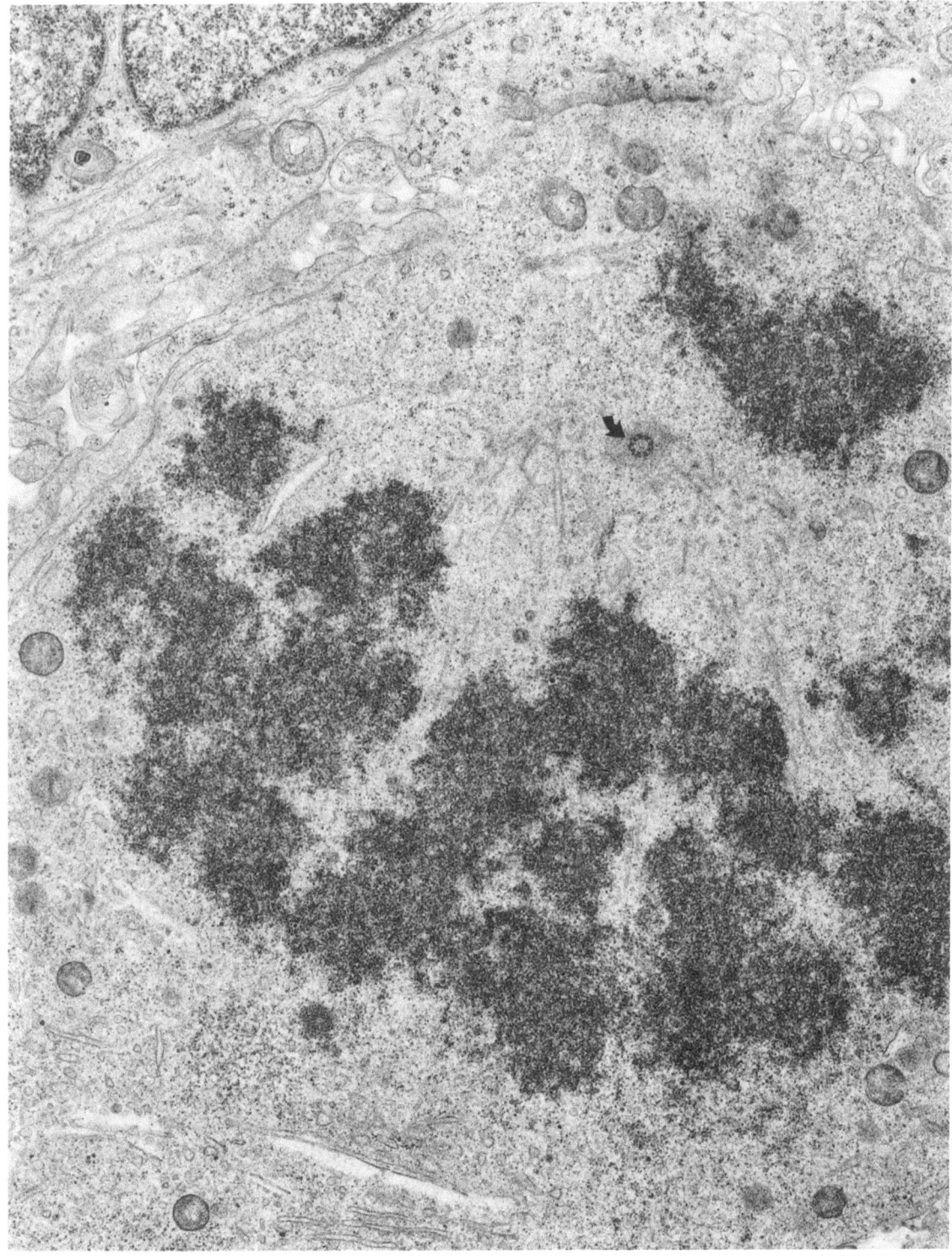

Fig. 9.9. *Medulloblastoma* (the same case as in Fig. 9.1). Higher magnification of Fig. 9.8. A transversely sectioned centriole (*arrow*), microtubules, and decondensed chromosomes are well visualized. × 13 800

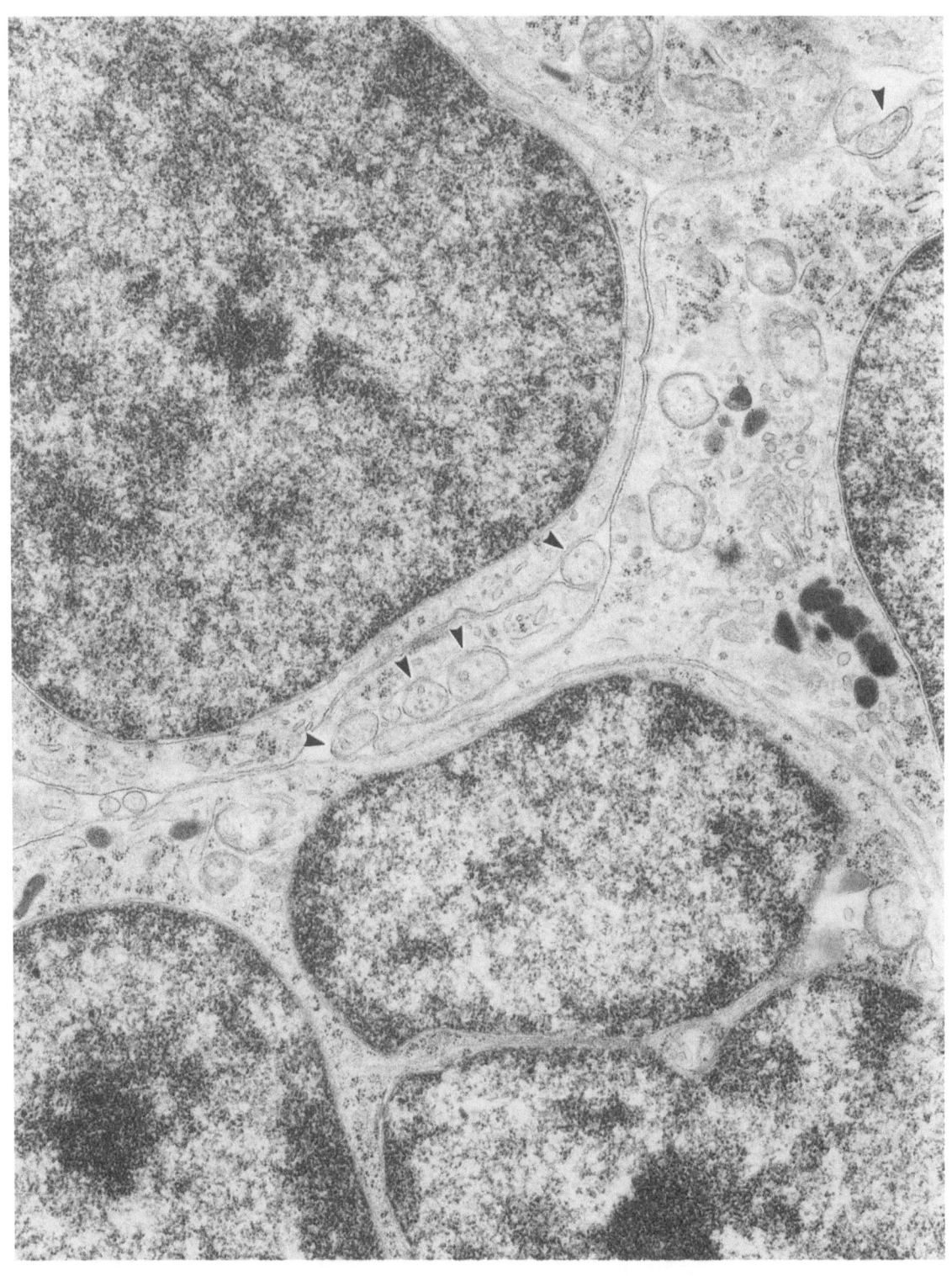

Fig. 9.10. *Medulloblastoma* (the same case as in Fig. 9.1). Cross sections of cell processes (*arrowheads*) are sometimes interspersed among solid sheets of tumor cells. × 21 000

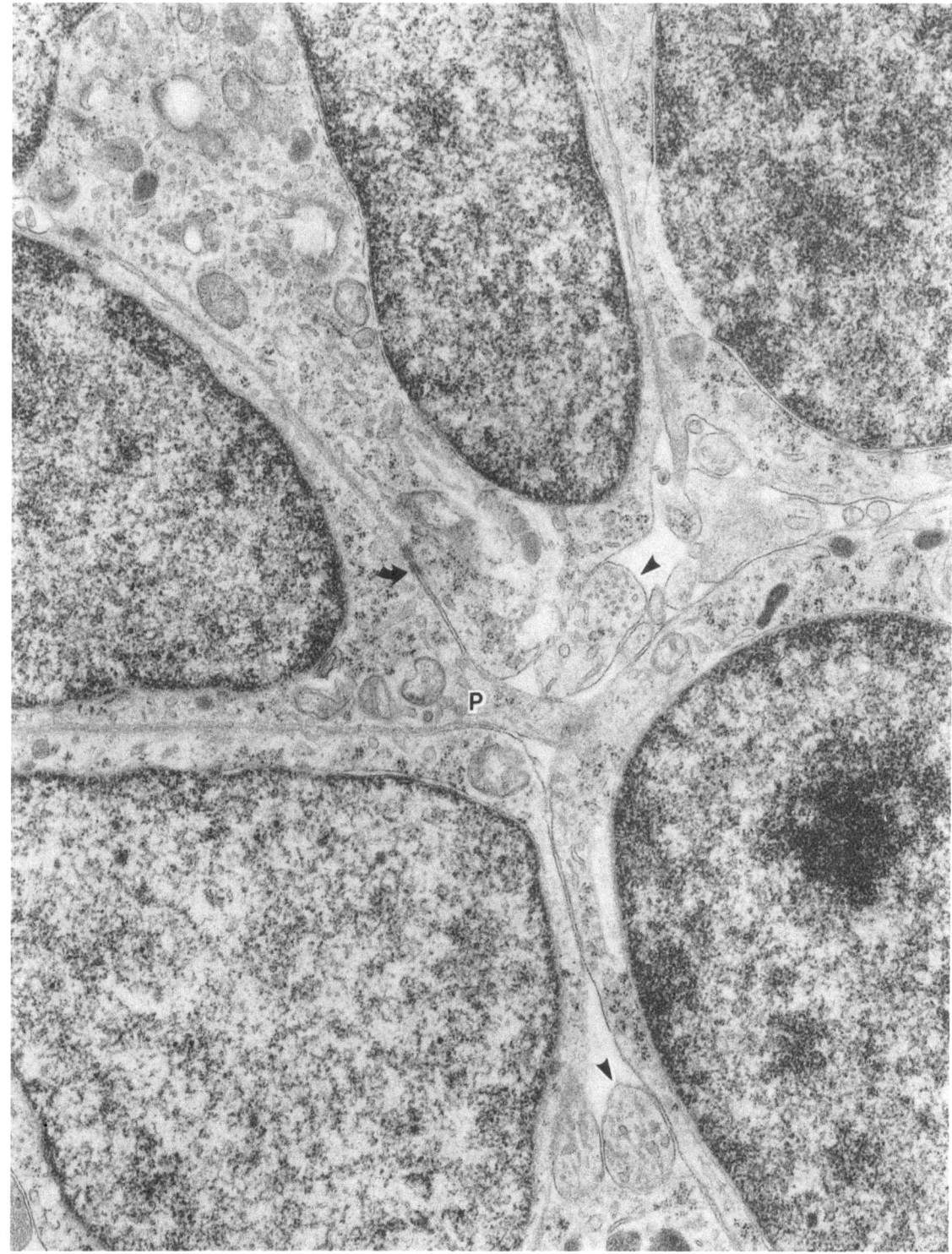

Fig. 9.11. *Medulloblastoma* (the same case as in Fig. 9.1). A cellular process (*P*) attaching to an other cell, a junctional apparatus (*arrow*), and some cross-sectioned processes (*arrowheads*) are seen. × 21 000

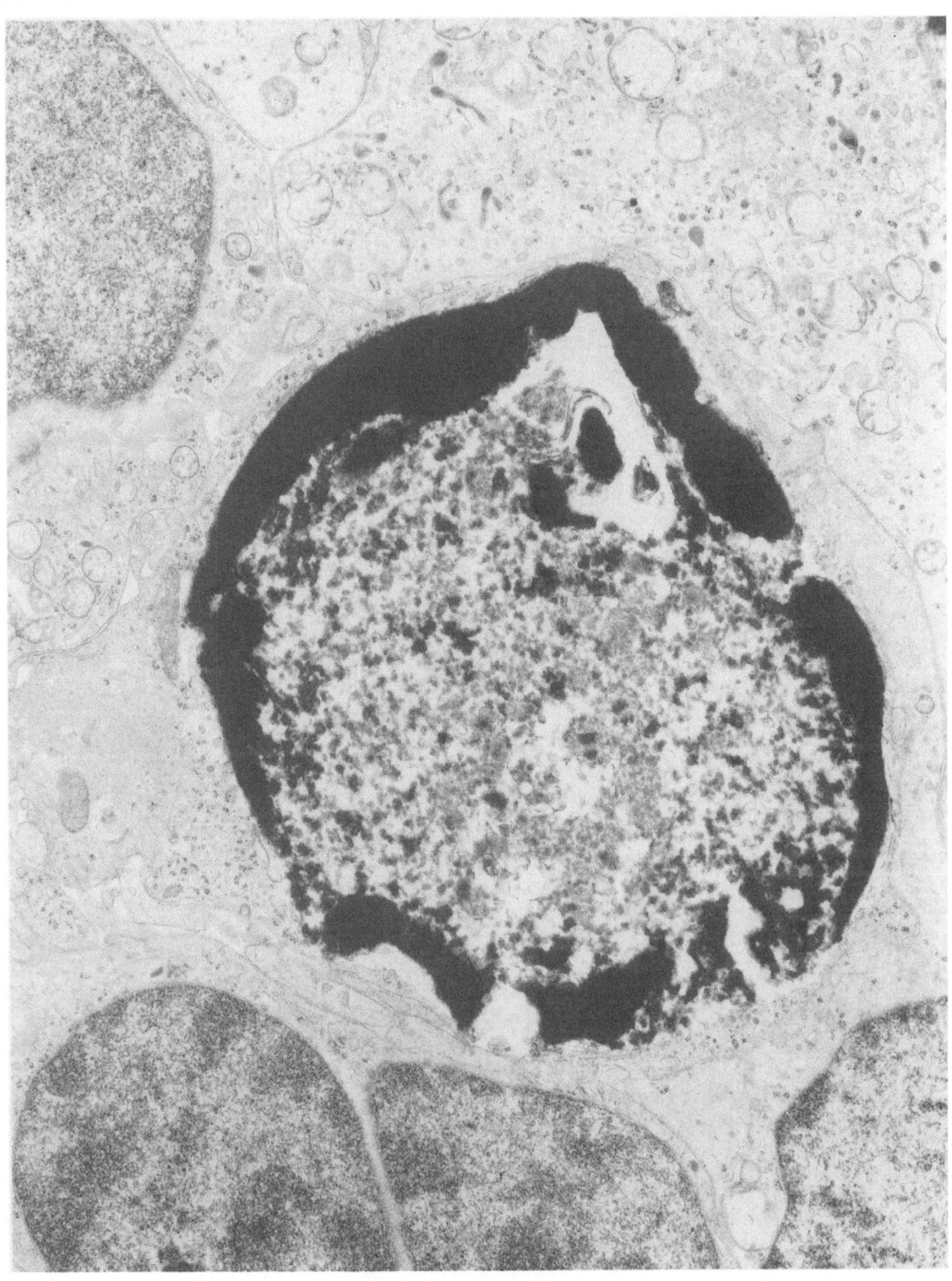

Fig. 9.12. *Medulloblastoma* (the same case as in Fig. 9.1). The central cell shows a pyknotic nucleus and lysing cytoplasm. Degenerating features of individual cells are not uncommon in this tumor. × 14 400

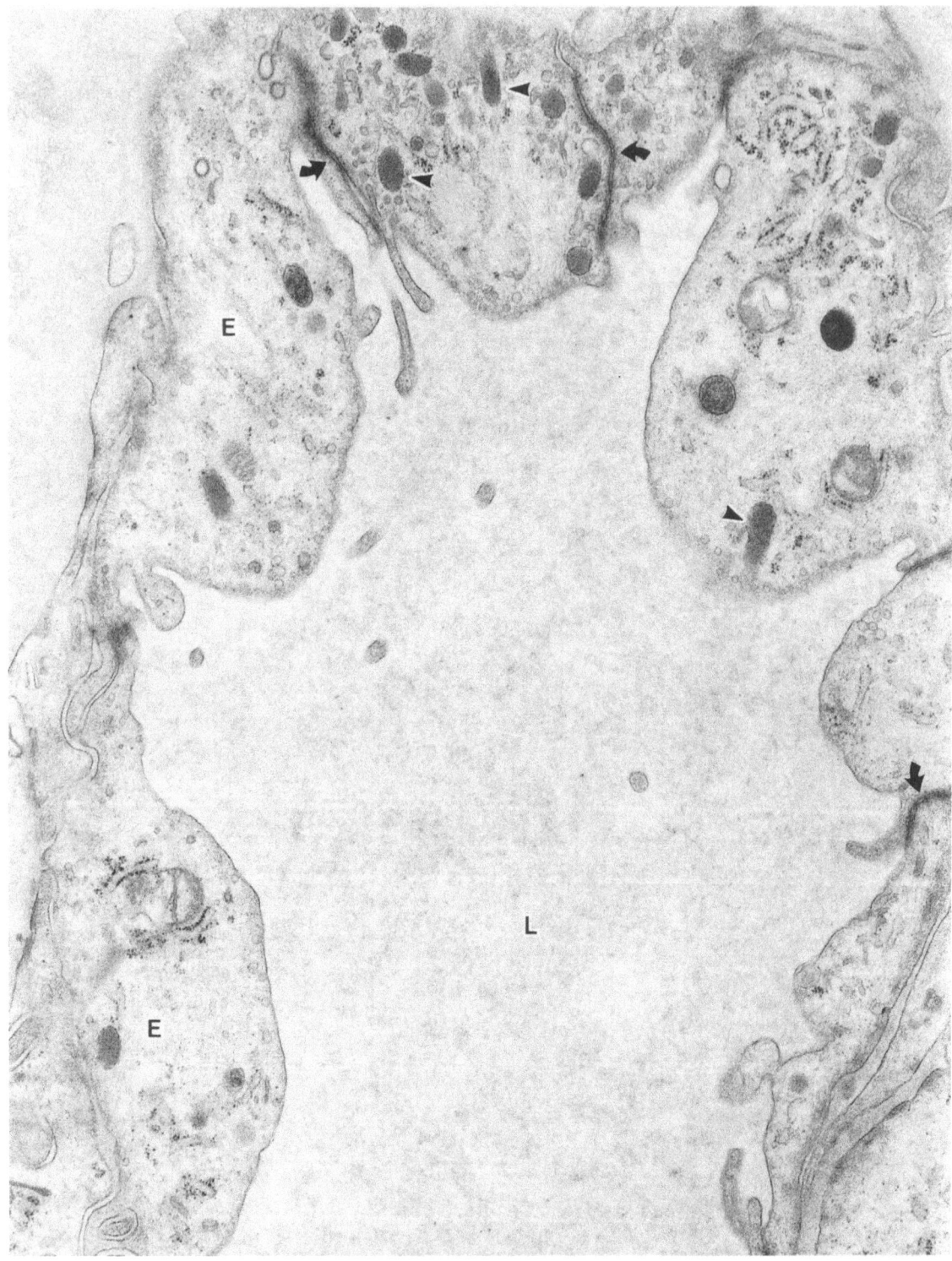

Fig. 9.13. A capillary in the medulloblastoma (the same case as in Fig. 9.1). Intercellular junctions (*arrows*) of the occluding type are seen between endothelial cells (*E*). Several Weibel-Palade bodies (*arrowheads*) are observed, indicating angiogenesis in the tumor. *L* capillary lumen. × 22 000

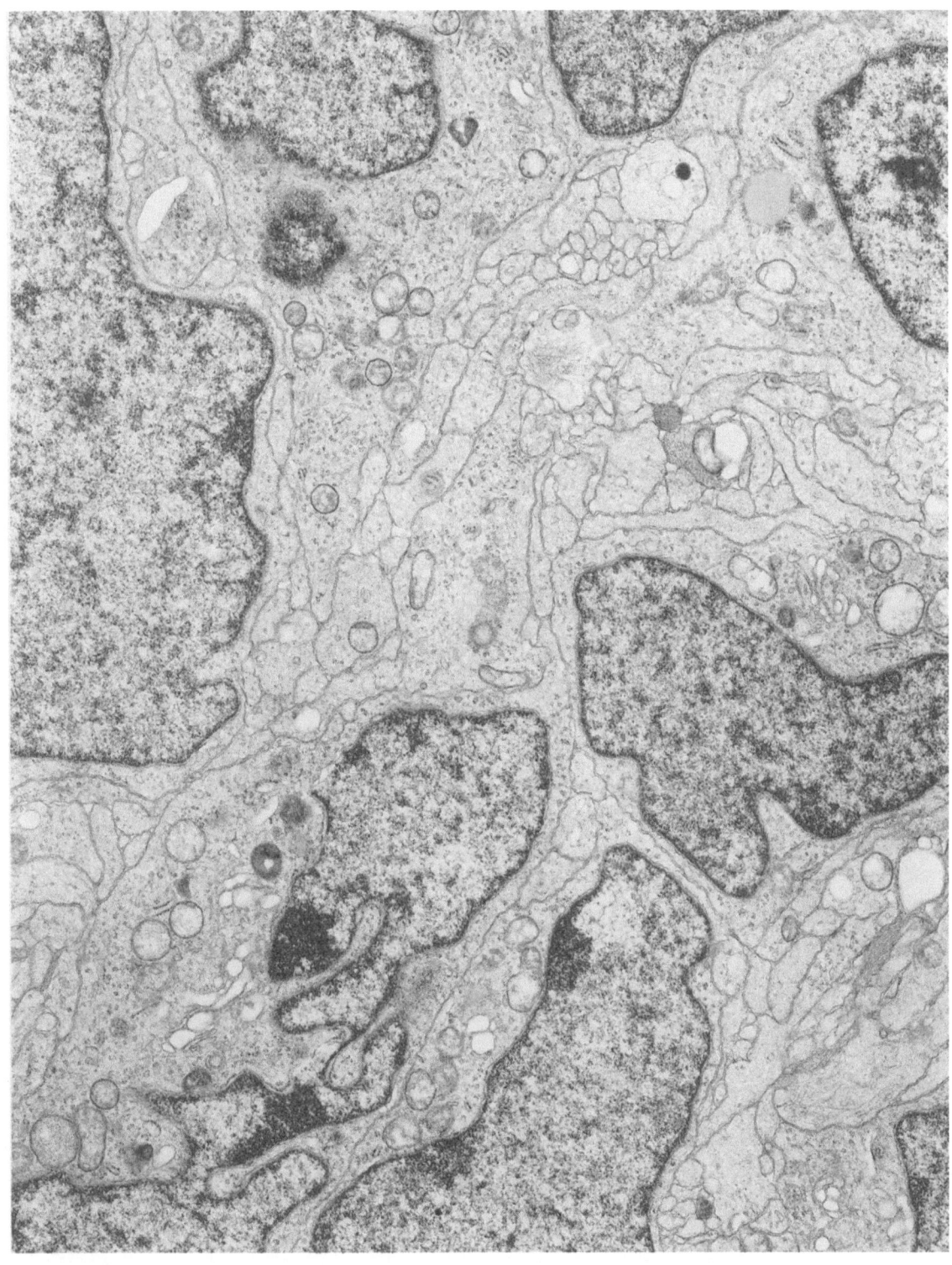

Fig. 9.14. *Medulloblastoma* (the same case as in Fig. 9.3). Transversely sectioned processes of tumor cells resemble a neuropil. × 12 200

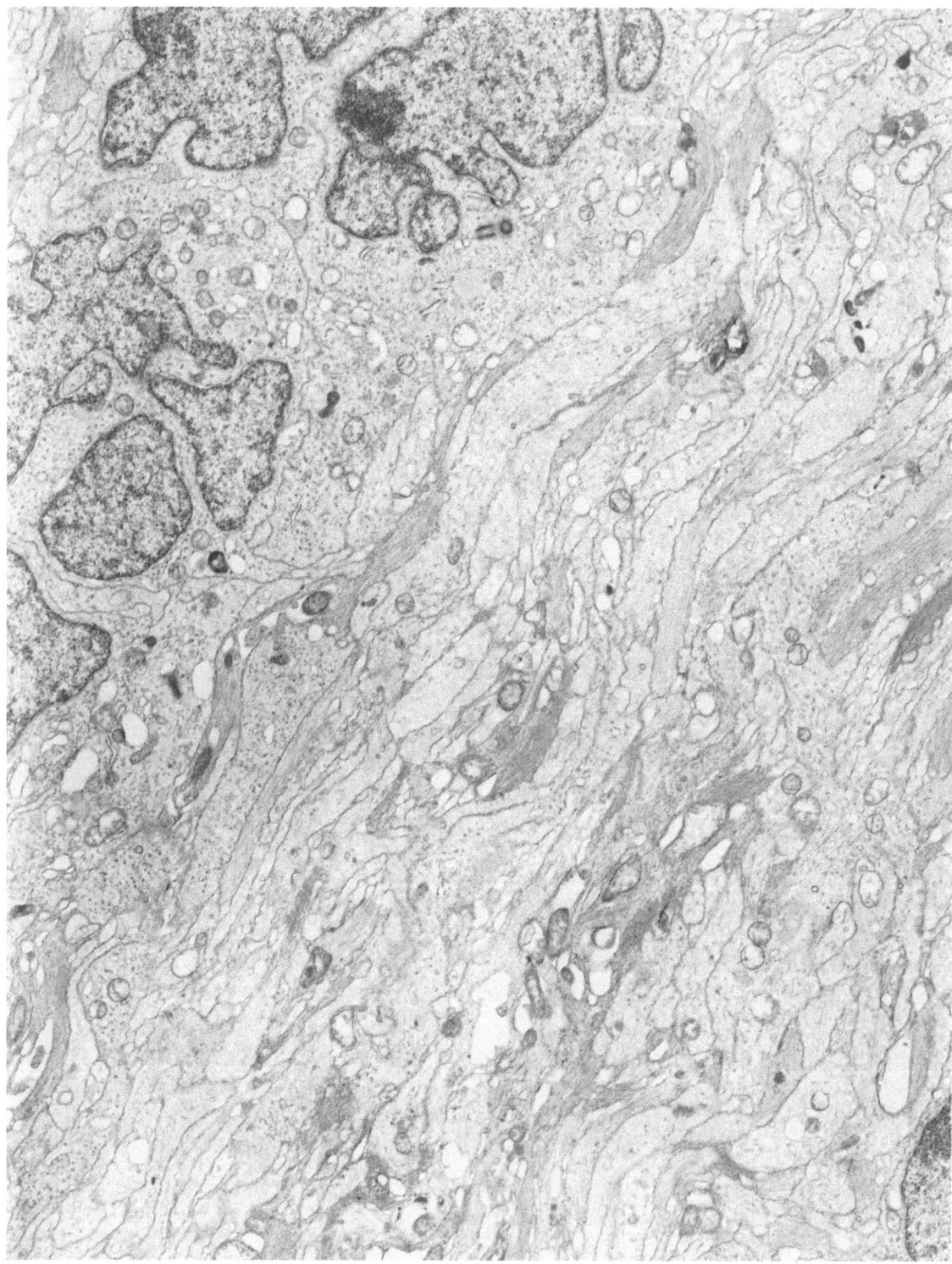

Fig. 9.15. *Medulloblastoma* (the same case as in Fig. 9.3). Longitudinally sectioned processes of tumor cells contain abundant intermediate filaments. No collagen is visible. × 8900

10. Ganglioglioma

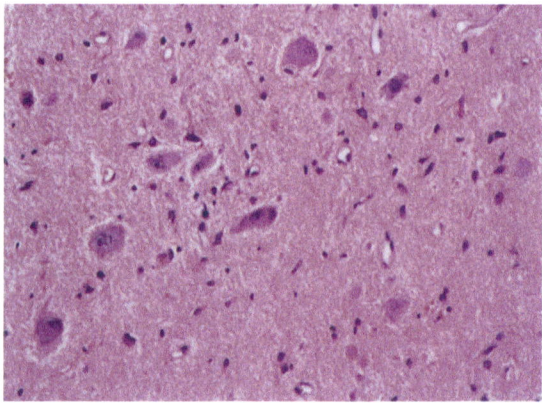

Fig. 10.1. *Ganglioglioma* of the left cerebellar hemisphere in a 10-month-old infant. The tumor consists of neoplastic neuronal cells of different size and shape as well as small glial cells, though the cellularity is low. H and E, × 80

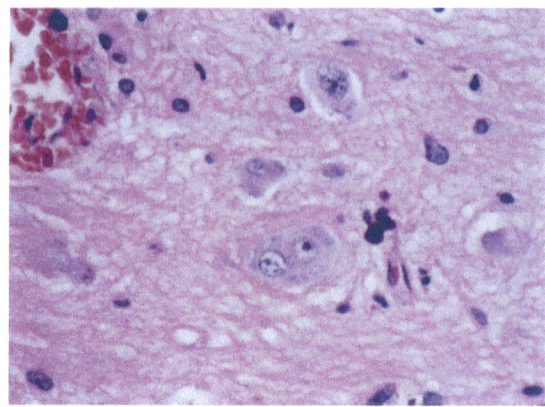

Fig. 10.2. *Ganglioglioma* (the same case as in Fig. 10.1). A binucleate neuronal cell is evident. Calcopherites are usually seen in the tumor. H and E, × 160

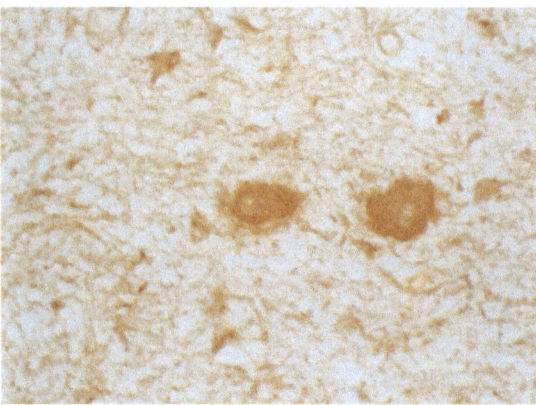

Fig. 10.3. *Ganglioglioma* (the same case as in Fig. 10.1). A positive immunohistochemical reaction for neuron-specific enolase (NSE) is localized in the cytoplasm of both the neuronal and glial cells. Indirect immunoperoxidase method without counterstain, × 160

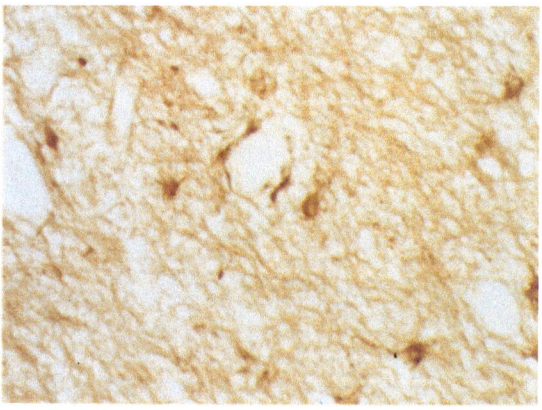

Fig. 10.4. *Ganglioglioma* (the same case as in Fig. 10.1). A positive reaction for glial fibrillary acidic protein (GFAP) is confined to the glial cytoplasm and processes; it is absent from the neuronal cells. Indirect immunoperoxidase method without counterstain, × 160

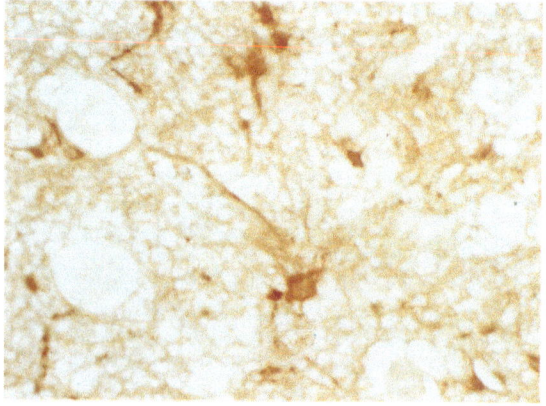

Fig. 10.5. *Ganglioglioma* (the same case as in Fig. 10.1). Positive staining for S-100 protein (β-subunit) is seen in the glial cells but not in the neuronal cells. Indirect immunoperoxidase method without counterstain, × 160

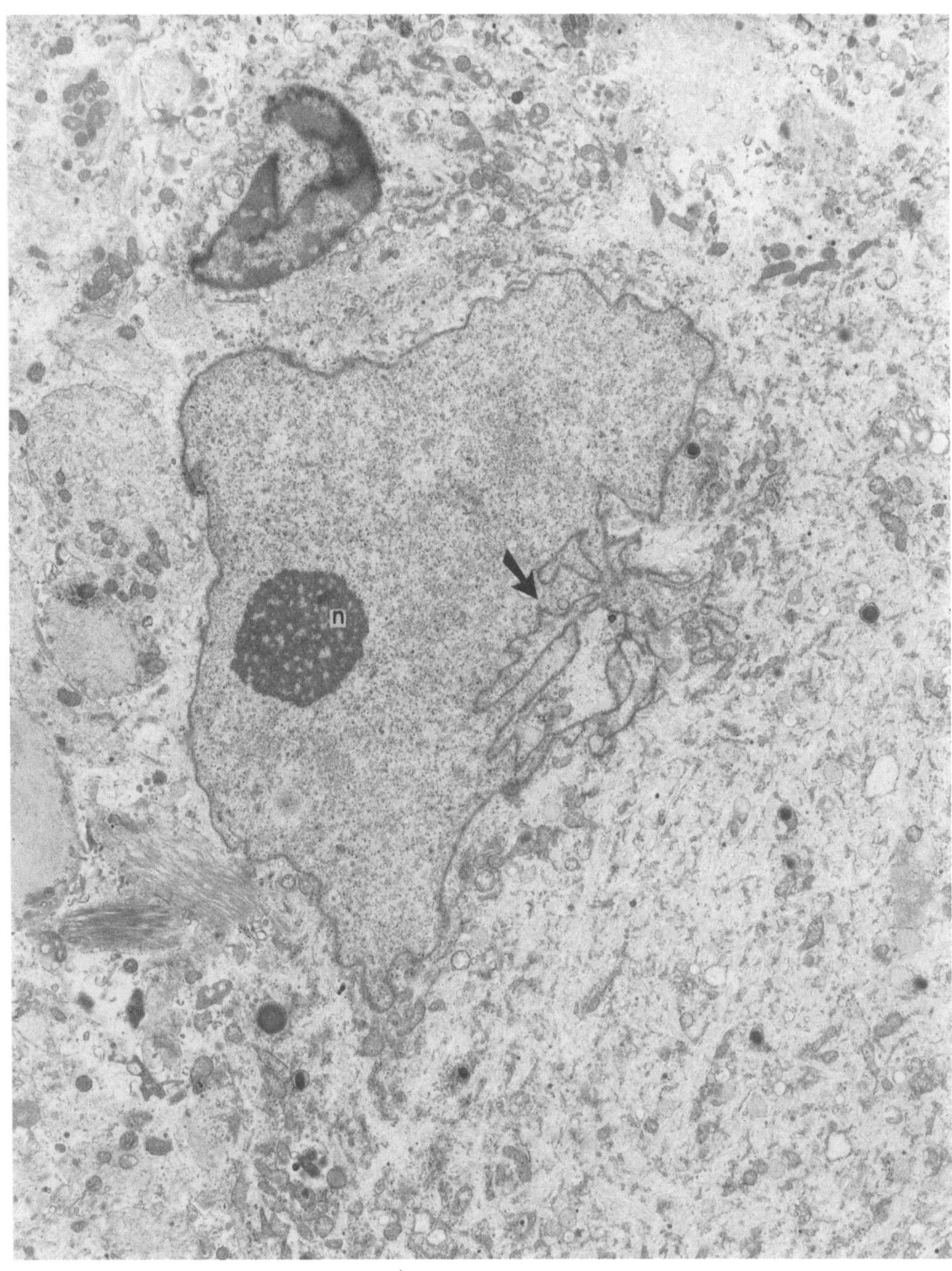

Fig. 10.6. *Ganglioglioma* (the same case as in Fig. 10.1). A ganglionic cell shows meandering invaginations of the nucleus (*arrow*) and a well-marginated nucleolus (*n*). The cytoplasm is filled with organelles, including intermediate filaments, microtubules, and some dense core vesicles. × 9800

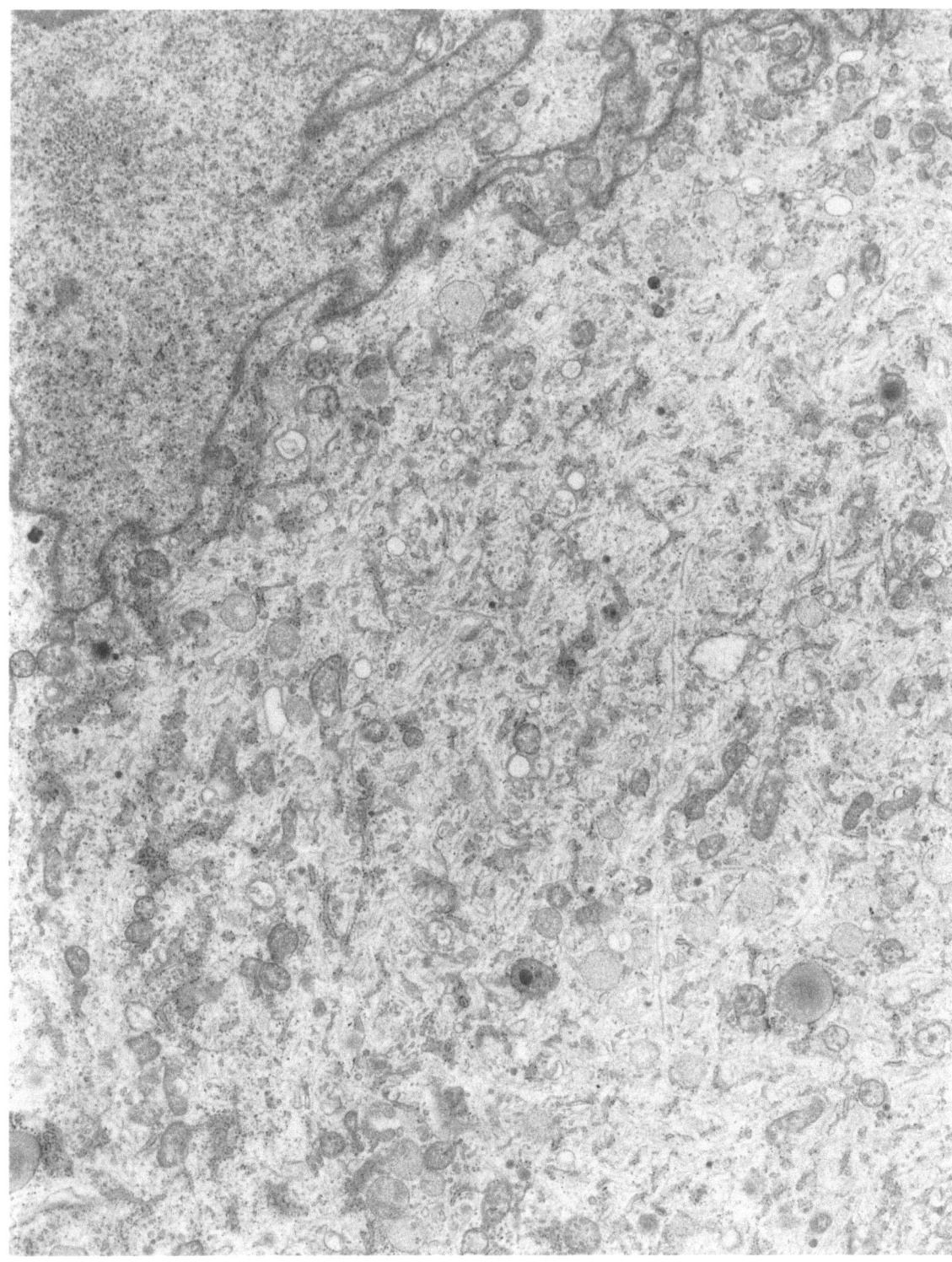

Fig. 10.7. *Ganglioglioma* (the same case as in Fig. 10.1). Higher magnification reveals details of the cytoplasm of a ganglionic cell in which intermediate filaments and microtubules are intermingled. × 14 000

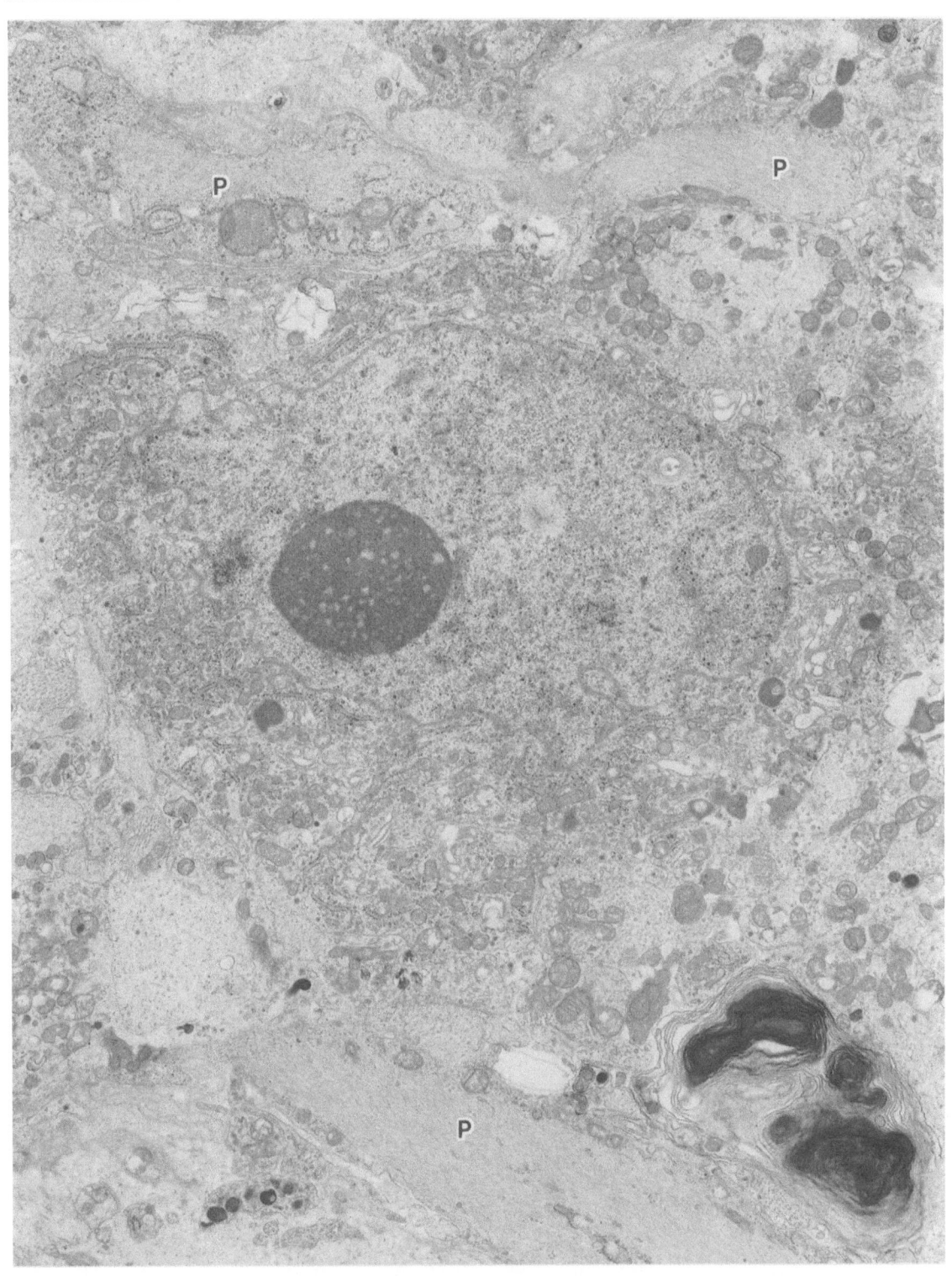

Fig. 10.8. *Ganglioglioma* (the same case as in Fig. 10.1). A ganglionic cell is surrounded by neoplastic astrocyte processes (*P*) containing abundant glial filaments. × 9800

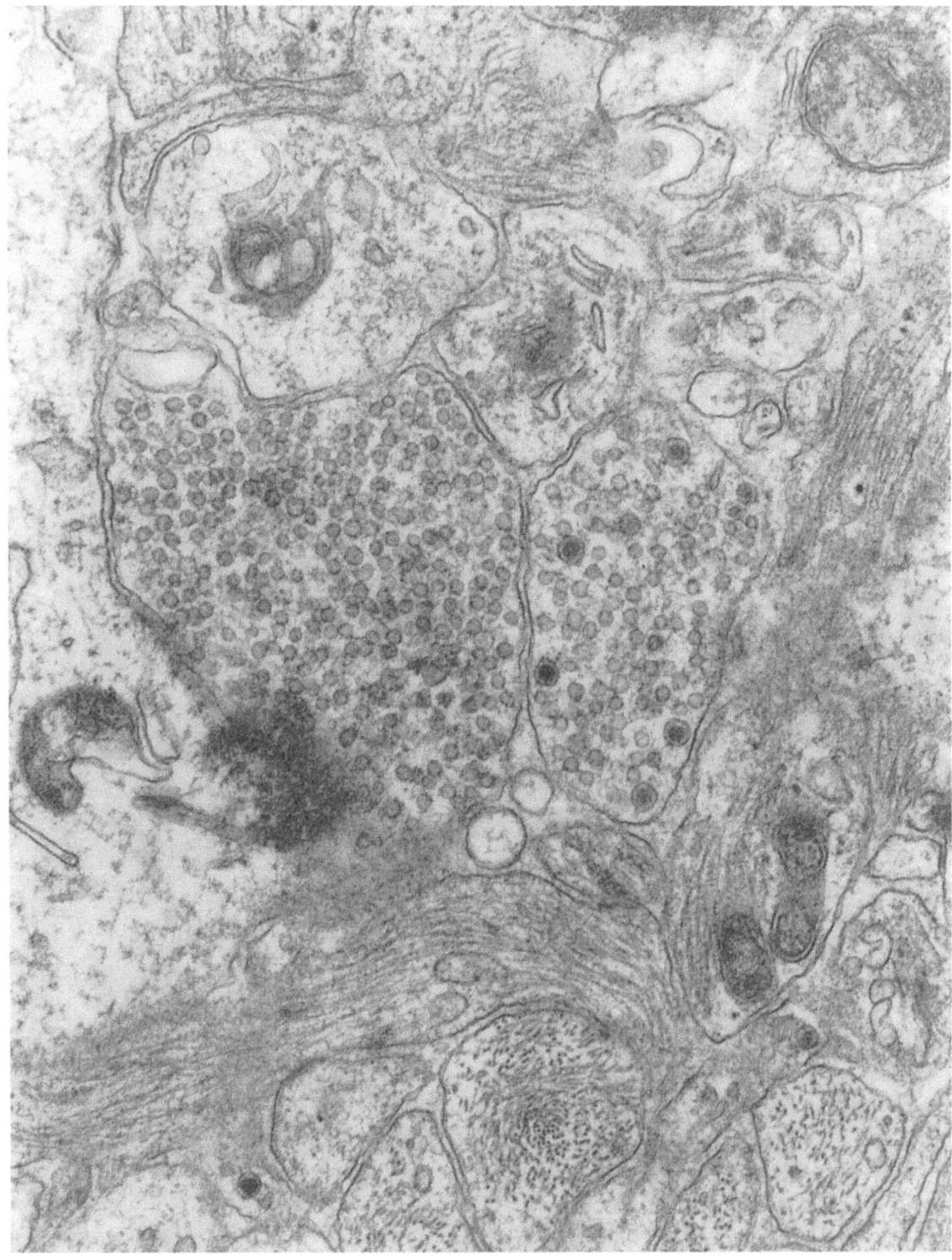

Fig. 10.9. *Ganglioglioma* (the same case as in Fig. 10.1). Transversely sectioned dendrite-like structures and axon terminals, the latter are filled with numerous small vesicles, measuring 70–90 nm in diameter, and some dense core vesicles, approximately 130 nm in diameter. × 38 000

11. Central Neurocytoma

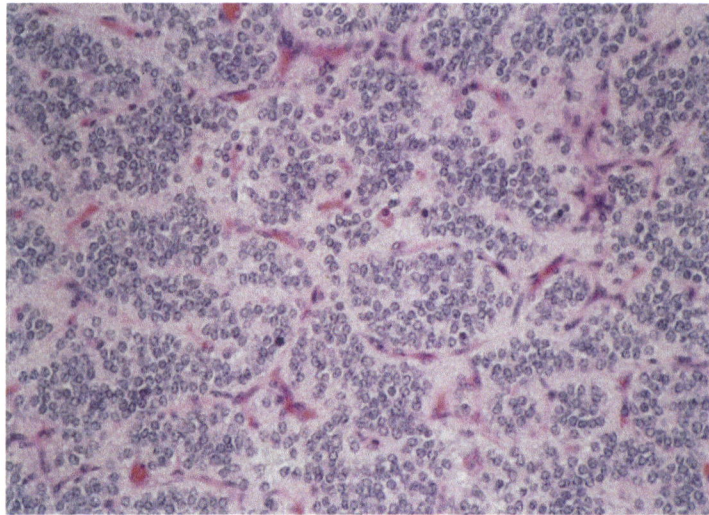

Fig. 11.1. *Central neurocytoma* which arose intraventricularly in a 22-year-old woman. Tumor cells with round nuclei are grouped, forming cell nests which are separated from each other by capillary stroma. H and E, × 80

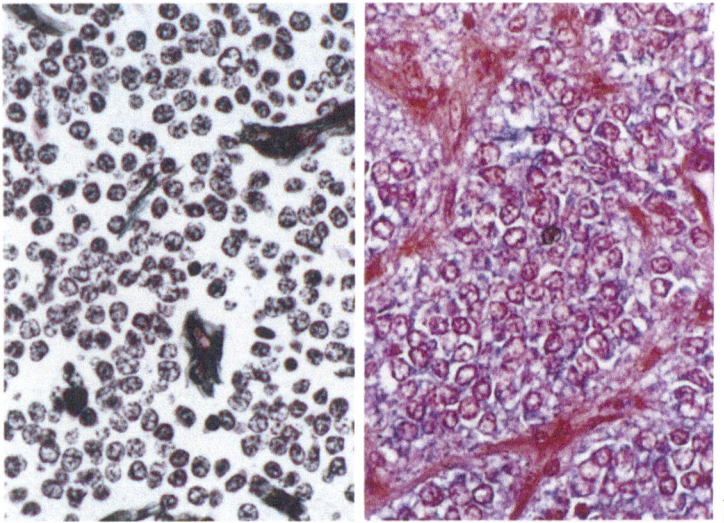

Fig. 11.2a, b. *Central neurocytoma* (the same case as in Fig. 11.1). Neither neuritic processes nor neuroglial fibers are present. **a** silver impregnation, × 160; **b** phosphotungstic acid hematoxylin, × 160

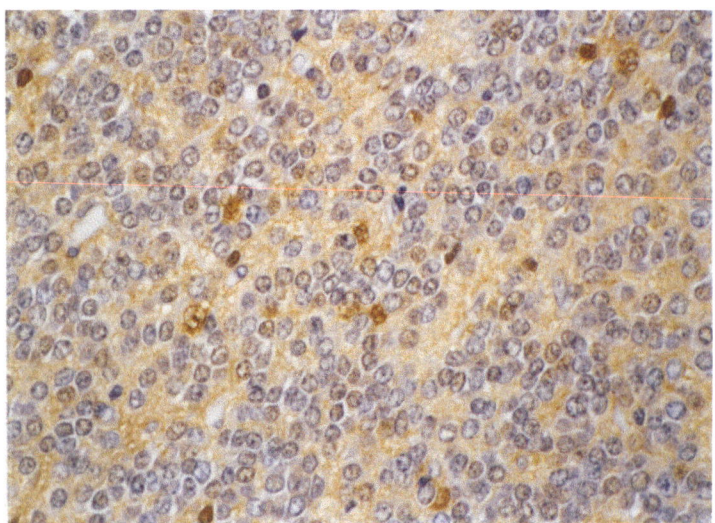

Fig. 11.3. *Central neurocytoma* (the same case as in Fig. 11.1). A weak, though unequivocally positive staining for S-100 protein is seen in both the cytoplasm and nuclei of some tumor cells. Indirect immunoperoxidase method counterstained with hematoxylin, × 160

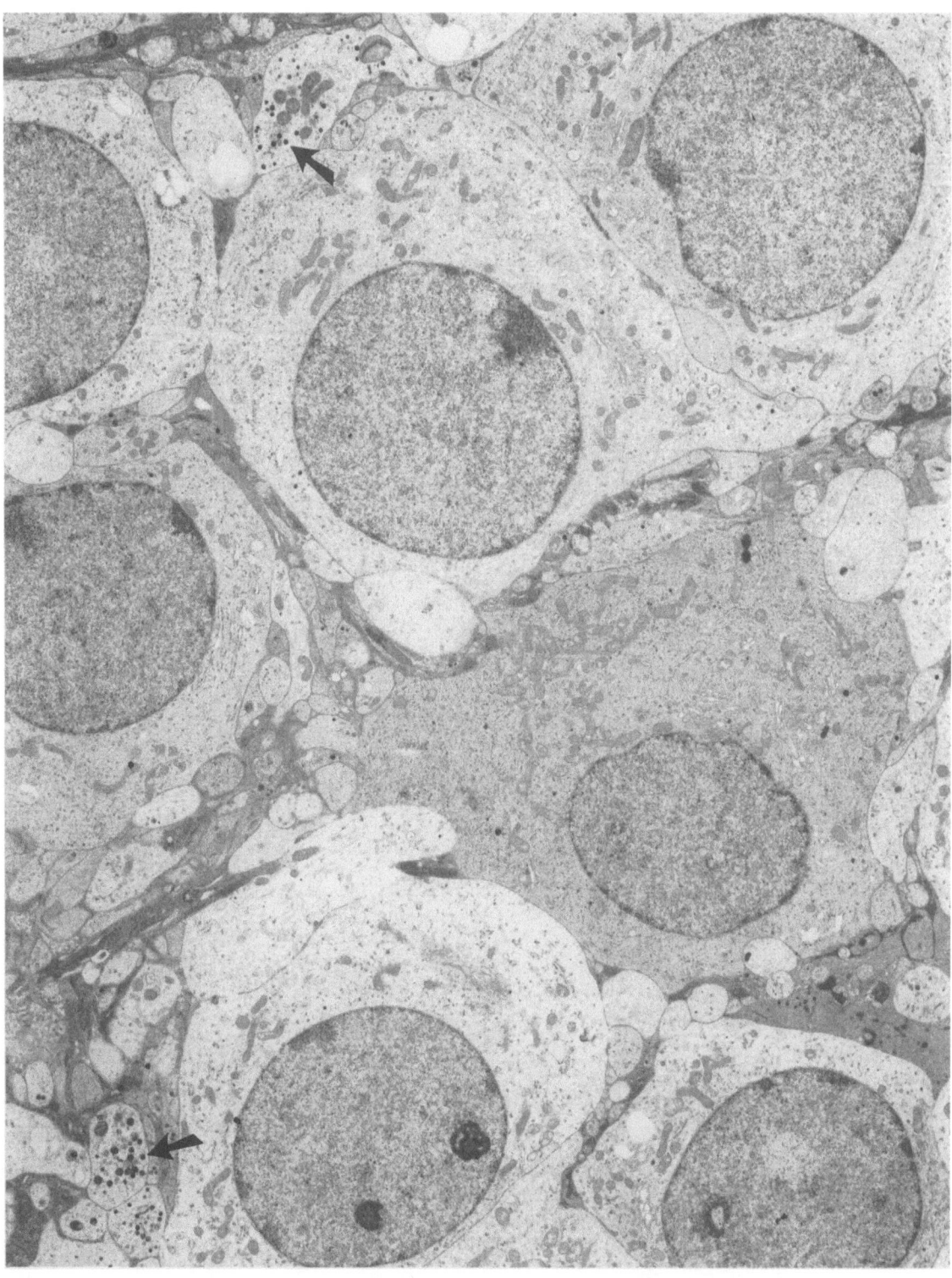

Fig. 11.4. *Central neurocytoma* (the same case as in Fig. 11.1). The tumor cells have a well-defined electron-lucent cytoplasm containing a considerable number of organelles. Small electron-dense granules (*arrows*), varying in size, are occasionally seen in the cell processes. × 6000

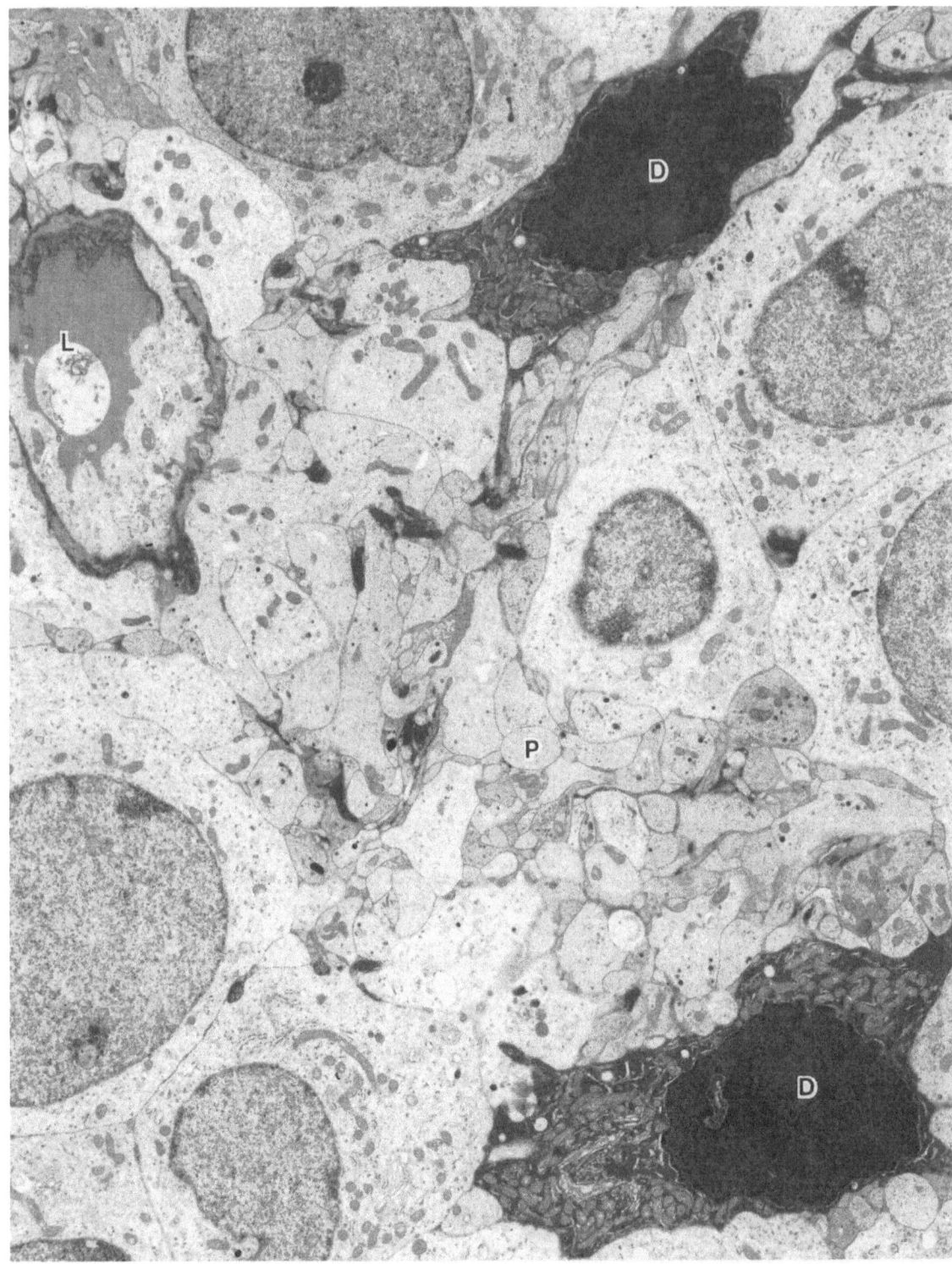

Fig. 11.5. *Central neurocytoma* (the same case as in Fig. 11.1). Uncharacterized "dark" cells (*D*) are often encountered in the tumor. There are many cell processes (*P*) sectioned transversely. *L* capillary lumen. × 6000

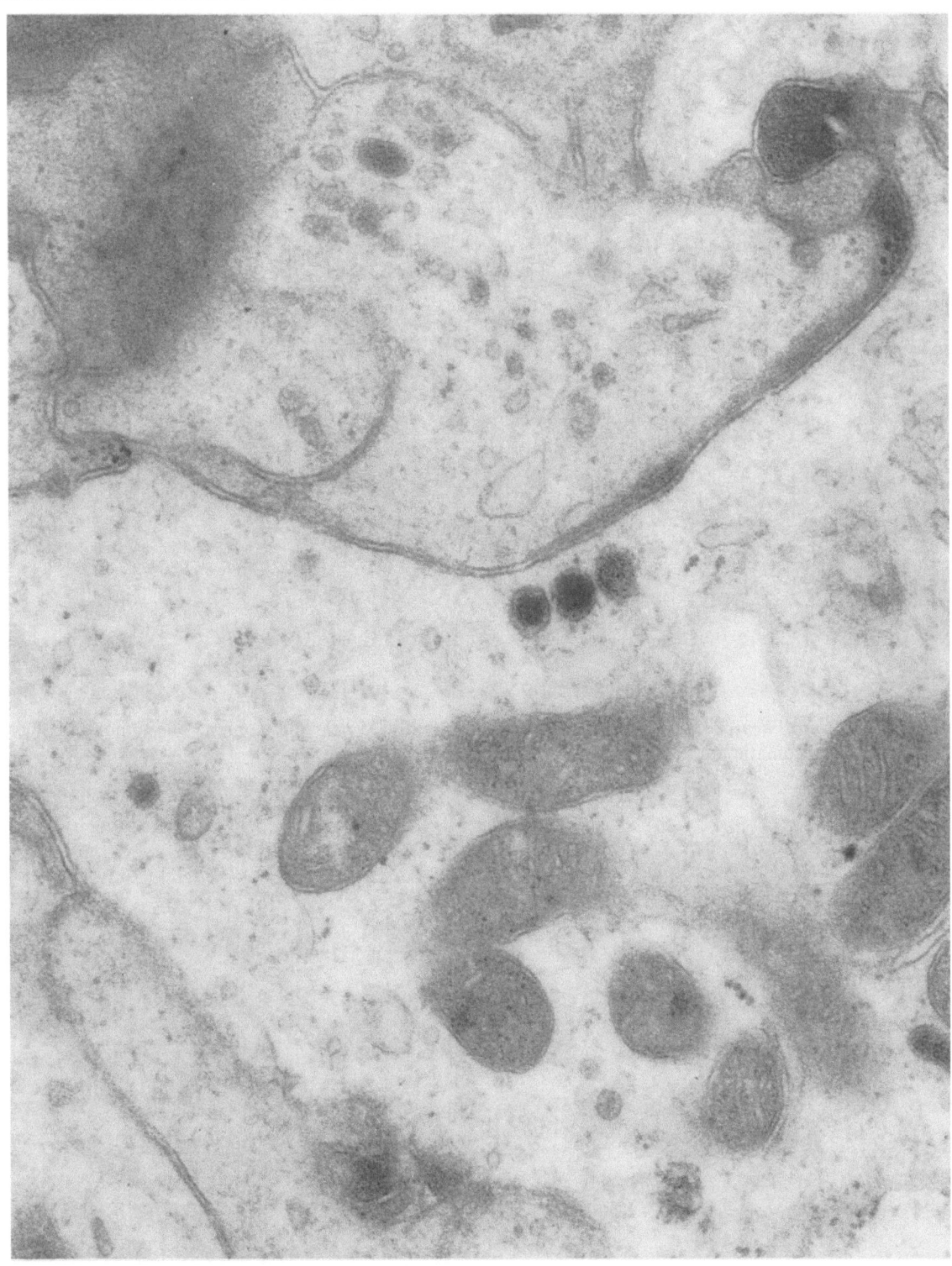

Fig. 11.6. *Central neurocytoma* (the same case as in Fig. 11.1). Higher magnification reveals dense core vesicles as well as a synapse-like structure, which are important diagnostic features in this tumor. × 42 000

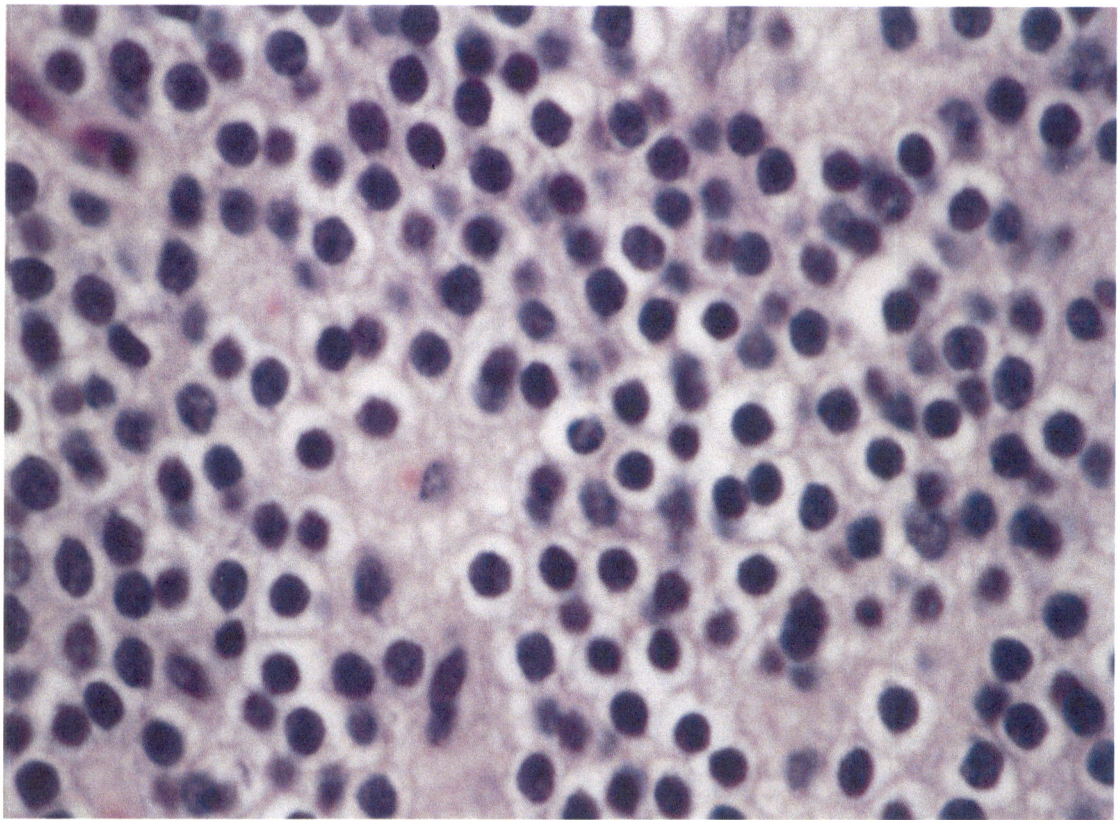

Fig. 11.7. *Central neurocytoma* arising intraventricularly in a 35-year-old woman. The tumor cells have round, hyperchromatic nuclei and display perinuclear halos. H and E, × 500

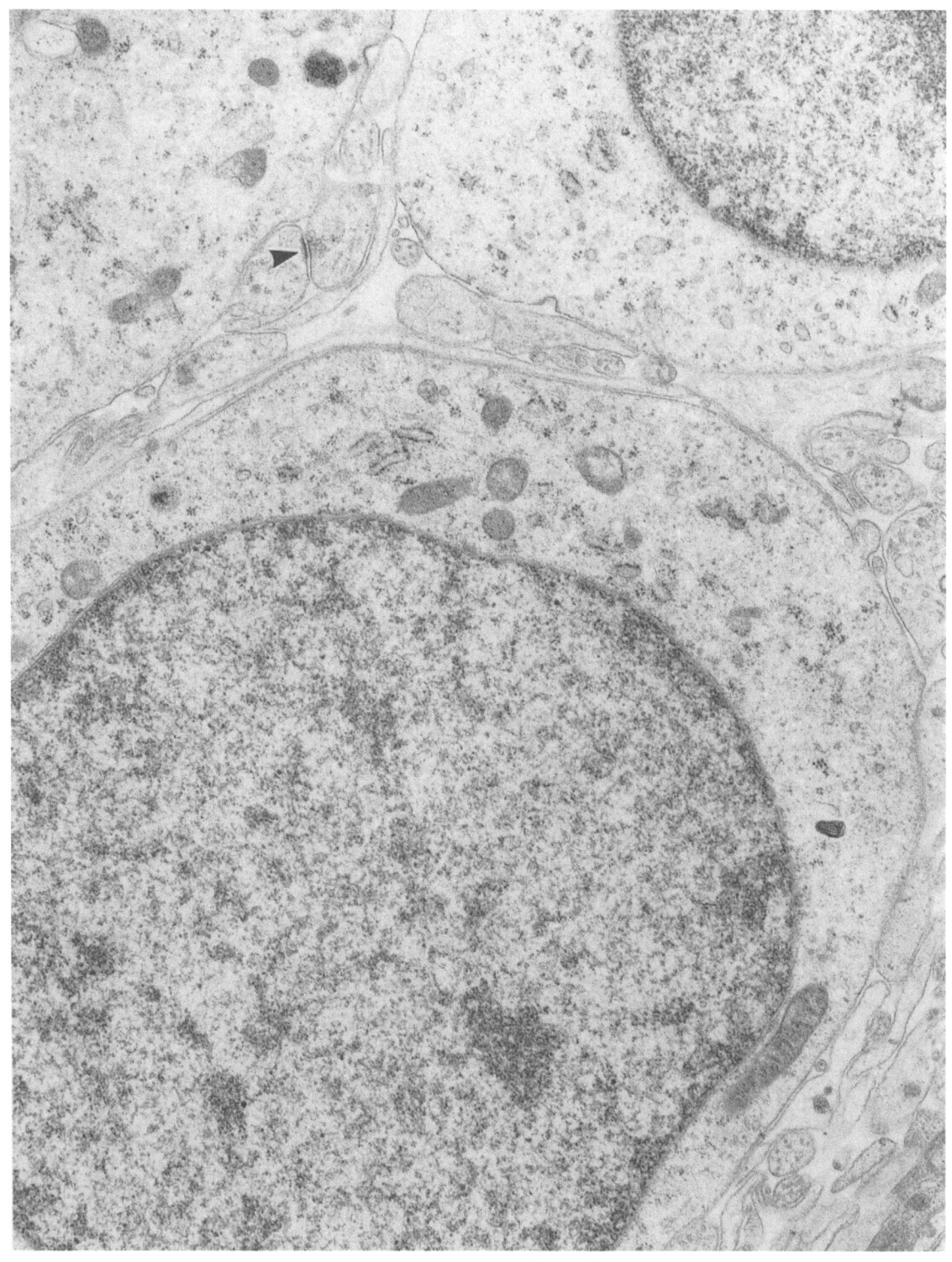

Fig. 11.8. *Central neurocytoma* (the same case as in Fig. 11.7). The tumor cell has a round nucleus and clear cytoplasm. A synapse-like structure (*arrowhead*) is seen. × 21 000

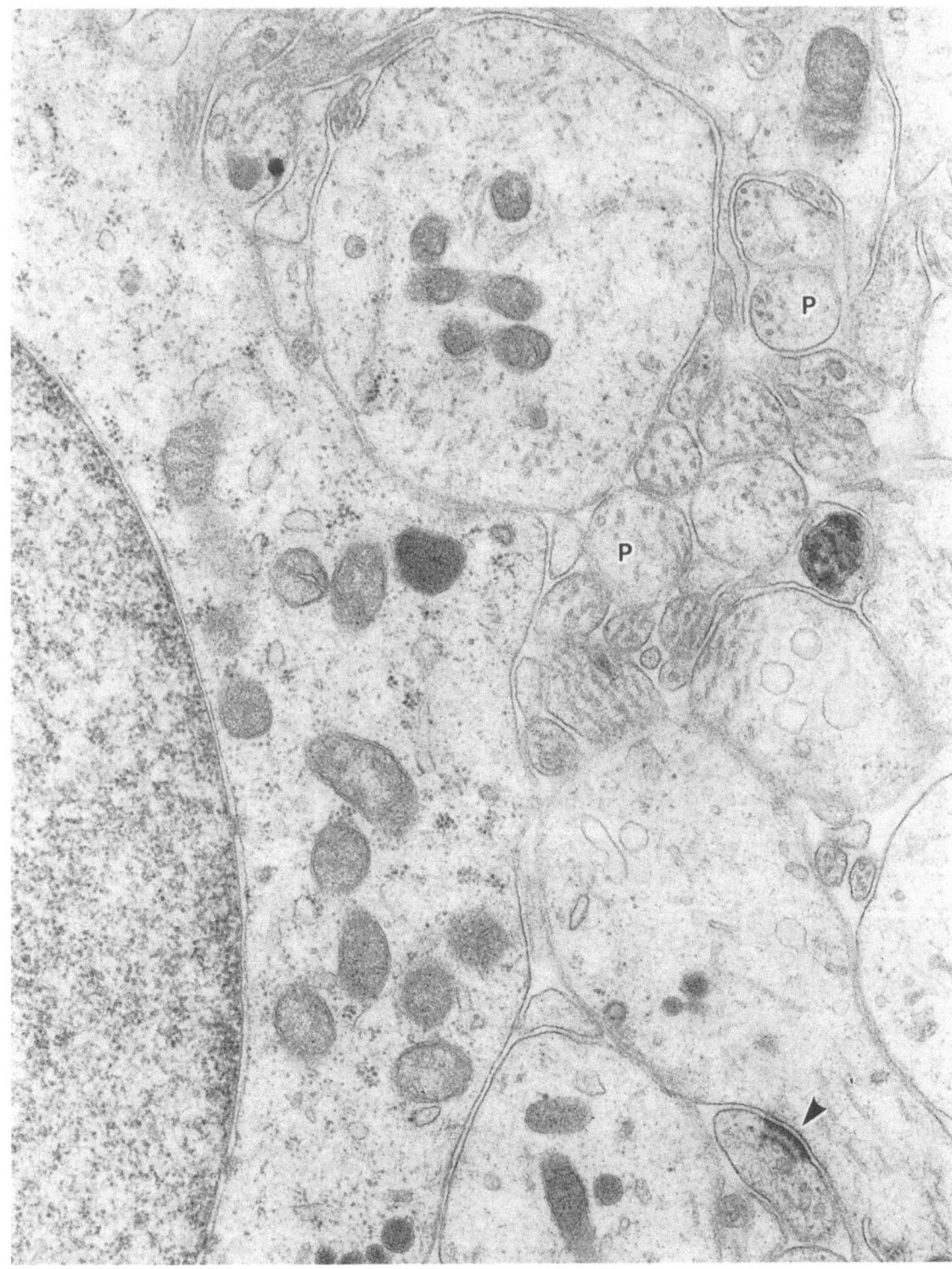

Fig. 11.9. *Central neurocytoma* (the same case as in Fig. 11.7). The cell processes (*P*) with microtubules and synapse-like structure (*arrowhead*) resemble a neuropil. × 35 000

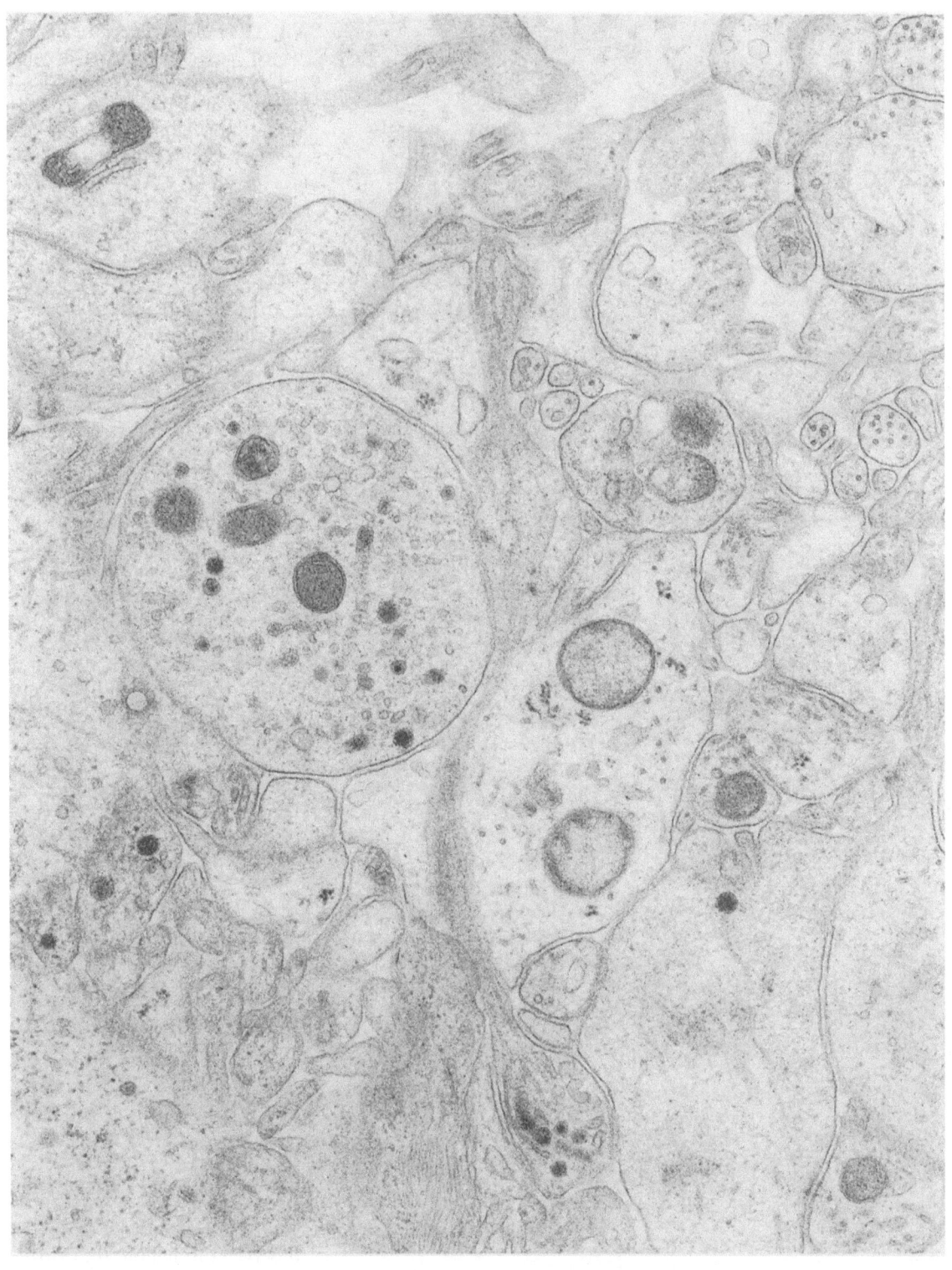

Fig. 11.10. *Central neurocytoma* (the same case as in Fig. 11.7). Dense core vesicles are often seen as the main diagnostic feature of this tumor. × 35 000

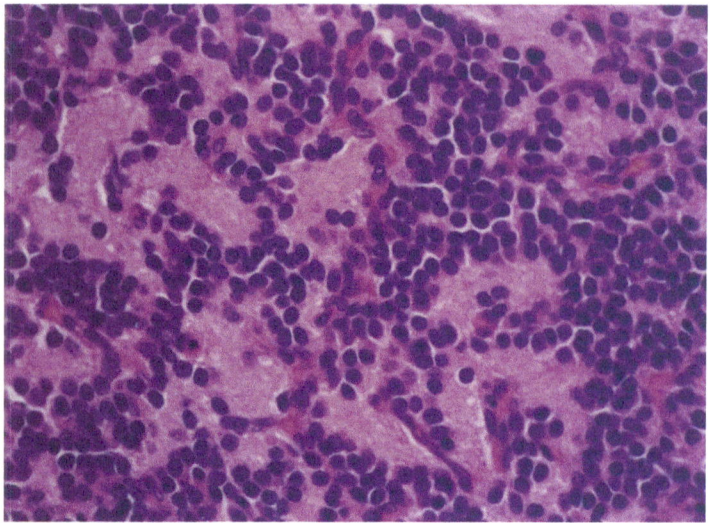

Fig. 11.11. *Central neurocytoma* which arose intraventricularly in a 42-year-old man. The tumor cells with hyperchromatic round nuclei show Homer-Wright rosettes. H and E, × 160

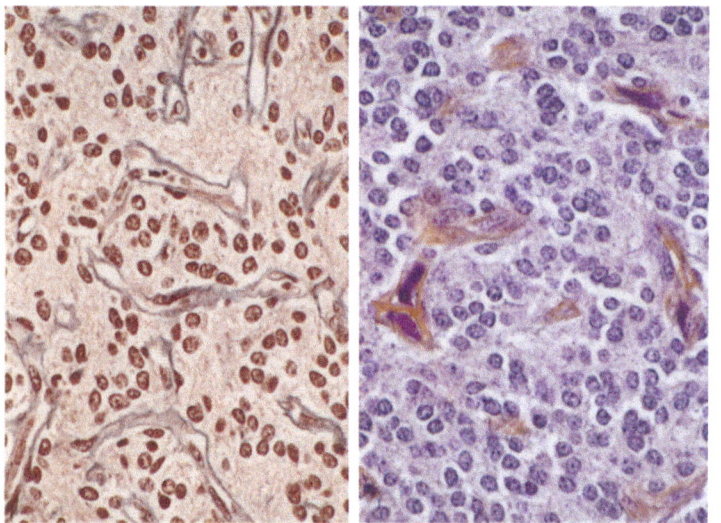

a   b

Fig. 11.12a, b. *Central neurocytoma* (the same case as in Fig. 11.11). Neither neuritic processes nor neuroglial fibers are evident. **a** Bodian, × 160; **b** phosphotungstic acid hematoxylin, × 160

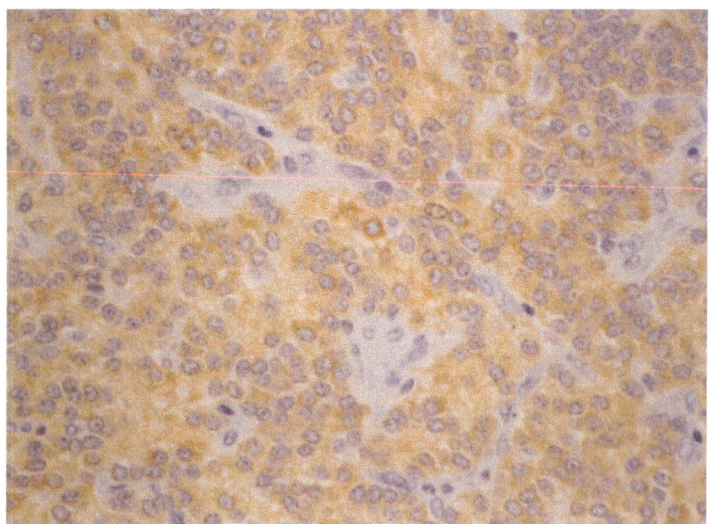

Fig. 11.13. *Central neurocytoma* (the same case as in Fig. 11.11). Weakly positive reaction for neuronspecific enolase (NSE) is observed throughout the cytoplasm of the tumor cells but not in the vascular stromal cells. Indirect immunoperoxidase method counterstained with hematoxylin, × 160

Fig. 11.14. *Central neurocytoma* (the same case as in Fig. 11.11). Sporadic positive staining for S-100 protein is seen in both the cytoplasm and nuclei of some tumor cells. Indirect immunoperoxidase method counterstained with hematoxylin, × 160

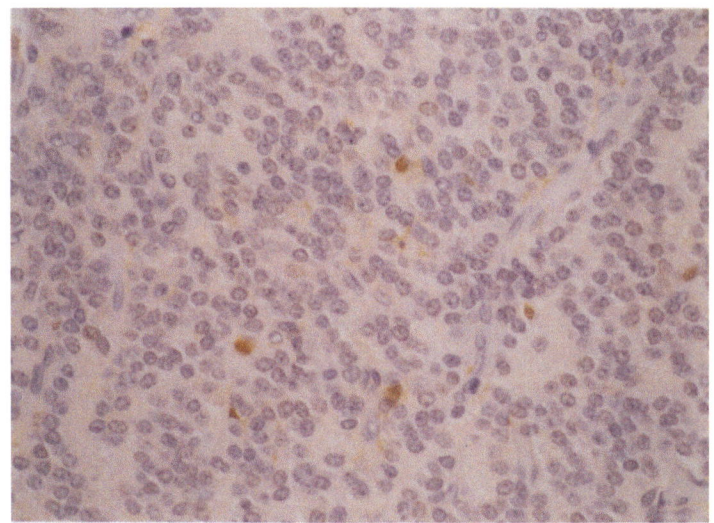

Fig. 11.15. *Central neurocytoma* (the same case as in Fig. 11.11). Glial fibrillary acidic protein (GFAP) is confined to the perivascular astrocytic endfeet and is absent from the tumor cells. Indirect immunoperoxidase method counterstained with hematoxylin, × 160

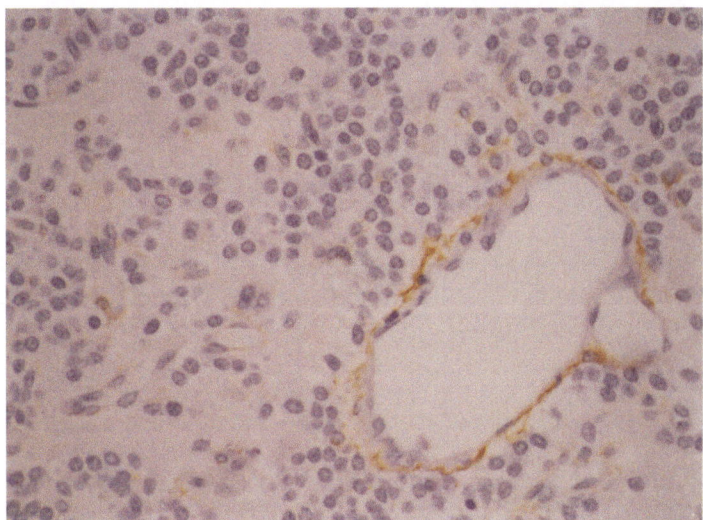

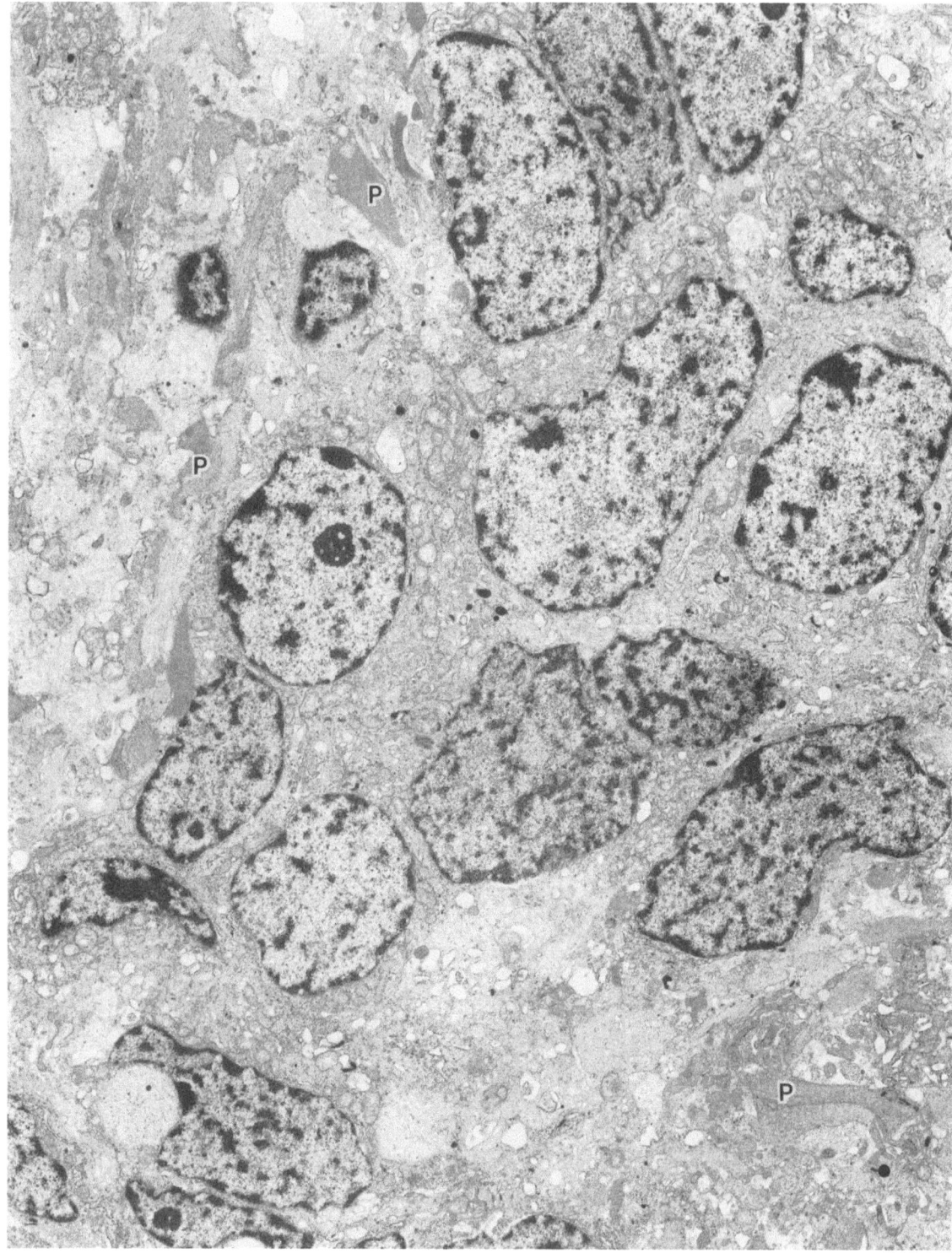

Fig. 11.16. *Central neurocytoma* (the same case as in Fig. 11.11). The tumor cells tend to form a cell nest, which is surrounded by astrocytic processes (*P*). × 5000

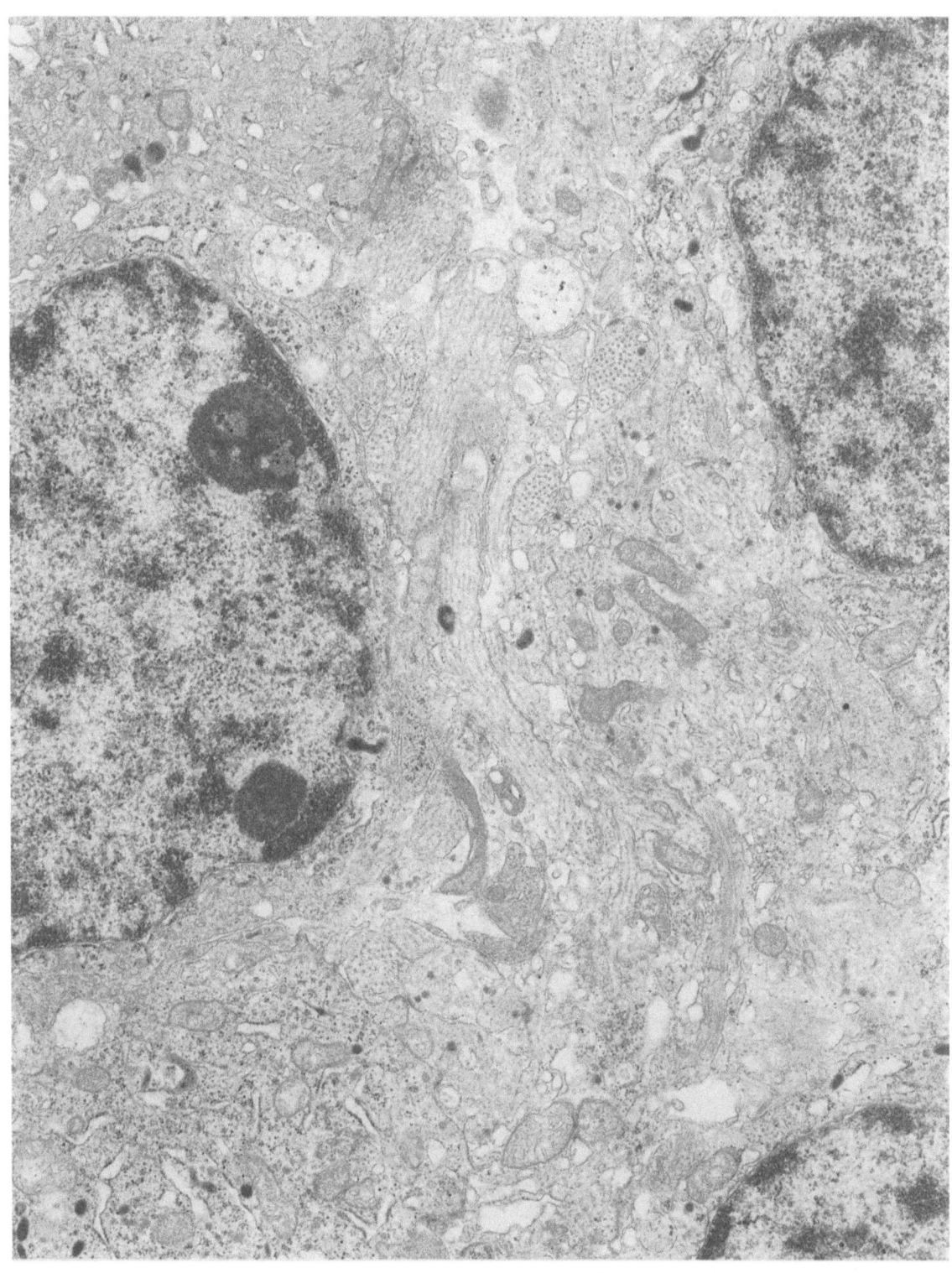

Fig. 11.17. *Central neurocytoma* (the same case as in Fig. 11.11). Intermingled processes of tumor cells resemble a neuropil. × 22 000

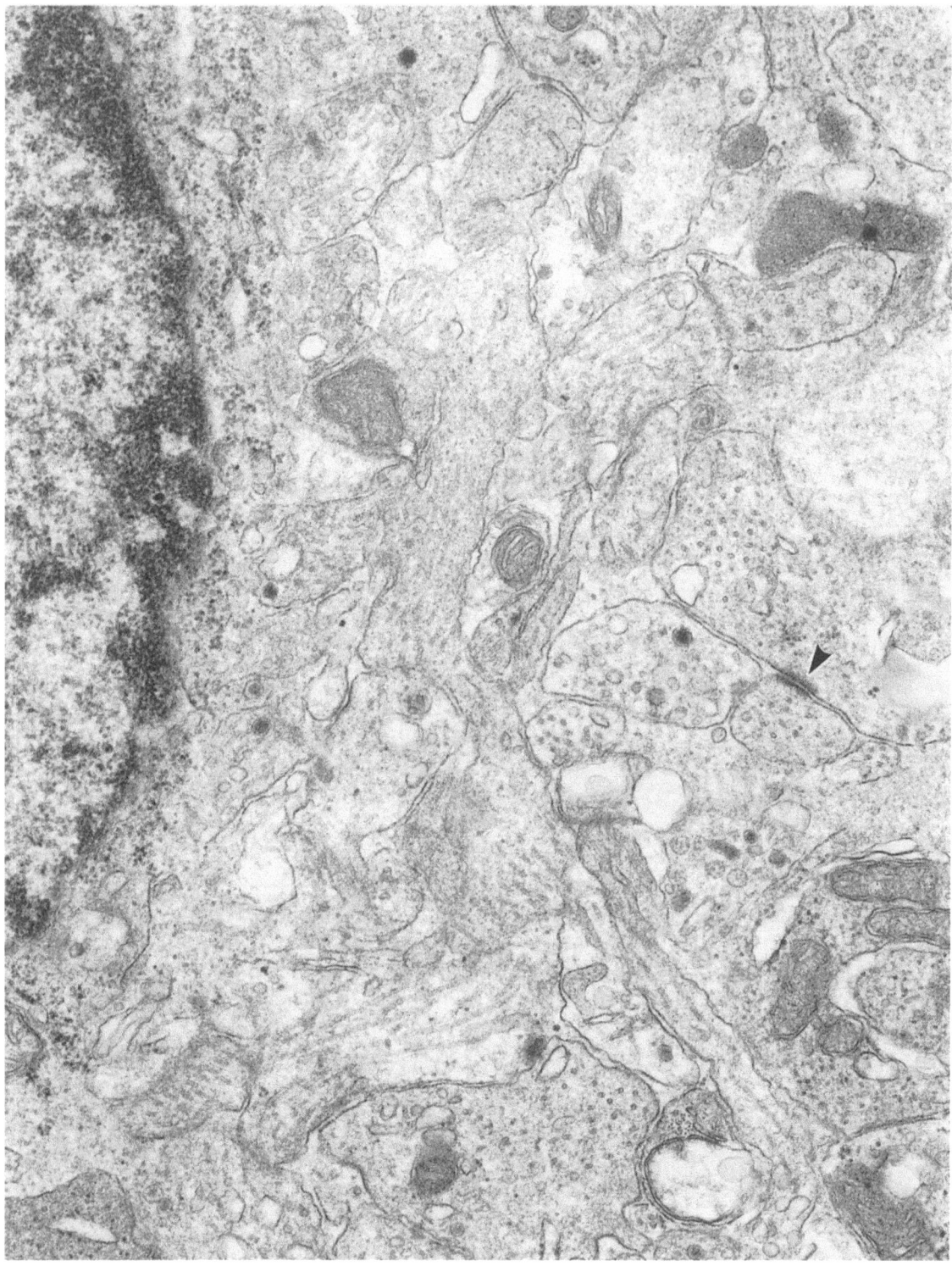

Fig. 11.18. *Central neurocytoma* (the same case as in Fig. 11.11). Both transversely and longitudinally sectioned processes of tumor cells display abundant microtubules and occasional dense core vesicles. A synapse-like structure (*arrowhead*) is also seen. × 35 000

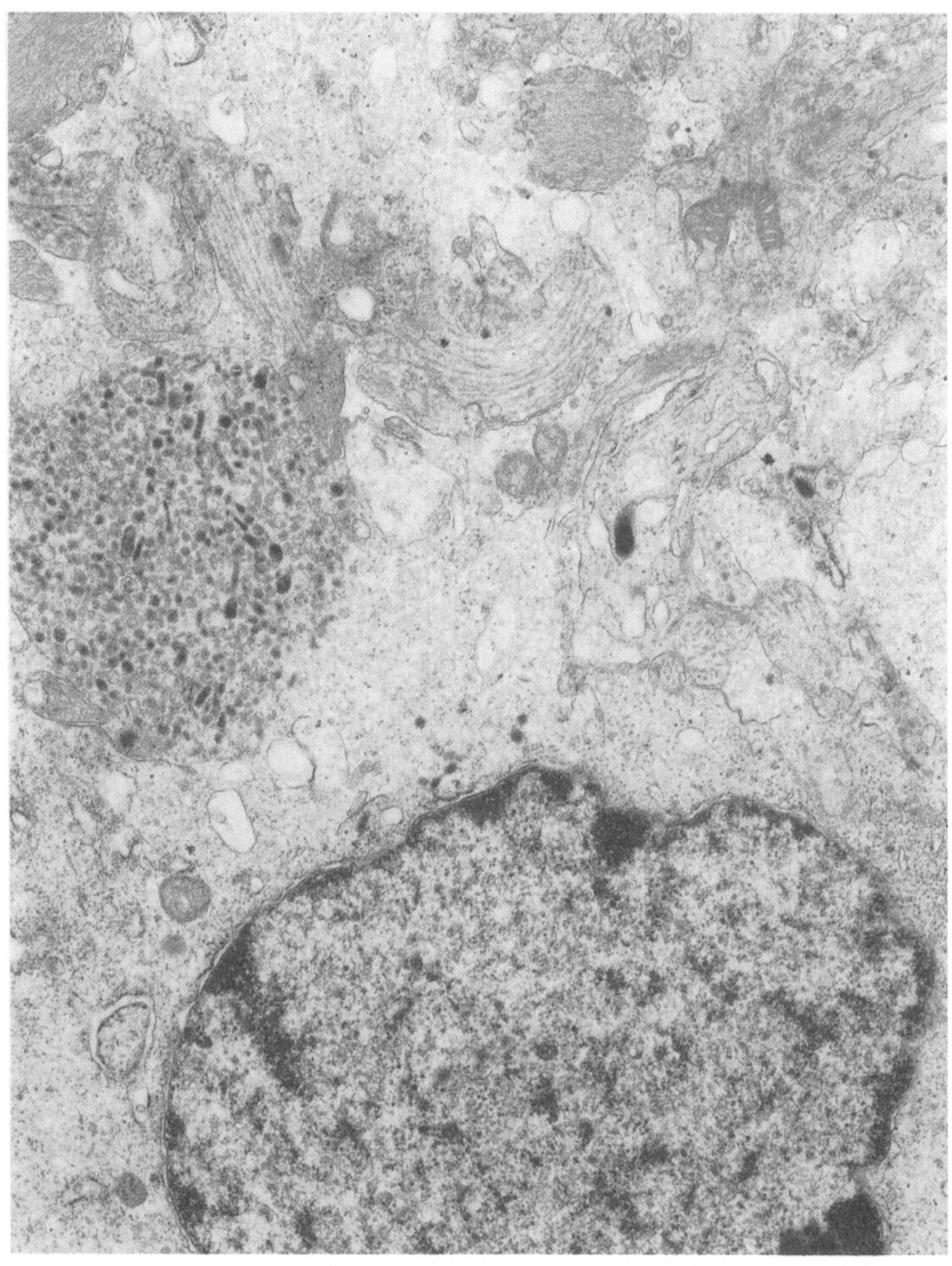

Fig. 11.19. *Central neurocytoma* (the same case as in Fig. 11.11). An intracytoplasmic clustering of electron-dense granules, 70–150 nm in diameter, is observed in a tumor cell. × 22 000

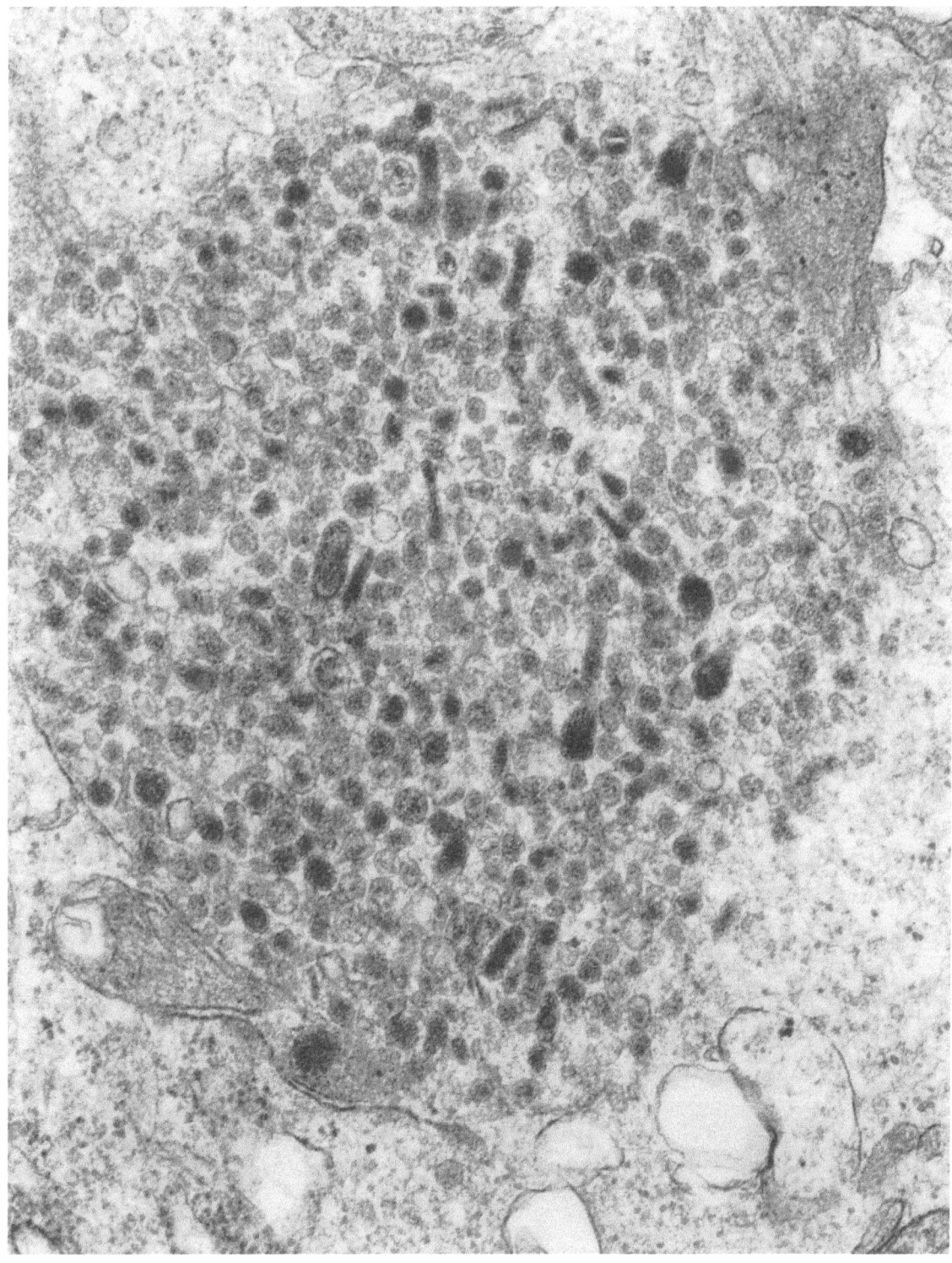

Fig. 11.20. *Central neurocytoma* (the same case as in Fig. 11.11). Higher magnification reveals dense granules of various size, shape, and electron density. × 55000

12. Cerebral Neuroblastoma

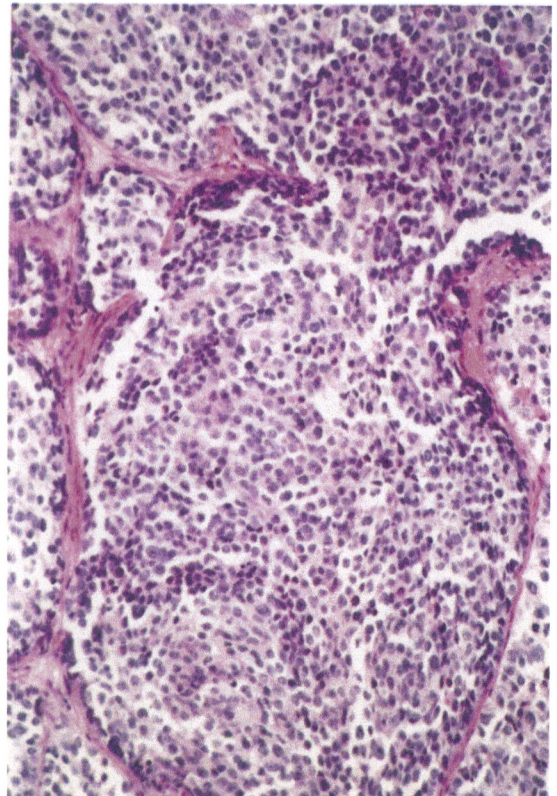

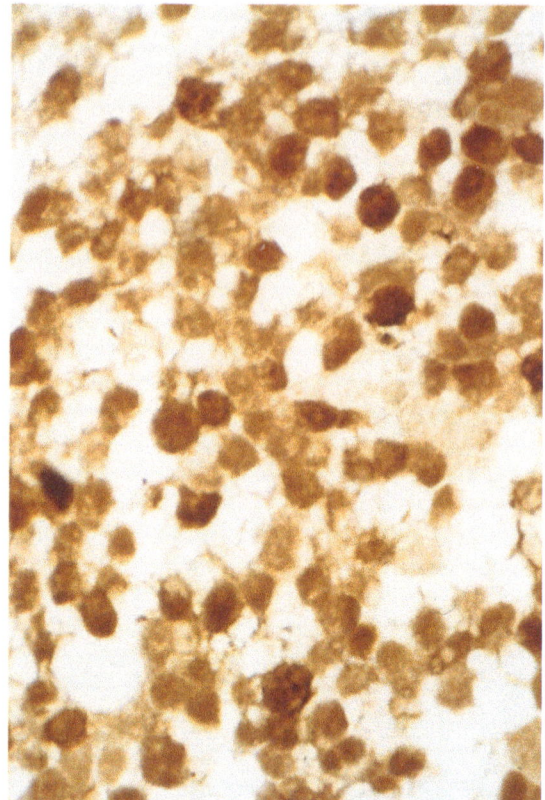

Fig. 12.1. *Cerebral neuroblastoma* of the left frontal lobe in an 8-year-old girl. The tumor is composed of lobulated sheets of closely packed small cells without any special arrangement. H and E, × 90

Fig. 12.2. *Cerebral neuroblastoma* (the same case as in Fig. 12.1). The tumor cells reveal positive staining for S-100 protein, particularly in the nuclei. Indirect immunoperoxidase method without counterstain, × 450

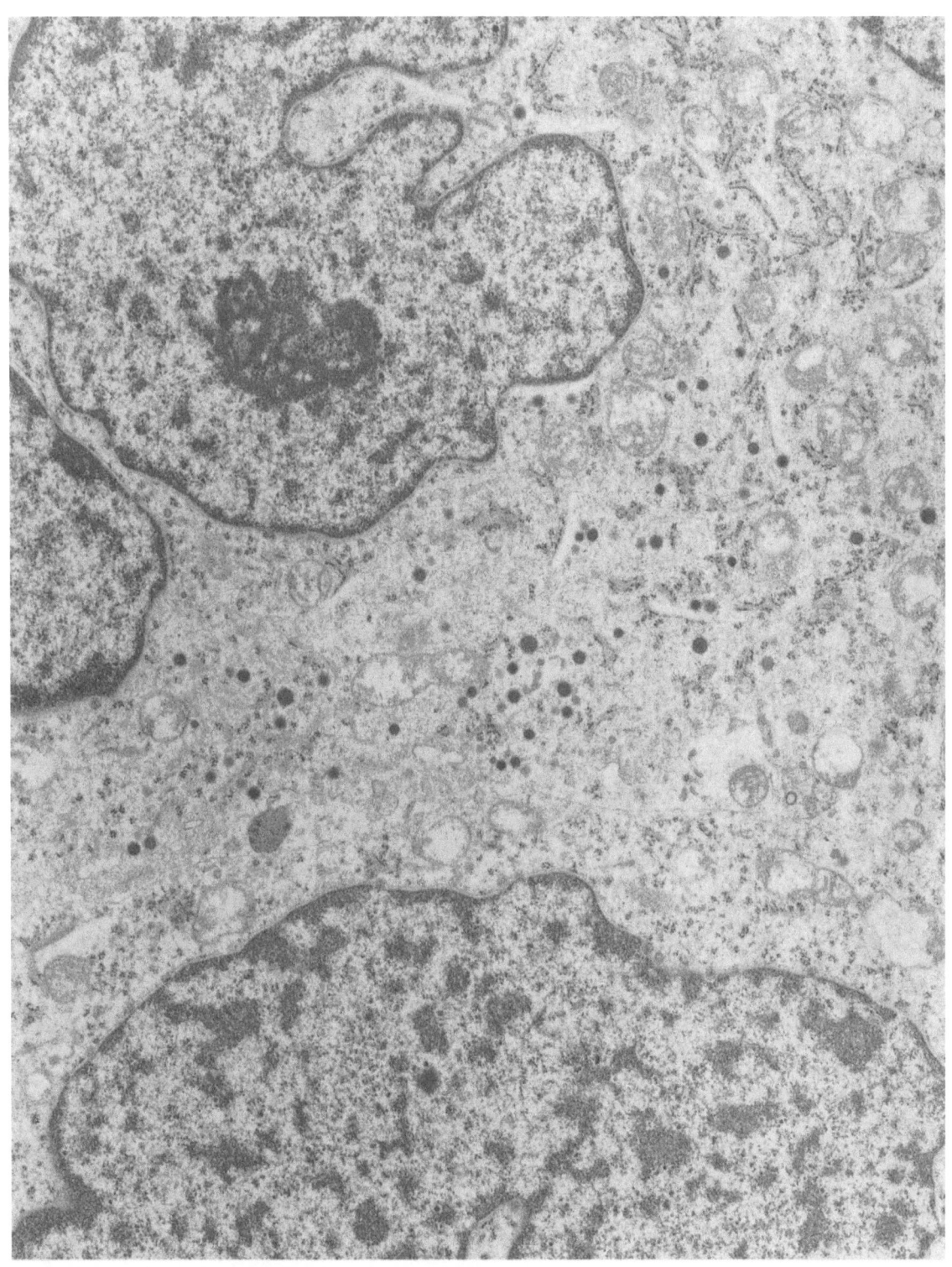

Fig. 12.3. *Cerebral neuroblastoma* (the same case as in Fig. 12.1). The tumor cells occasionally display dense core vesicles, 120–170 nm in diameter, in the cytoplasm. × 17 000

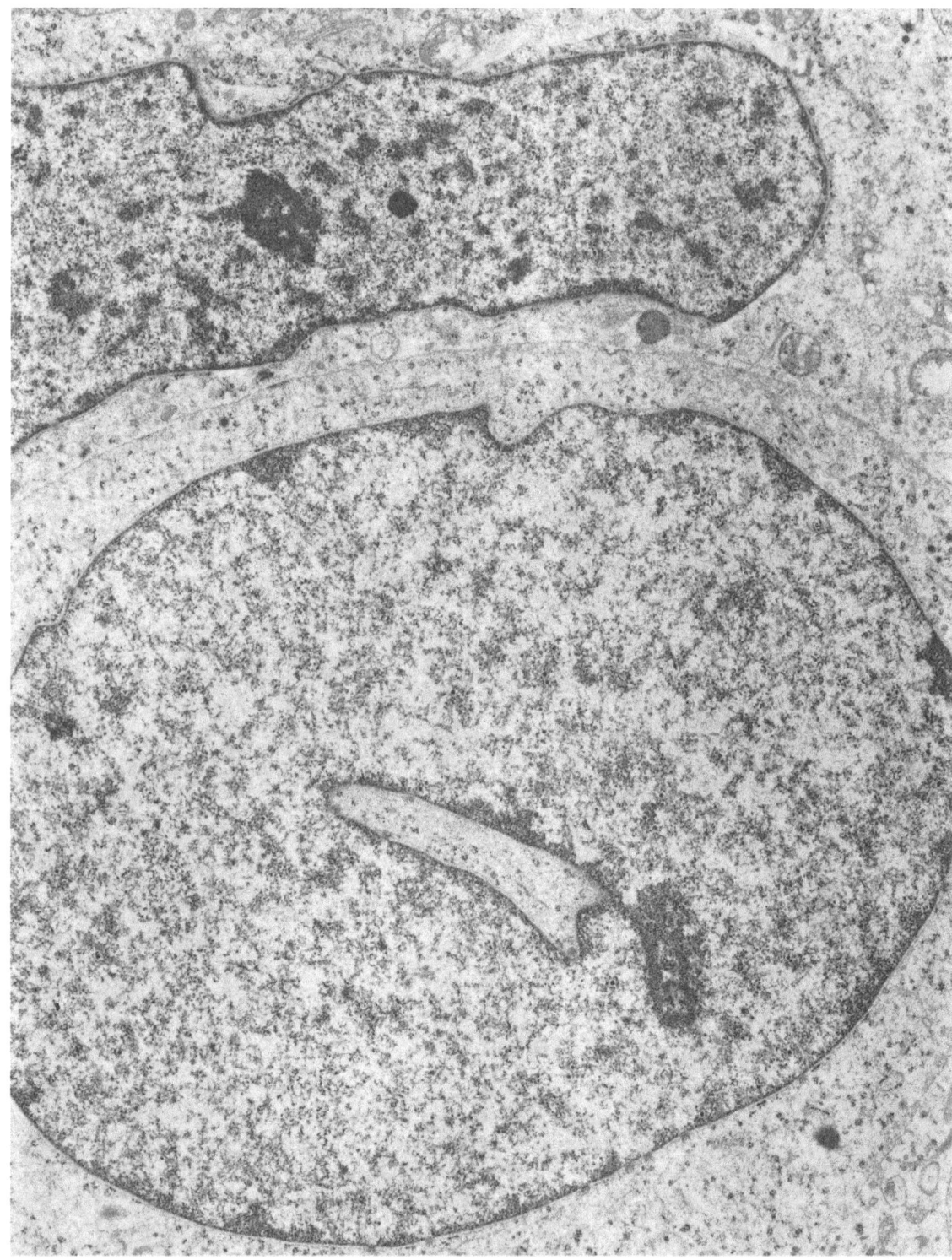

Fig. 12.4. *Cerebral neuroblastoma* (the same case as in Fig. 12.1). A tumor cell with a round nucleus shows a nuclear pseudoinclusion containing a cytoplasmic structure. × 14 700

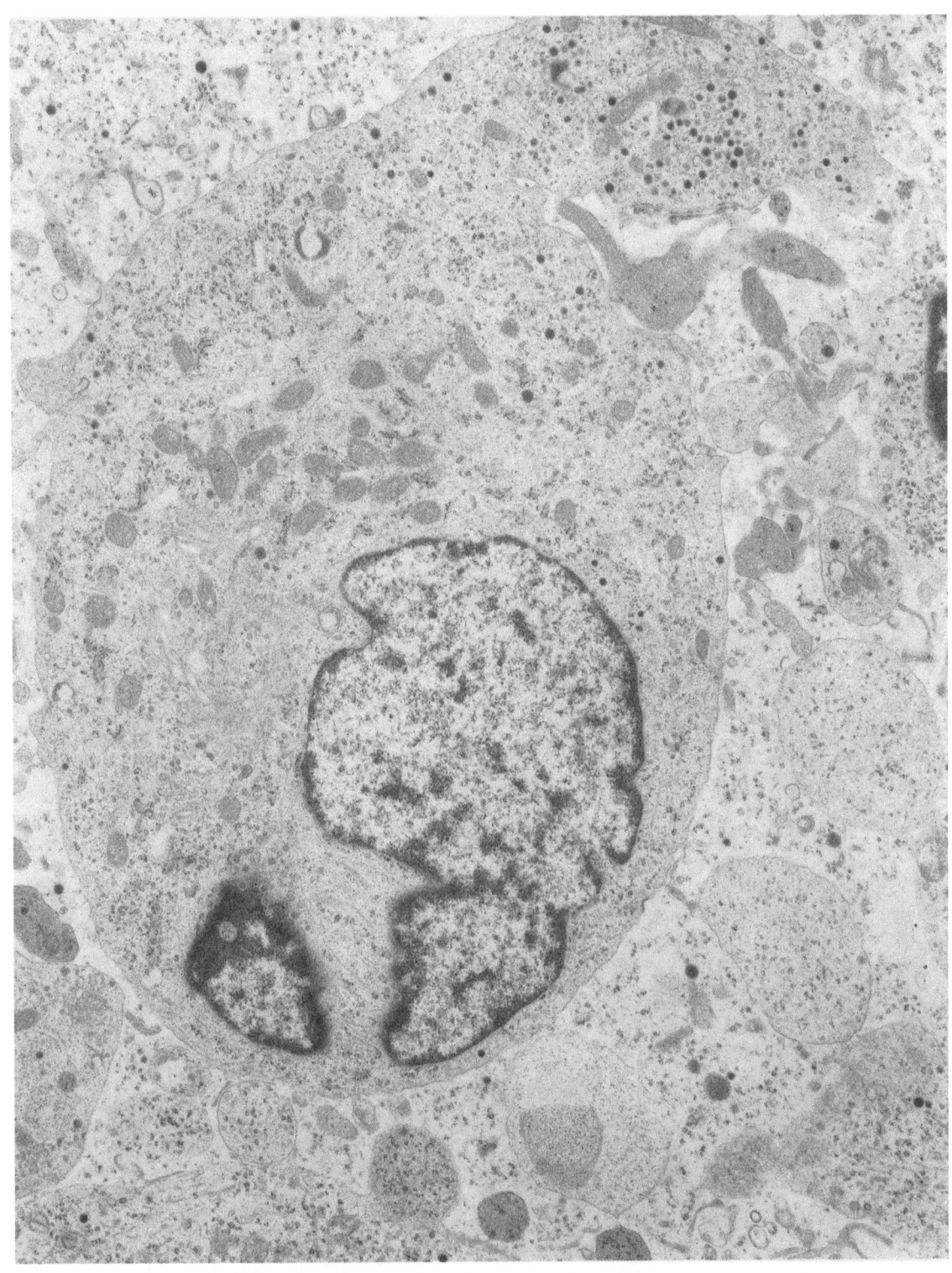

Fig. 12.5. *Cerebral neuroblastoma* (the same case as in Fig. 12.1). The tumor cell has a process containing many dense core vesicles, resembling an axon. × 10 000

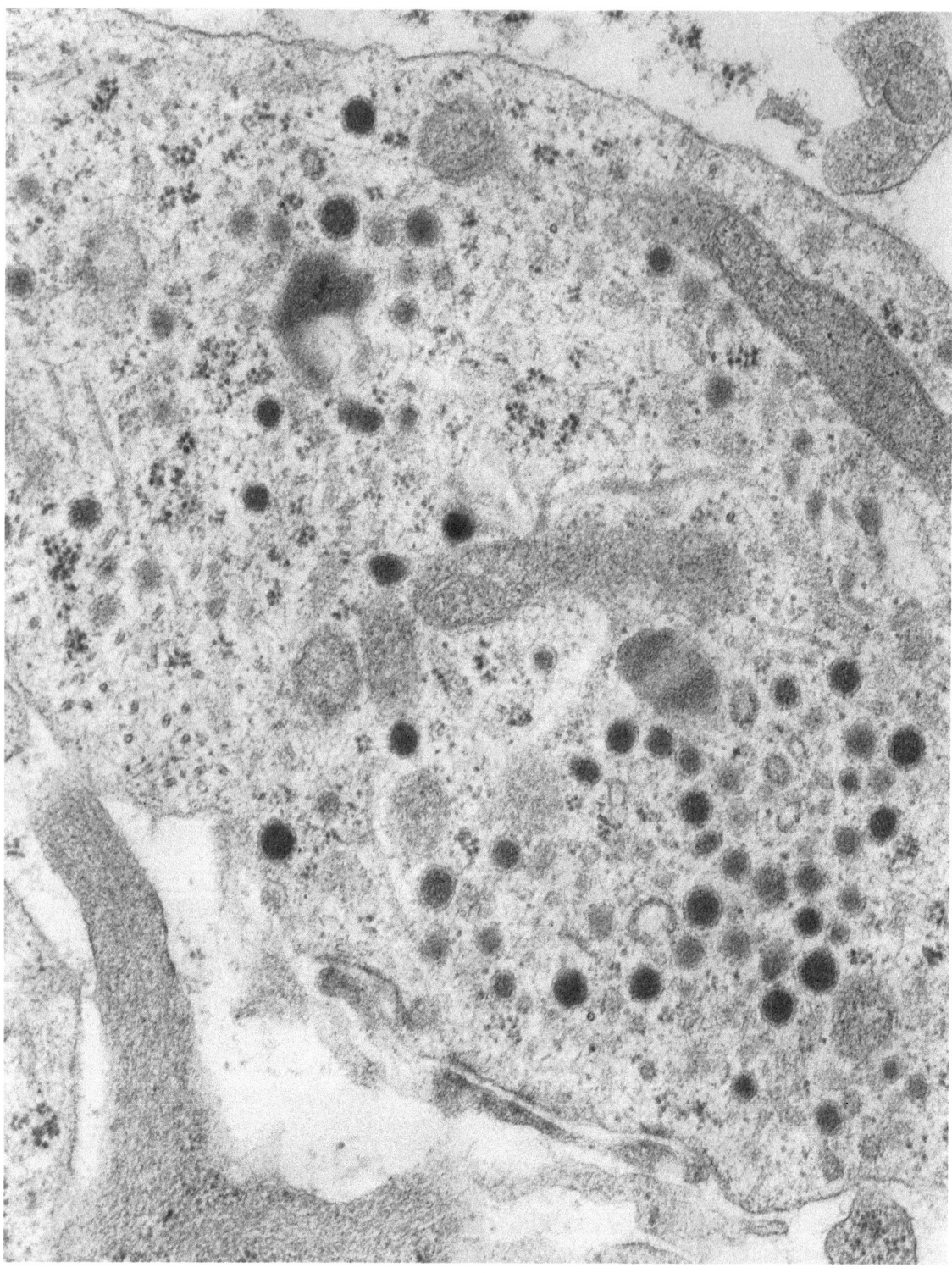

Fig. 12.6. *Cerebral neuroblastoma* (the same case as in Fig. 12.1). Higher magnification of Fig. 12.5 discloses details of the dense core vesicles. × 40 000

13. Olfactory Neuroblastoma (Esthesioneuroblastoma)

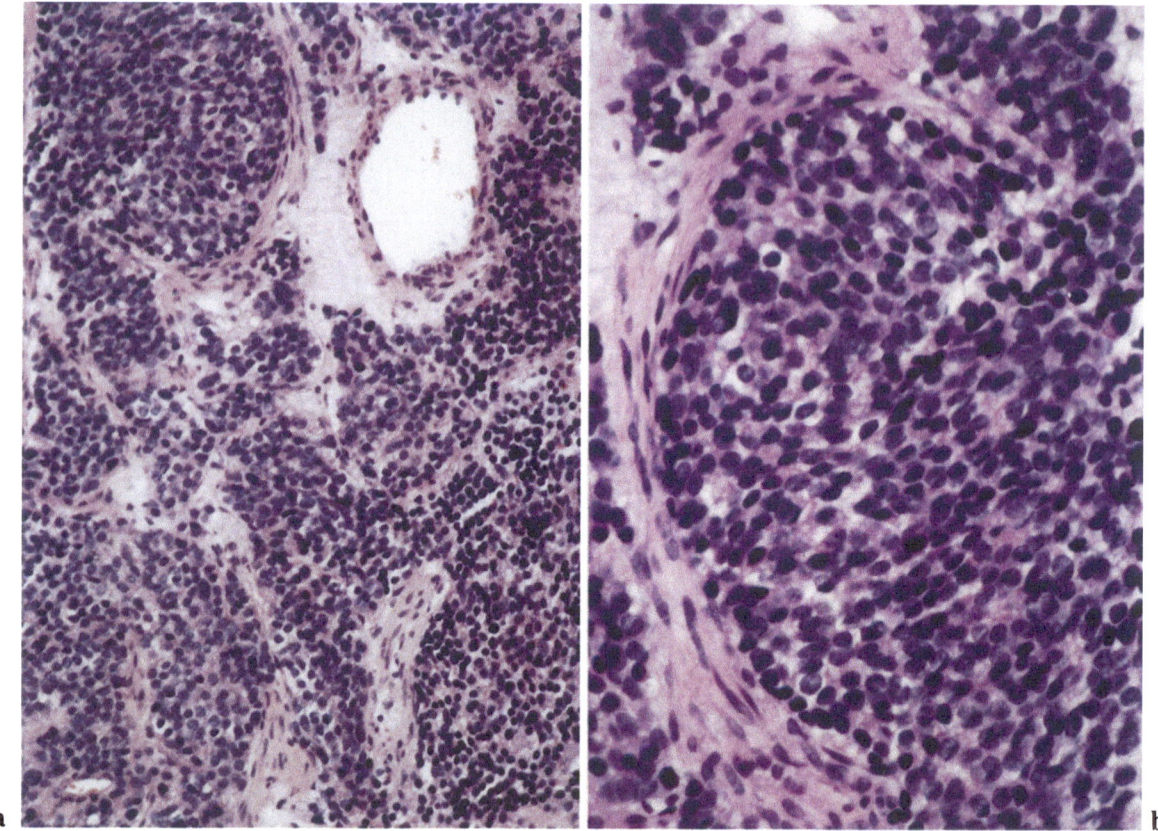

Fig. 13.1a, b. *Olfactory neuroblastoma* (esthesioneuroblastoma) arising from the cribriform plate in a 48-year-old man. The tumor consists of relatively small polygonal cells with hyperchromatic, round to oval nuclei and scant cytoplasm. The tumor cells are closely packed with fibrous stroma. H and E; **a** × 90, **b** × 180

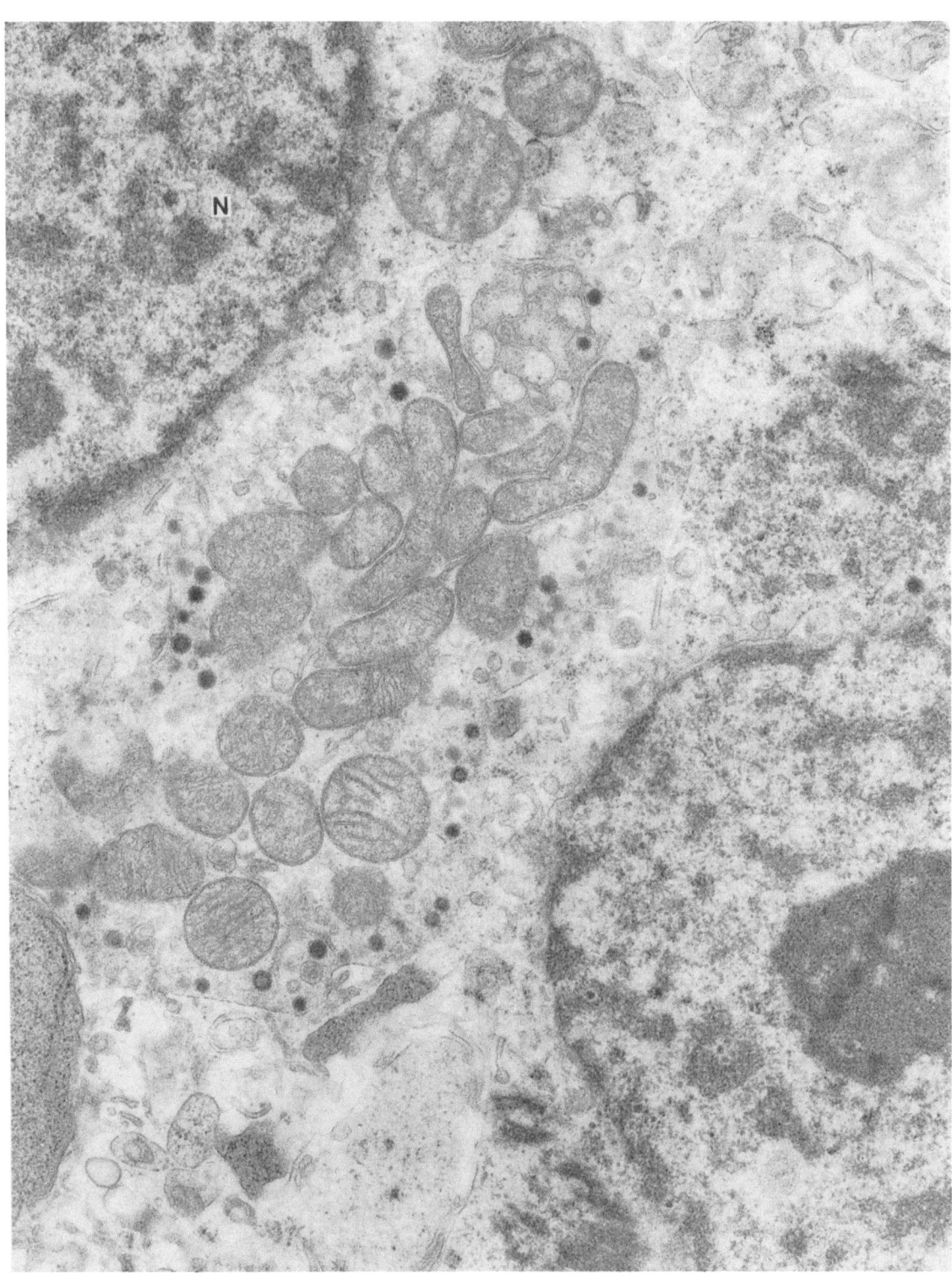

Fig. 13.2. *Olfactory neuroblastoma* (the same case as in Fig. 13.1). There are numerous mitochondria and dense core vesicles, 110–130 nm in diameter, in the cytoplasm of a tumor cell. *N* nucleus. × 27 000

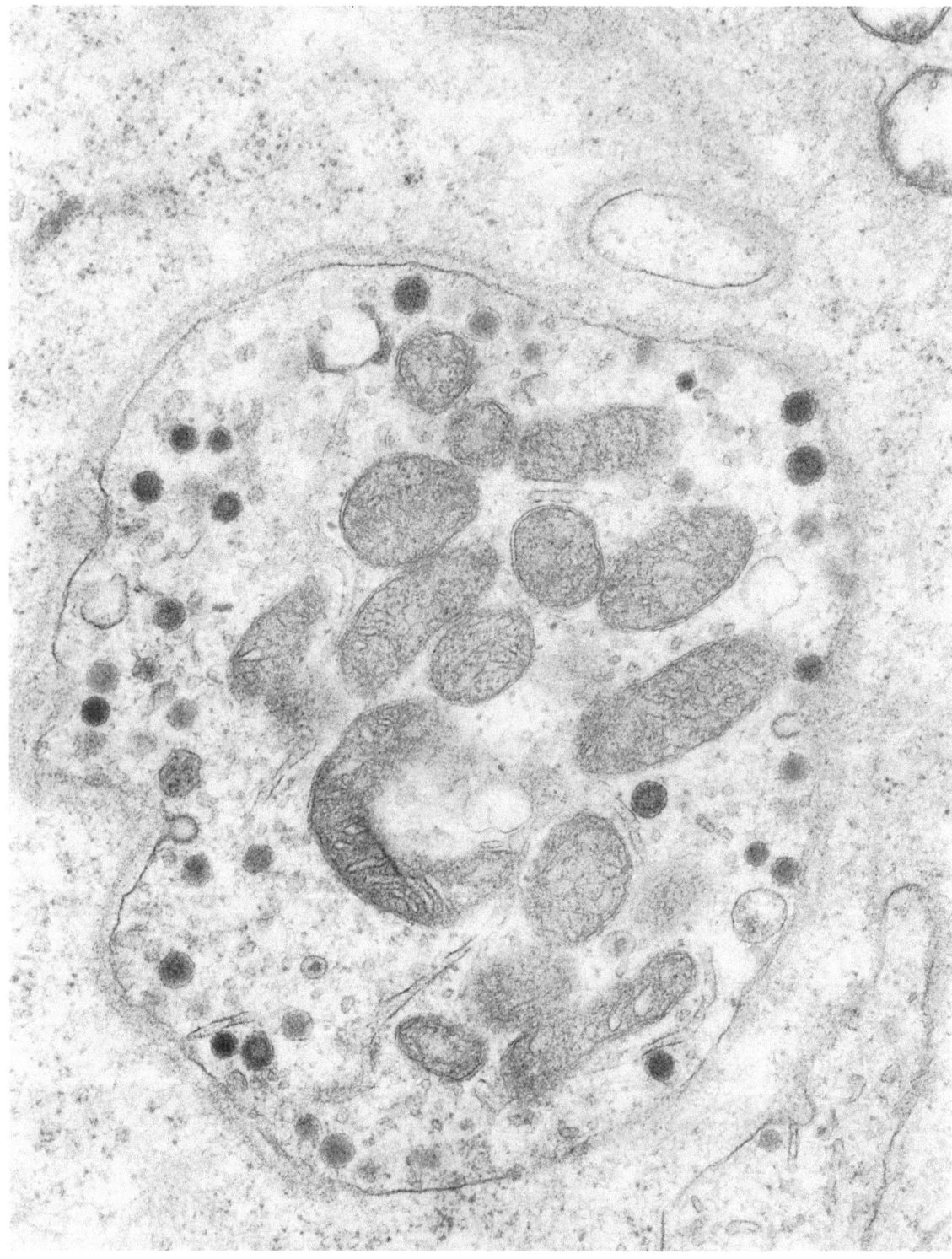

Fig. 13.3. *Olfactory neuroblastoma* (the same case as in Fig. 13.1). Membrane-associated dense core vesicles as well as mitochondria are conspicuous in the transversely sectioned neuritic process of a tumor cell. × 40 000

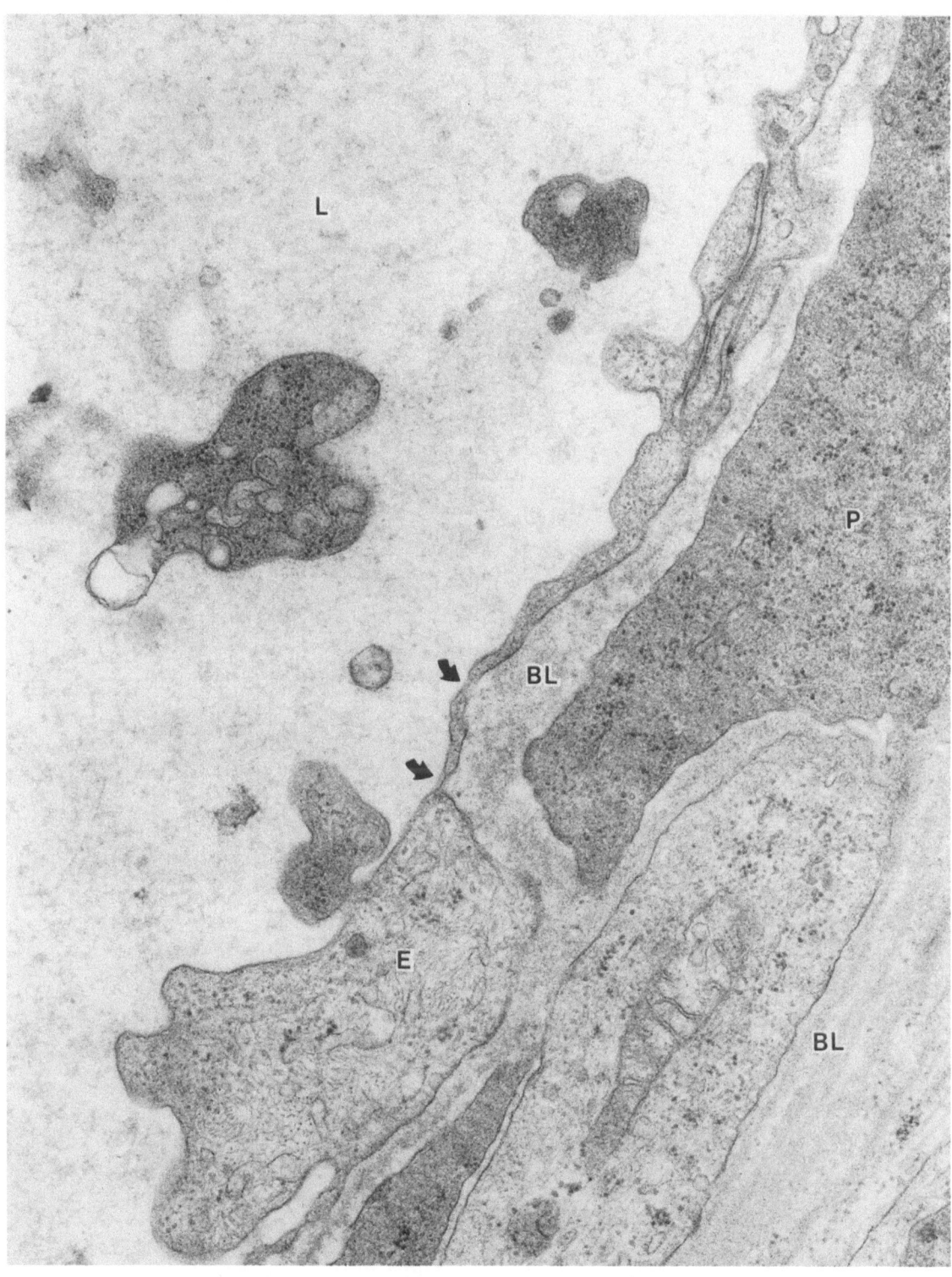

Fig. 13.4. *Olfactory neuroblastoma* (the same case as in Fig. 13.1). Higher magnification reveals the endothelial fenestrations (*arrows*) of a capillary in the tumor. *L* capillary lumen, *E* endothelial cell, *P* pericyte, *BL* basal lamina. × 38 000

14. Primitive Neuroectodermal Tumor (PNET)

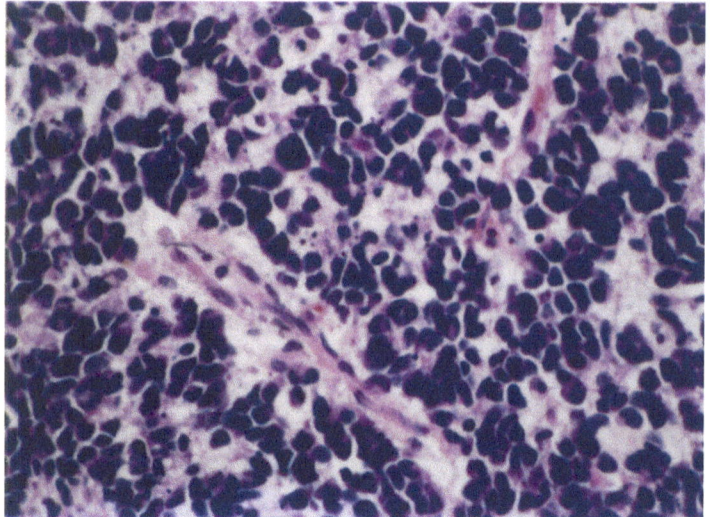

Fig. 14.1. *Primitive neuroectodermal tumor* (PNET) of the right parietal lobe in a 7-year-old girl. The tumor consists of cells with hyperchromatic nuclei in great disarray. H and E, × 160

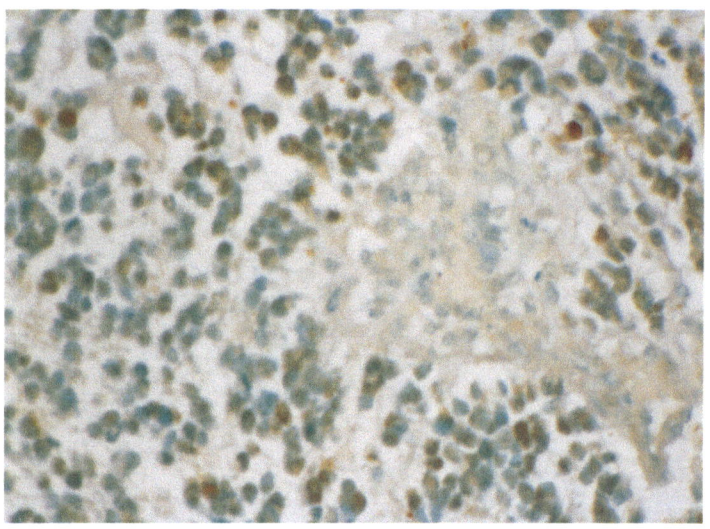

Fig. 14.2. *Primitive neuroectodermal tumor* (the same case as in Fig. 14.1). The positive staining for S-100 protein is weak and varies in intensity among the tumor cells. Peroxidase antiperoxidase method counterstained with methyl green, × 160

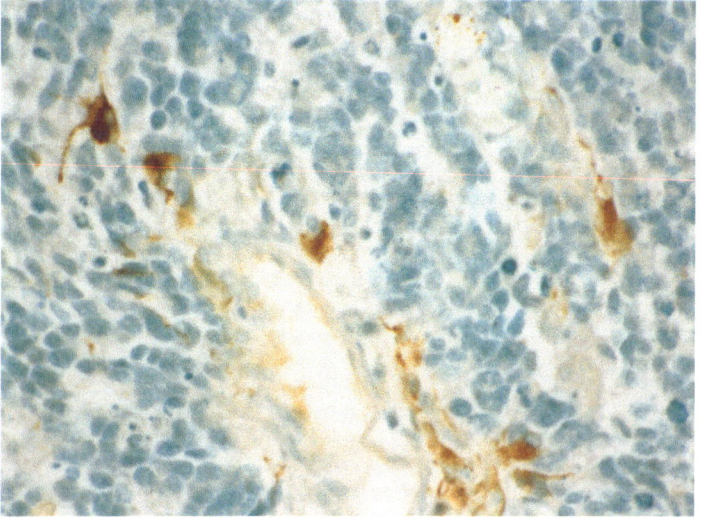

Fig. 14.3. *Primitive neuroectodermal tumor* (the same case as in Fig. 14.1). Glial fibrillary acidic protein (GFAP) is positive in the perivascular entrapped astrocytes but not in the tumor cells. Peroxidase antiperoxidase method counterstained with methyl green, × 160

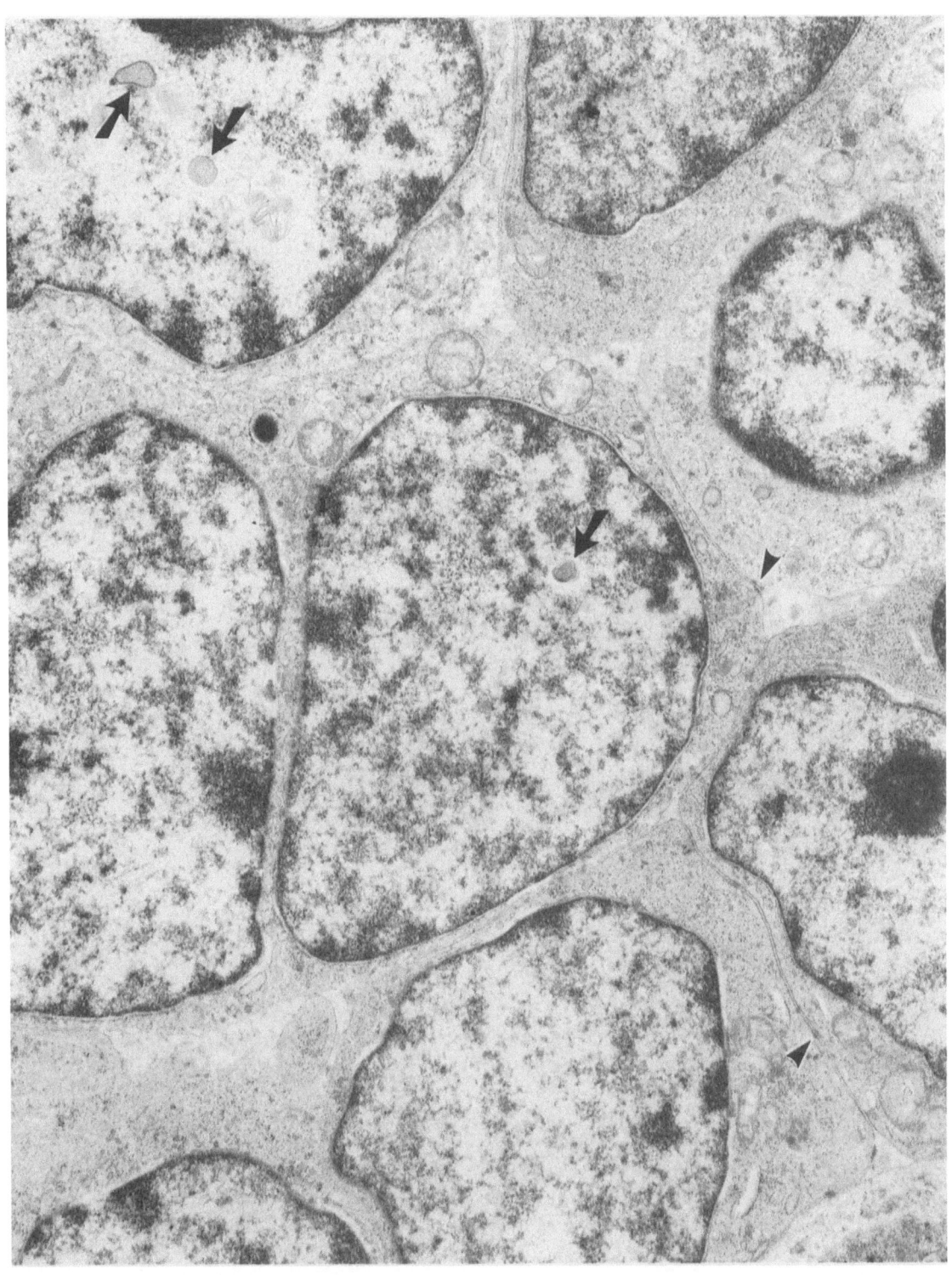

Fig. 14.4. *Primitive neuroectodermal tumor* (the same case as in Fig. 14.1). Closely packed undifferentiated cells are indistinguishable from those of a medulloblastoma. There are nuclear inclusions (*arrows*) and desmosomes (*arrowheads*). × 14 000

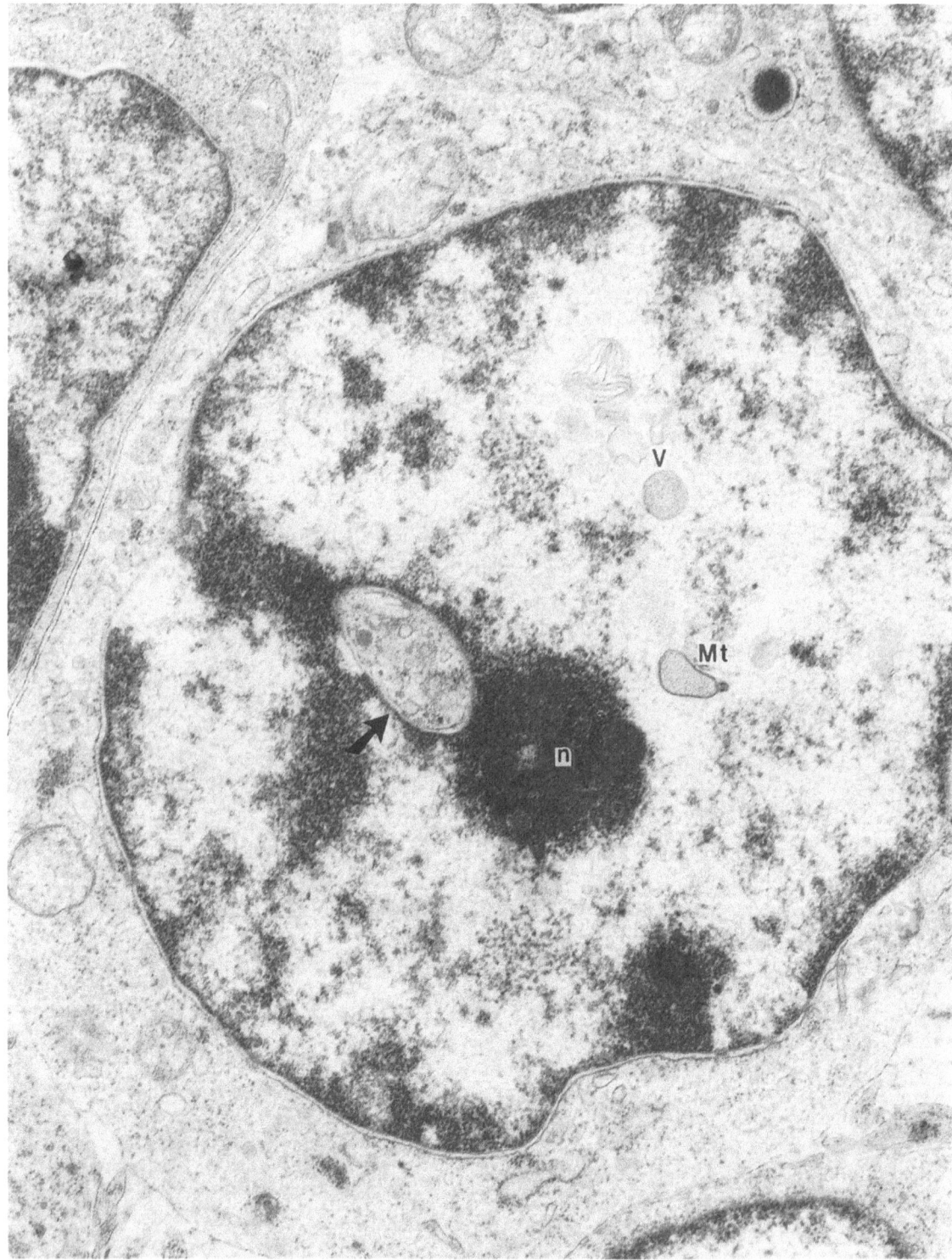

Fig. 14.5. *Primitive neuroectodermal tumor* (the same case as in Fig. 14.1). The tumor cell occasionally shows a nuclear pseudoinclusion delimited by nuclear membranes (*arrow*). Intranuclear mitochondria (*Mt*) and vesicular structure (*V*) are also seen. *n* nucleolus. × 24 000

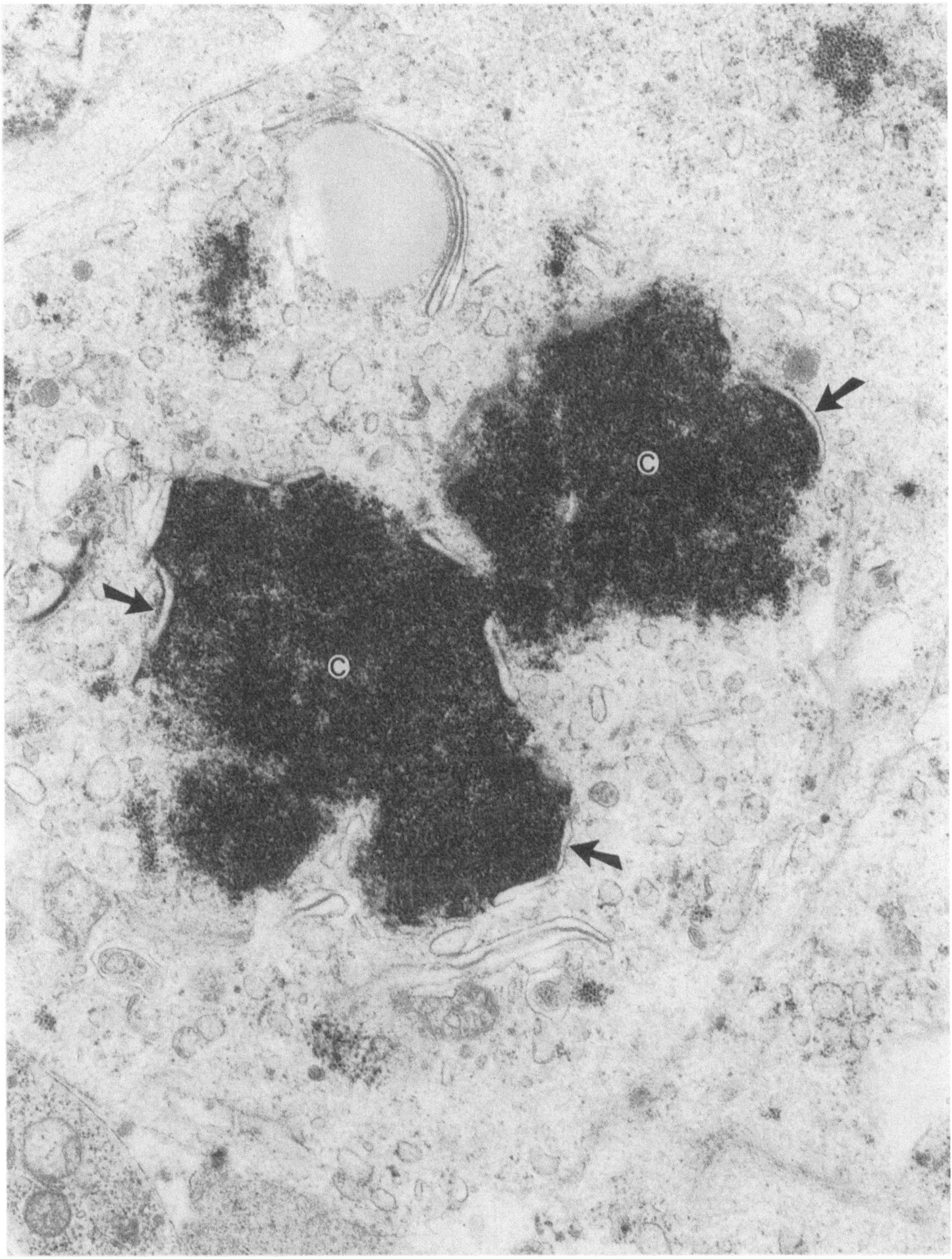

Fig. 14.6. *Primitive neuroectodermal tumor* (the same case as in Fig. 14.1). A tumor cell in telophase is reforming nuclear membranes (*arrows*) around individual chromosomes (*C*). × 27 000

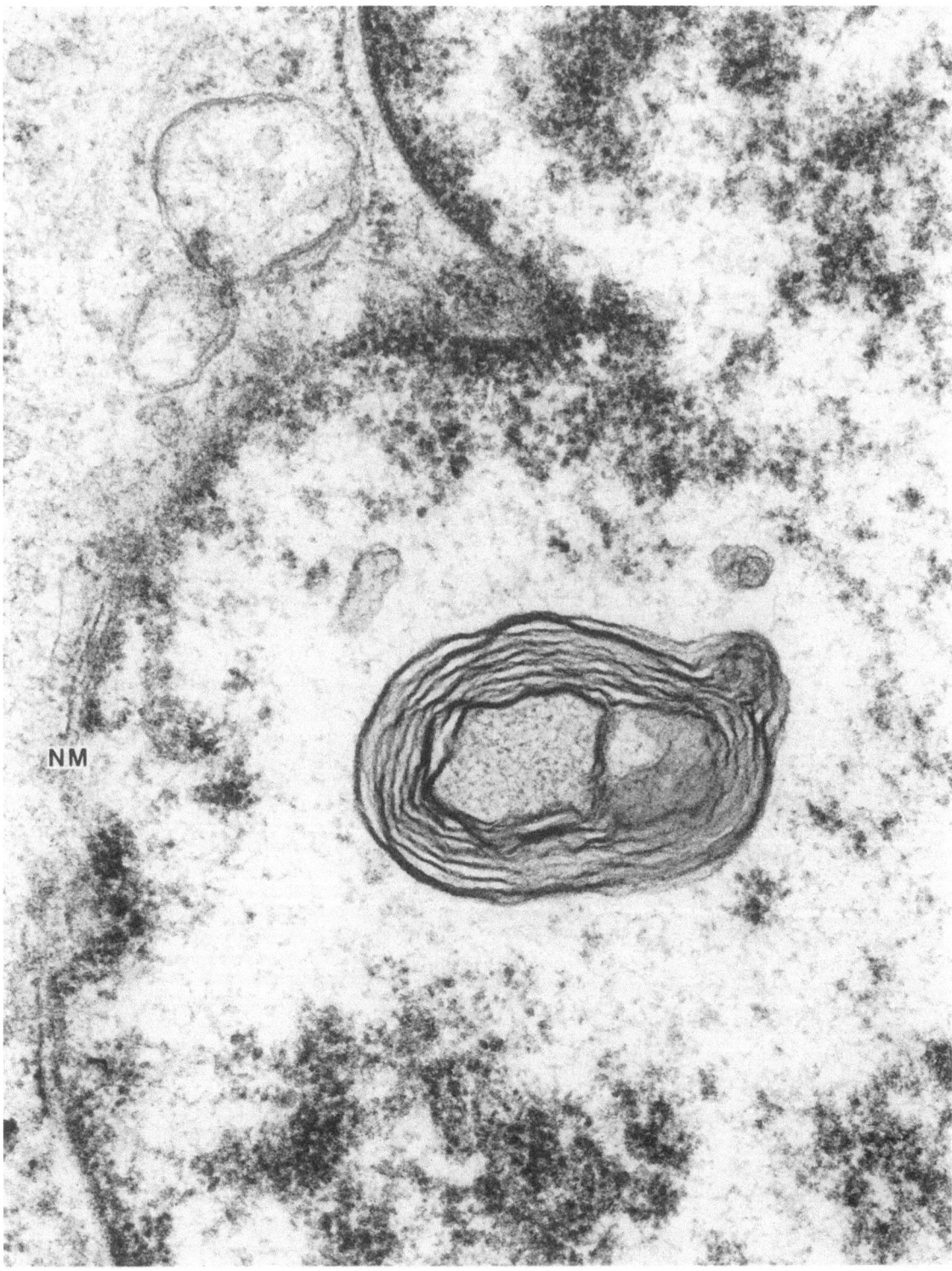

Fig. 14.7. *Primitive neuroectodermal tumor* (the same case as in Fig. 14.1). A laminated membranous structure (myelinosome) is seen lying in the nuclear matrix of a tumor cell. *NM* nuclear membranes. × 68 000

15. Pineocytoma

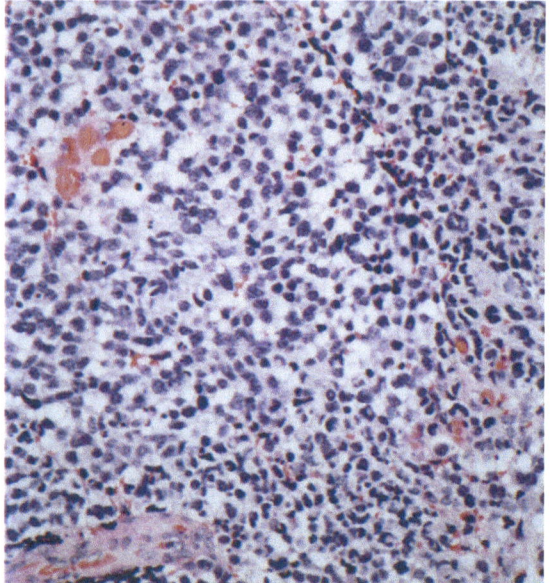

Fig. 15.1. *Pineocytoma* in a 3-year-old girl. The tumor consists of small cells of similar appearance with ill-defined fibrillary cytoplasm and a tendency toward a lobular arrangement. H and E, × 90

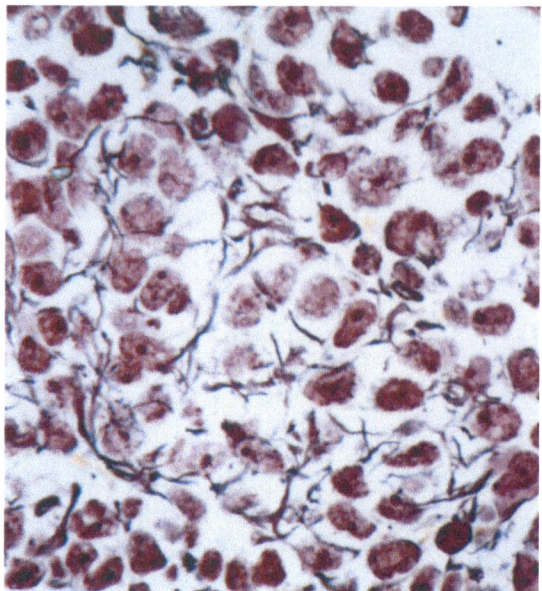

Fig. 15.2. *Pineocytoma* (the same case as in Fig. 15.1). Axonal processes are occasionally seen. Bodian, × 360

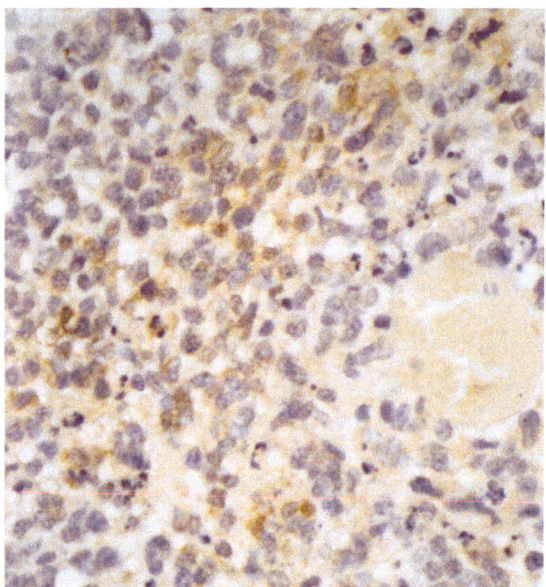

Fig. 15.3. *Pineocytoma* (the same case as in Fig. 15.1). Weakly positive staining for neuron-specific enolase (NSE) is localized in the cytoplasm of the tumor cells. Indirect immunoperoxidase method counterstained with hematoxylin, × 180

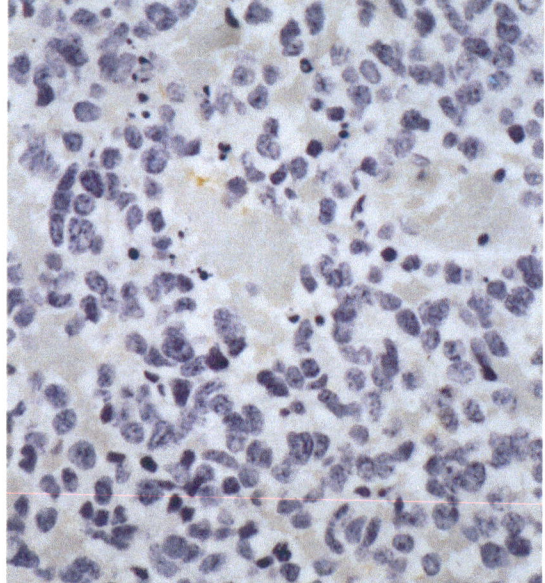

Fig. 15.4. *Pineocytoma* (the same case as in Fig. 15.1). The tumor cells reveal no positive reaction for glial fibrillary acidic protein (GFAP). Indirect immunoperoxidase method counterstained with hematoxylin, × 180

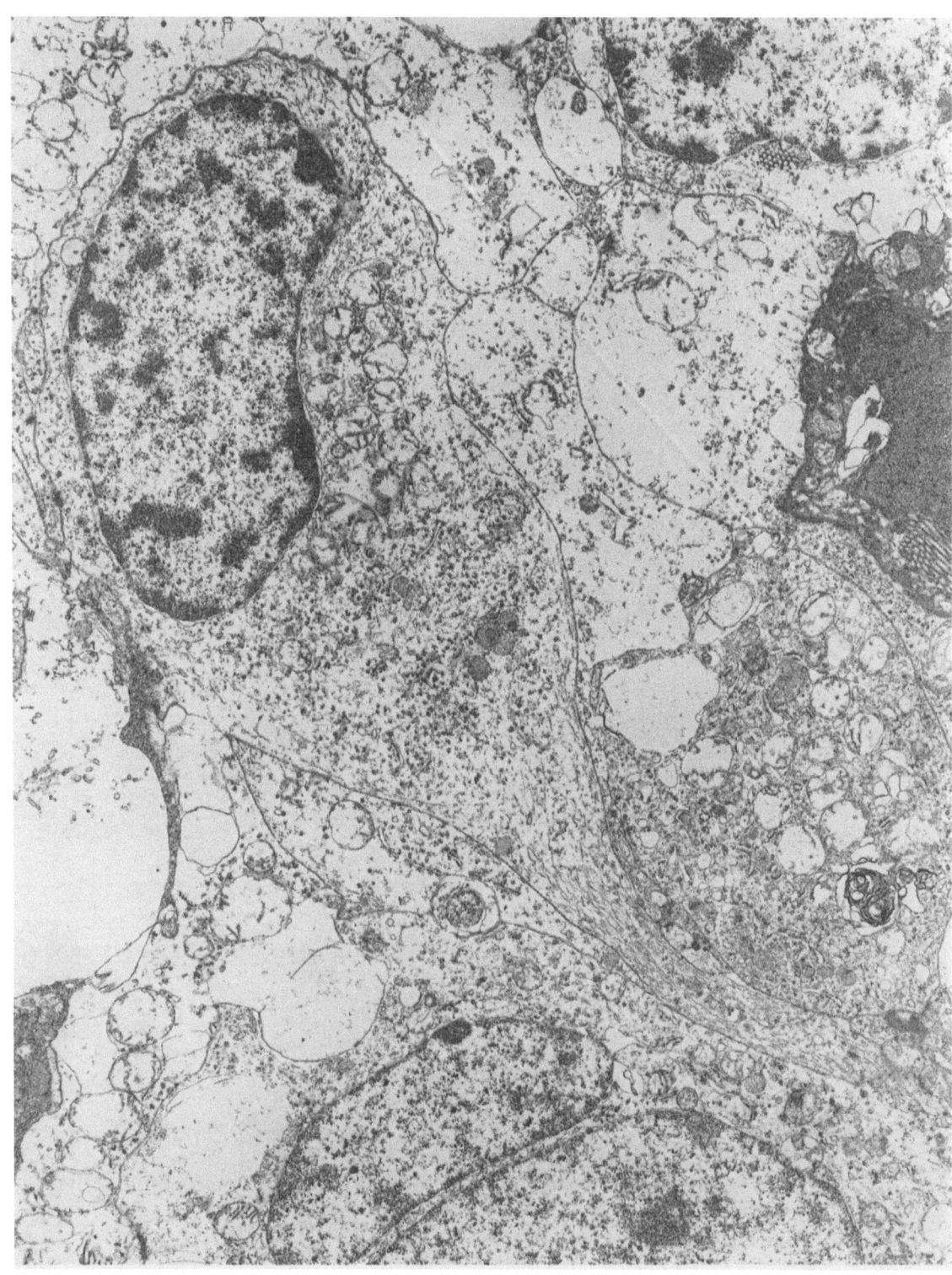

Fig. 15.5. *Pineocytoma* (the same case as in Fig. 15.1). A tumor cell shows the longitudinally sectioned process which resembles an axon. Formalin fixed, × 12000

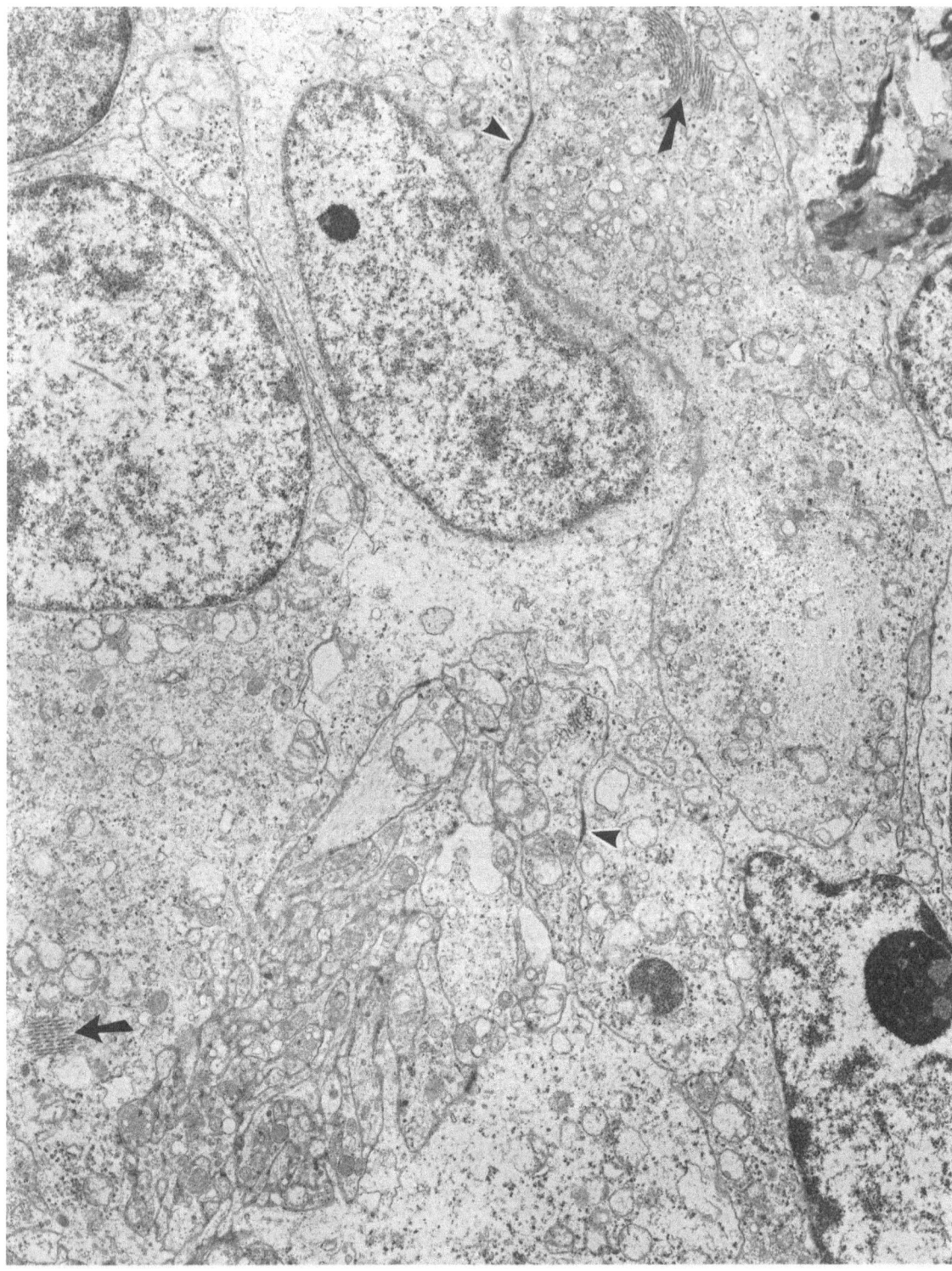

Fig. 15.6. *Pineocytoma* (the same case as in Fig. 15.1). The tumor cells with round to oval nuclei have abundant organelles. The cross-sectioned processes of tumor cells resemble a neuropil. Zonula occludens (*arrowheads*) and uncharacterized membranous structures (*arrows*) are also discernible. Formalin fixed, × 12 000

16. Germinoma

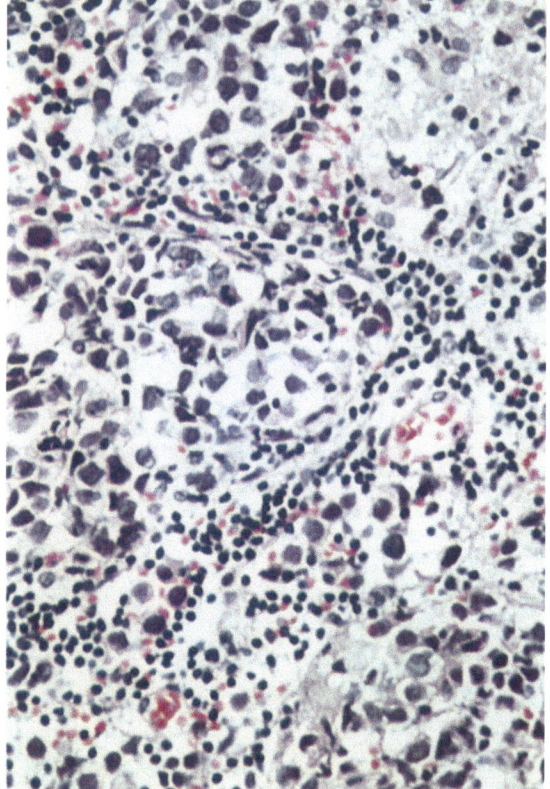

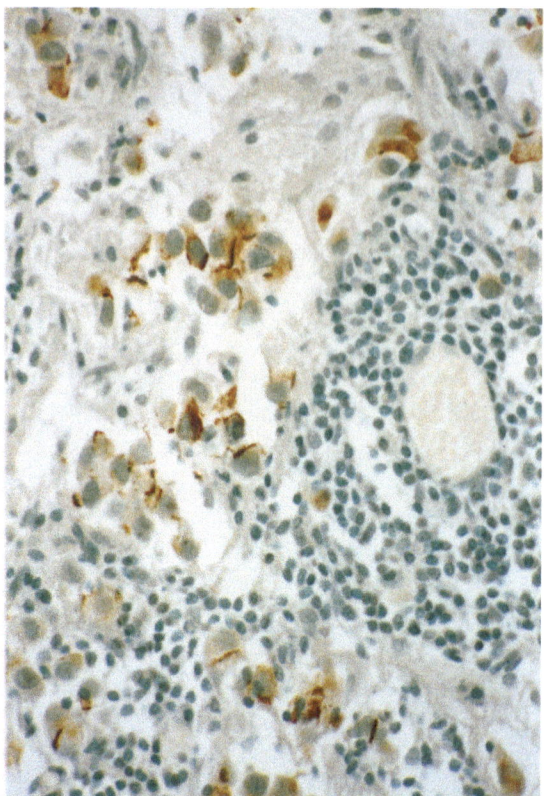

Fig. 16.1. Pineal *germinoma* in an 8-year-old boy. The tumor consists of large polygonal cells with vesicular nuclei and numerous lymphocytes. H and E, × 90

Fig. 16.2. Pineal *germinoma* (the same case as in Fig. 16.1). Immunohistochemical examination shows a positive reaction for placental alkaline phosphatase exclusively in the large polygonal cells, suggesting their germ cell origin. Peroxidase antiperoxidase method counterstained with methyl green, × 90

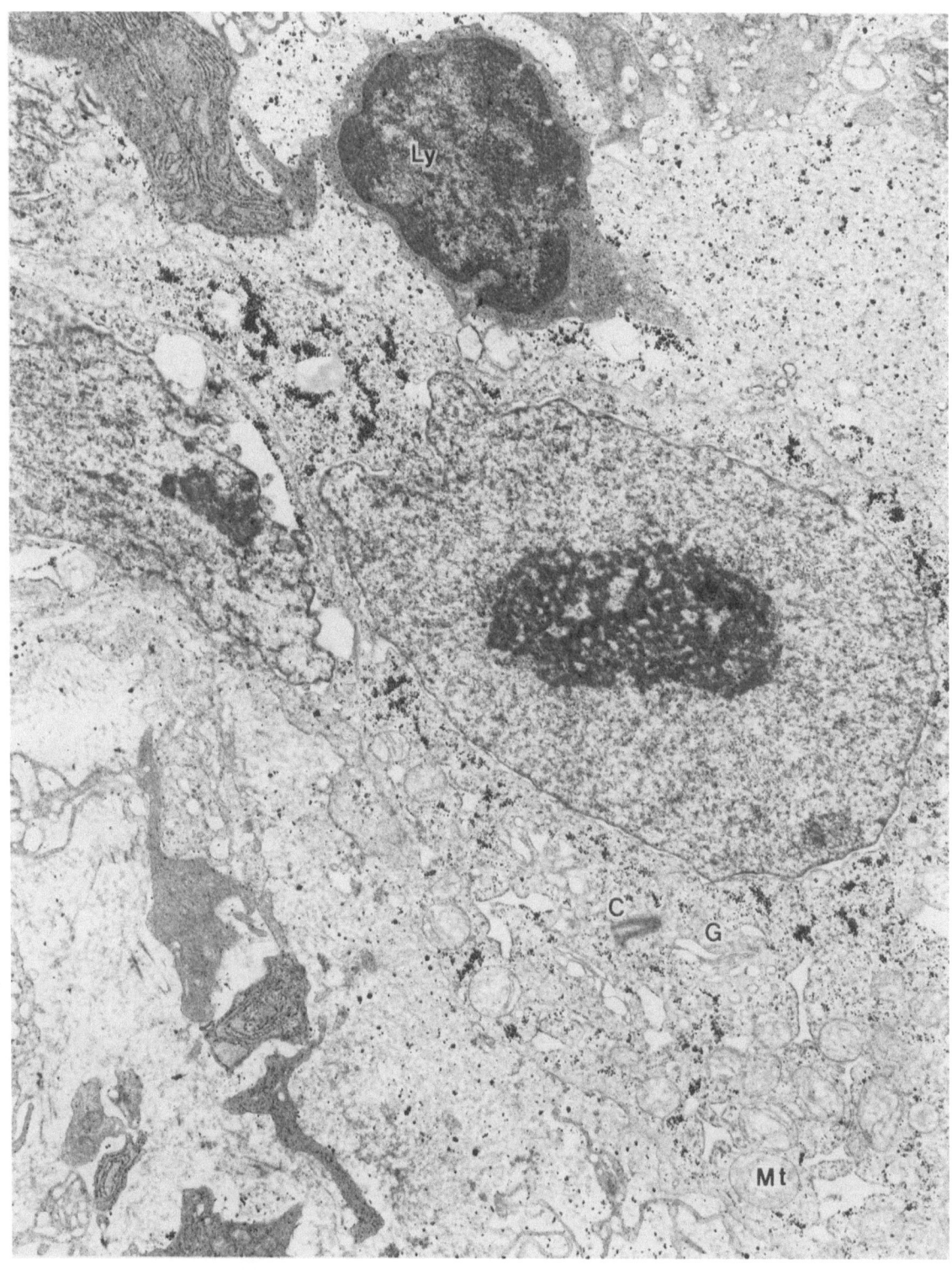

Fig. 16.3. Pineal *germinoma* in a 14-year-old boy. The germinoma cell has an ovoid nucleus with uniform granular chromatin and an elongated nucleolus with reticular nucleolonema. The cytoplasm is rich in organelles, including mitochondria (*Mt*), Golgi apparatus (*G*), and a centriole (*C*). The electron-dense granules are glycogen. Adjacent to the germinoma cell, a lymphocyte (*Ly*) is present. × 12 800

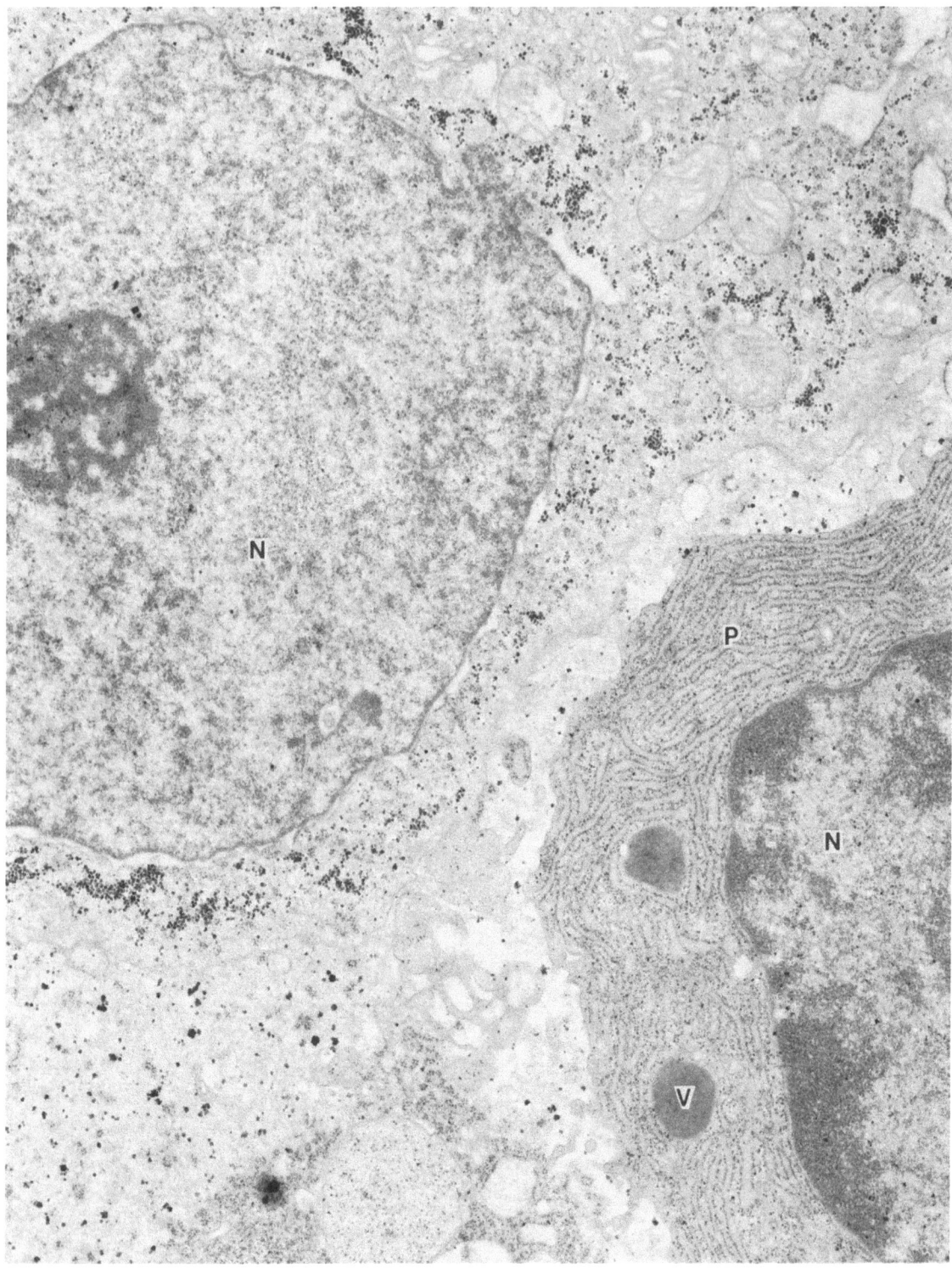

Fig. 16.4. Pineal *germinoma* (the same case as in Fig. 16.1). The germinoma cell (*upper left*) has many mitochondria with peculiar cristae. Intracytoplasmic glycogen is present either as electron-dense granules, approximately 15–30 nm in diameter (β-particles), or as collections of such granules (α-particles). A plasmacye (*P*) is easily discernible by the abundant arrays of rough endoplasmic reticulum and the electron-dense vesicles (*V*), probably containing the secretory product. *N* nucleus. × 20 000

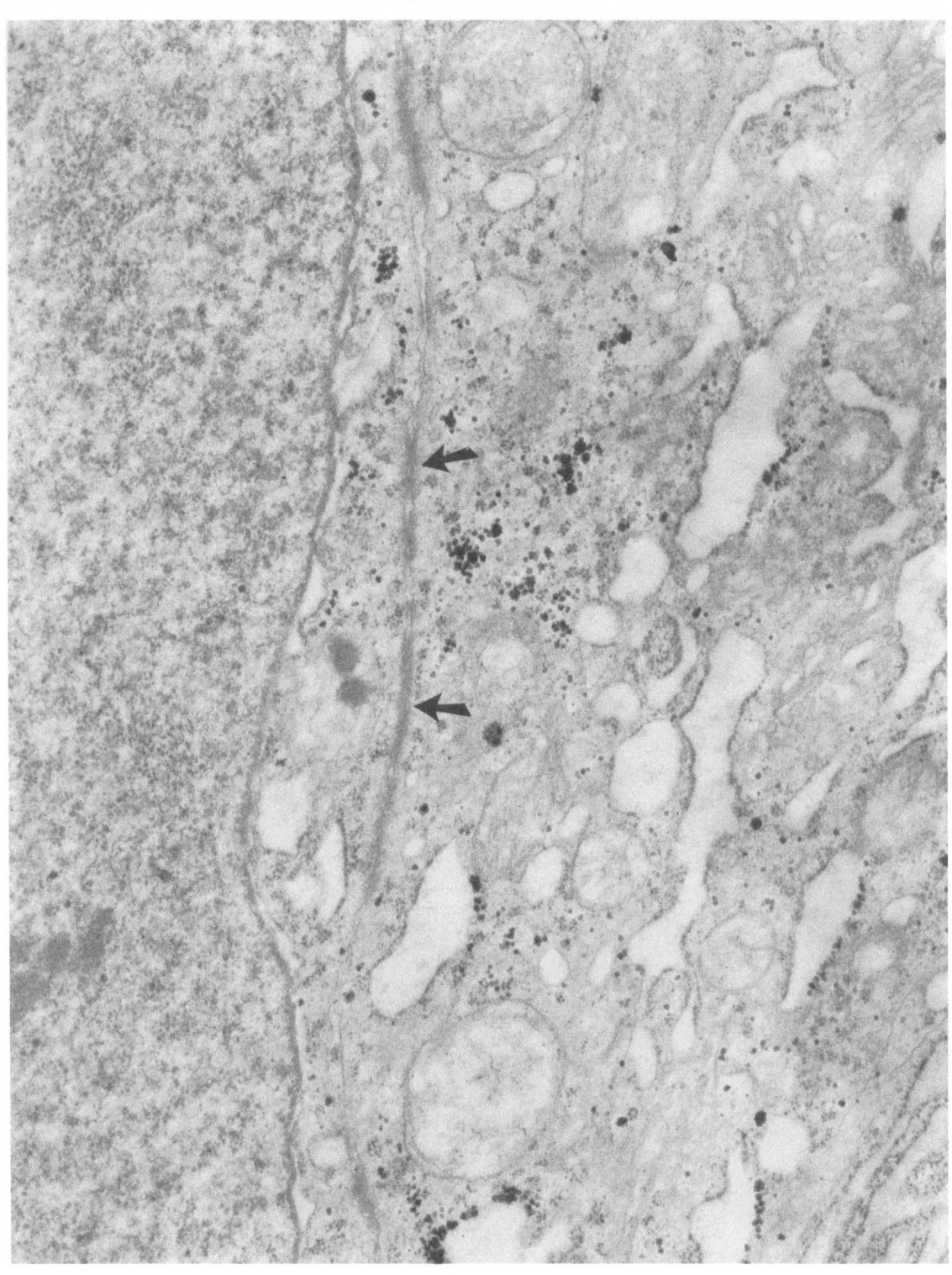

Fig. 16.5. Pineal *germinoma* (the same case as in Fig. 16.1). Desmosomes (*arrows*) are sometimes observed between the germinoma cells. The electron-dense granules are glycogen. × 30 000

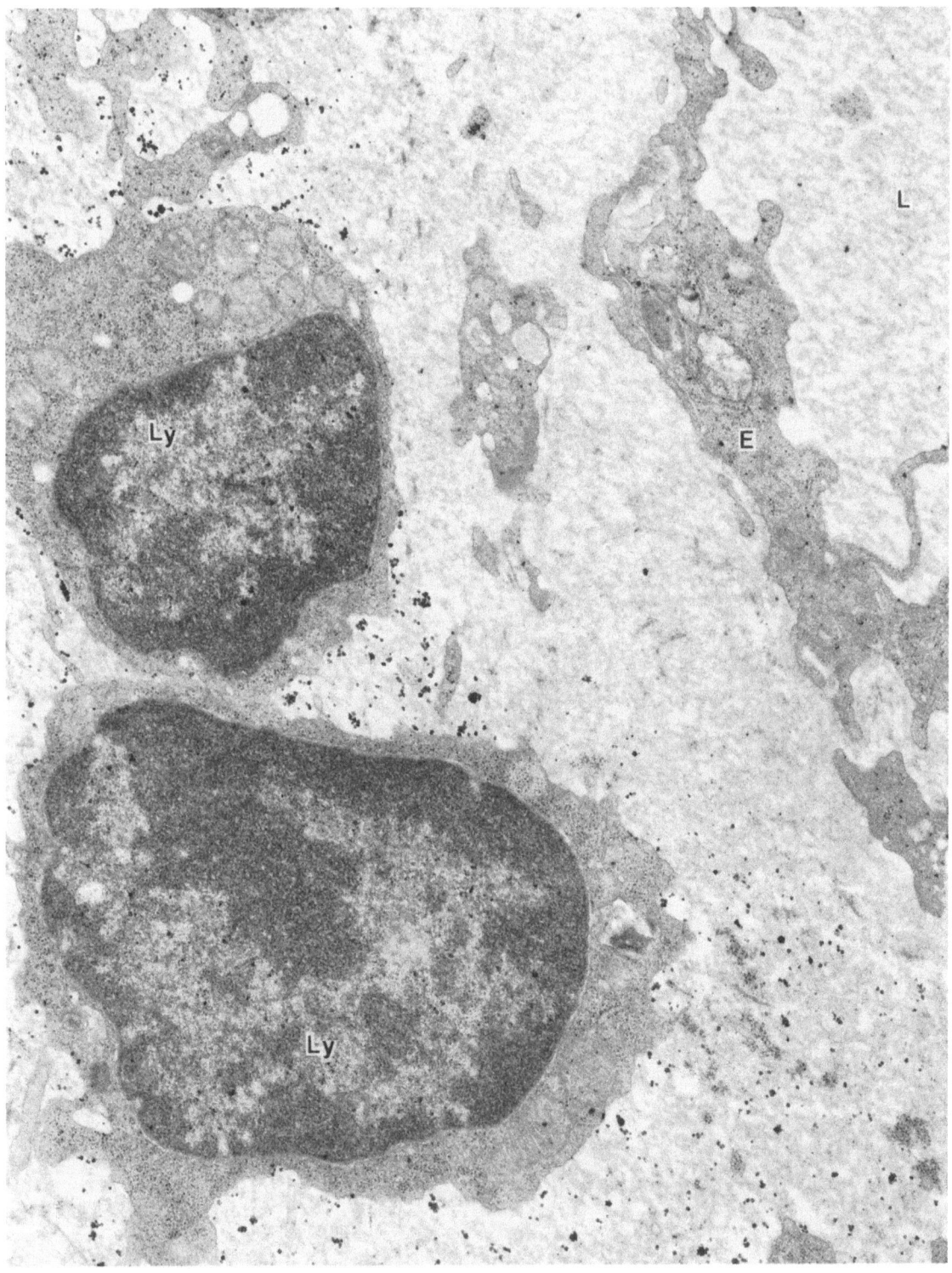

Fig. 16.6. Pineal *germinoma* (the same case as in Fig. 16.1). Nonneoplastic lymphocytes (*Ly*) are seen in the perivascular fluid space of the tumor. Note the glycogen in the extracellular space. *L* capillary lumen, *E* endothelial cell. × 24 000

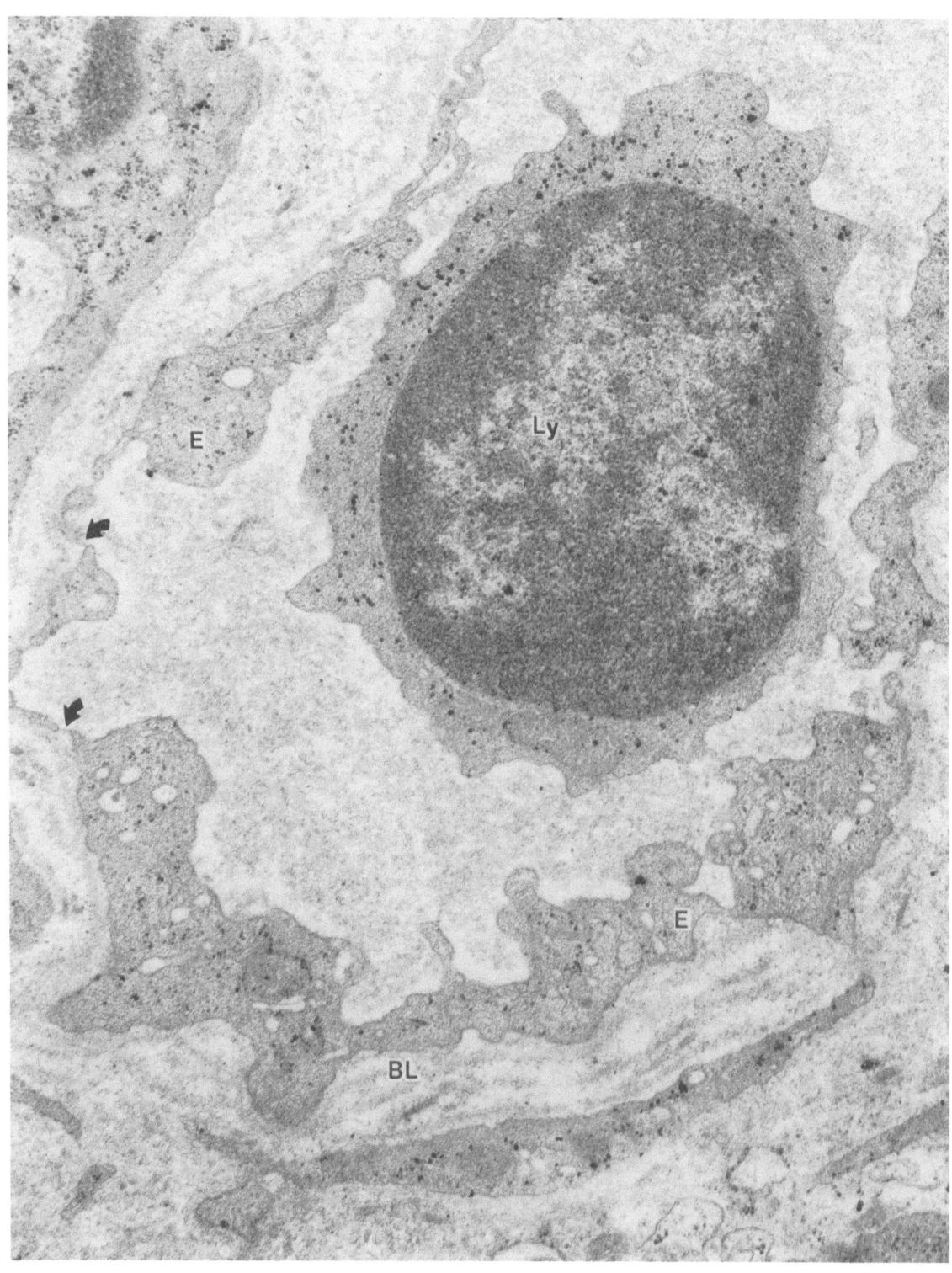

Fig. 16.7. Pineal *germinoma* (the same case as in Fig. 16.1). A blood capillary with a lymphocyte (*Ly*) shows endothelial fenestrations (*arrows*). *BL* basal lamina, *E* endothelial cell. × 33 600

17. Teratoma and Teratoid Tumor

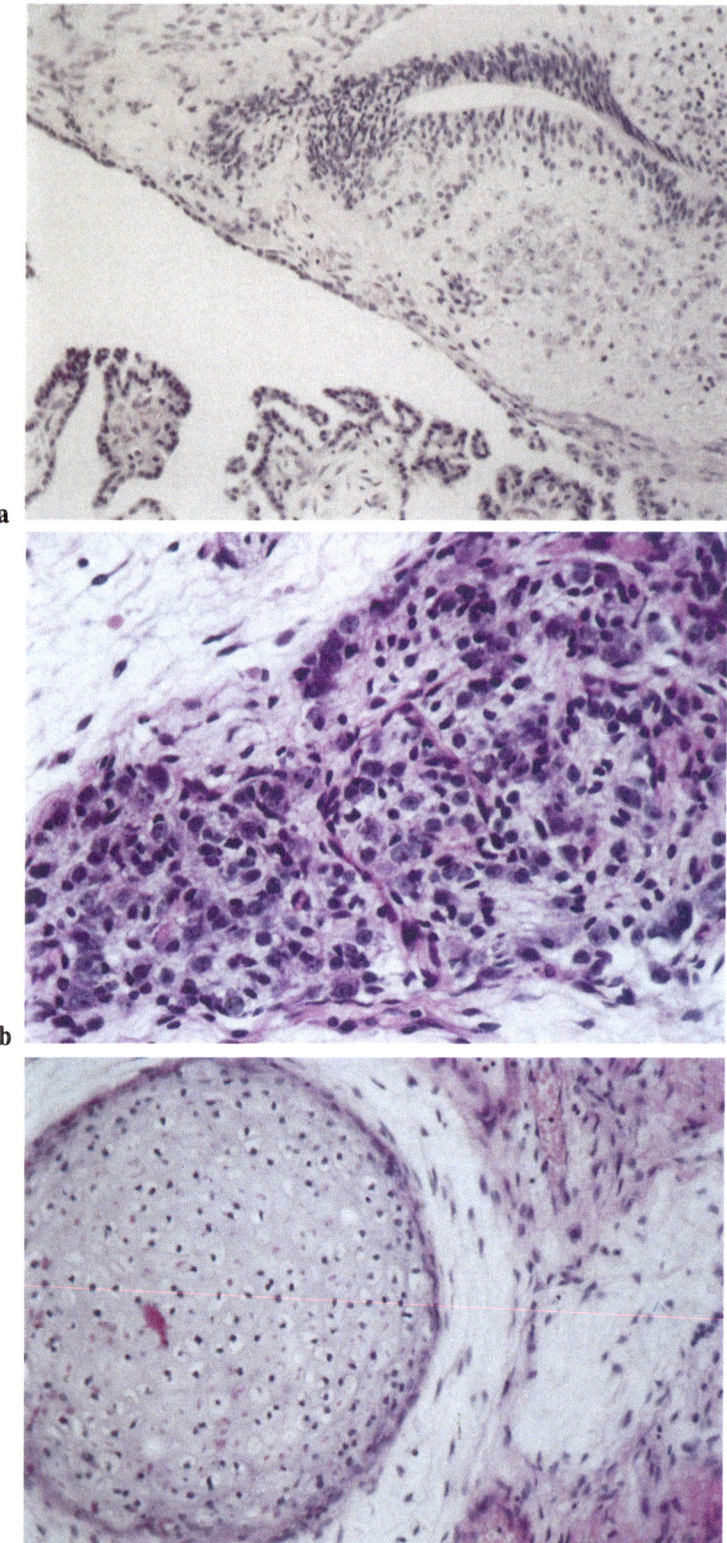

Fig. 17.1a–c. Pineal *teratoma* in a 9-year-old boy. The tumor is composed of a histological variety of tissues such as the choroid plexus and ependymal canal-like structures (**a**), ganglion cells with satellite cells (**b**), and chondrocytes (**c**). H and E; **a** × 80, **b** × 160, **c** × 80

Fig. 17.2a–c. Pineal *teratoma* (the same case in Fig. 17.1). Figures a, b, c are comparable sections to Fig. 17.1a, b, c, respectively, and reveal positive staining for S-100 protein. Indirect immunoperoxidase method counterstained with methyl green (except for **a**); **a** × 80, **b** × 160, **c** × 80

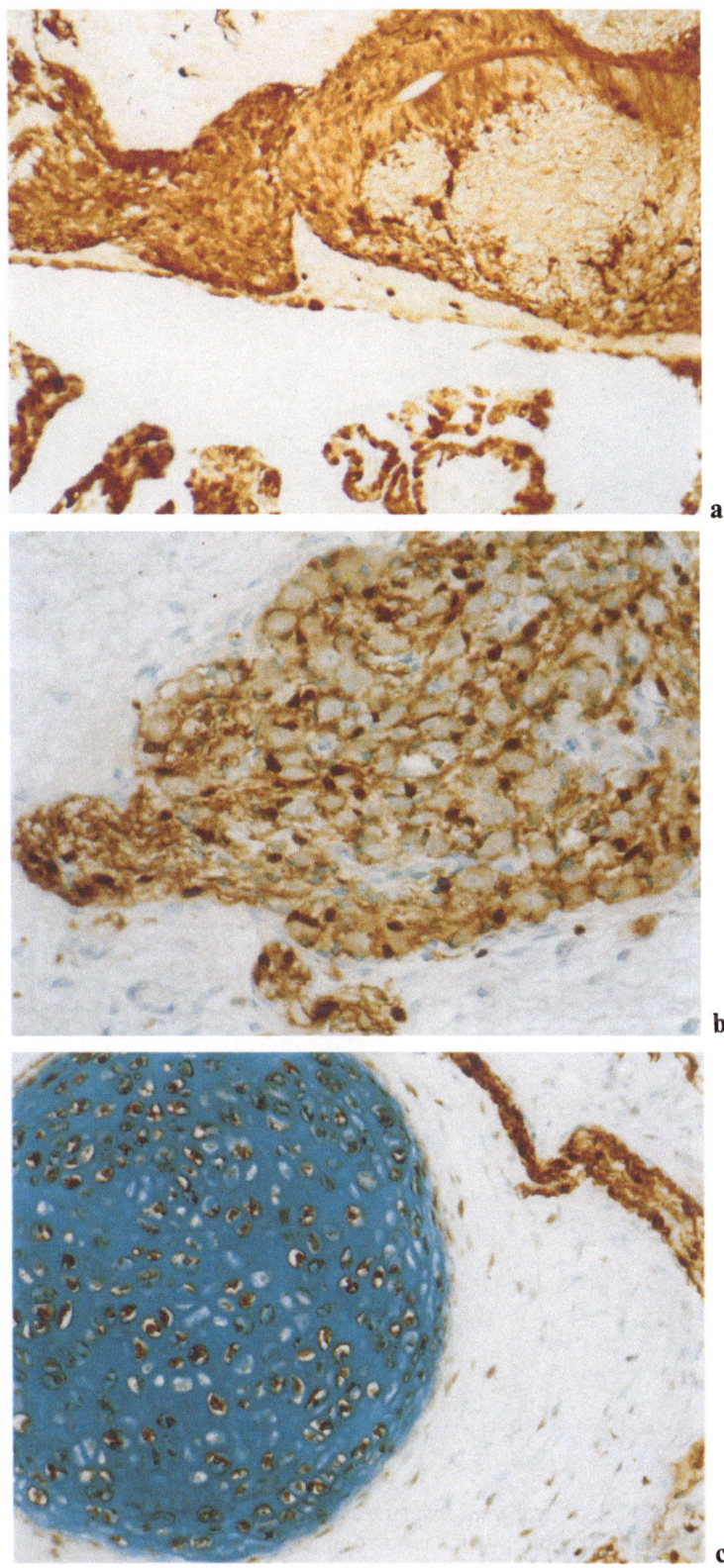

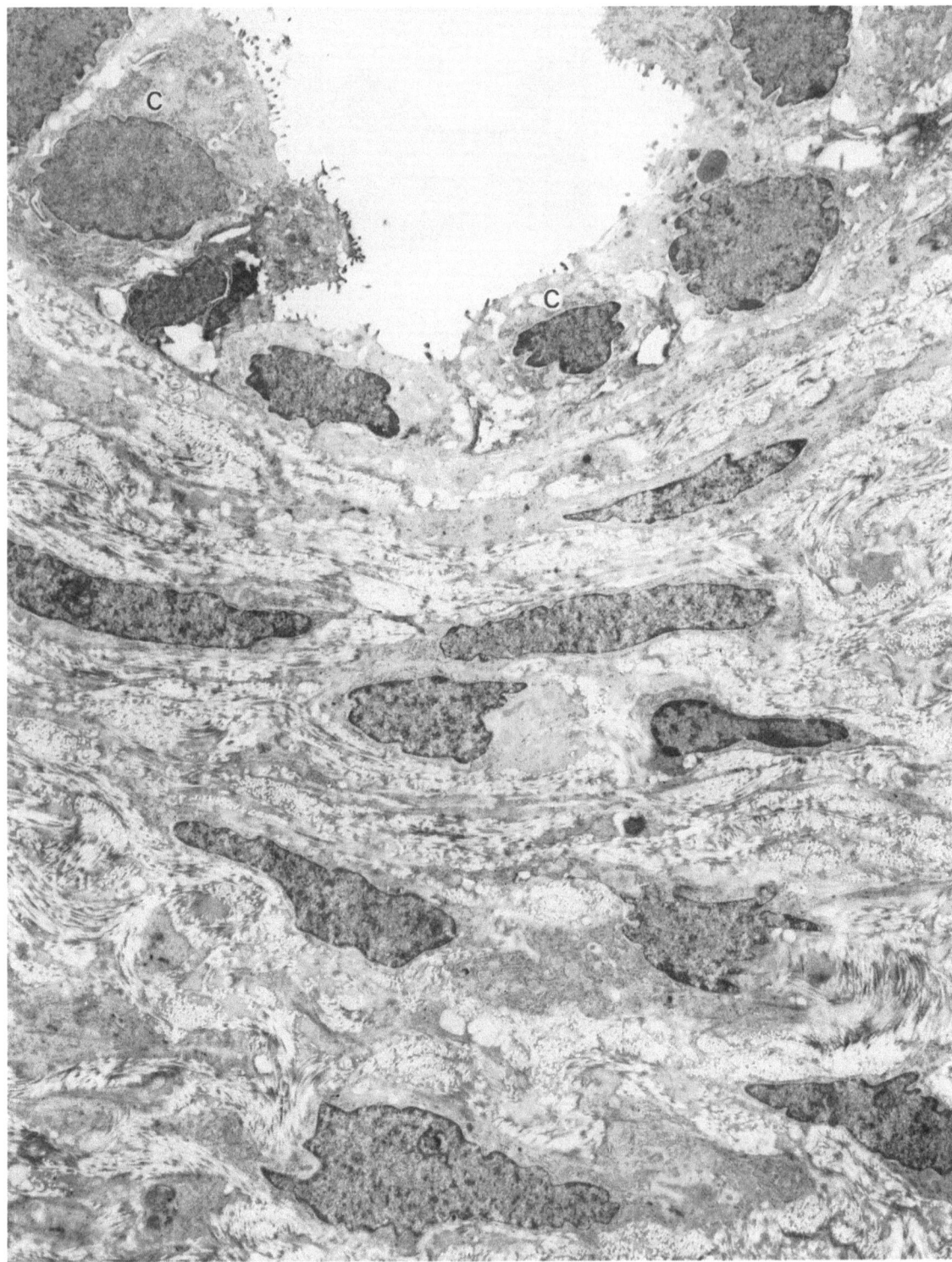

Fig. 17.3. Pineal *teratoma* (the same case as in Fig. 17.1). The tumor shows cuboidal cells (*C*), forming a tubular structure, which is surrounded by many fibroblasts with abundant collagen fibers. × 4700

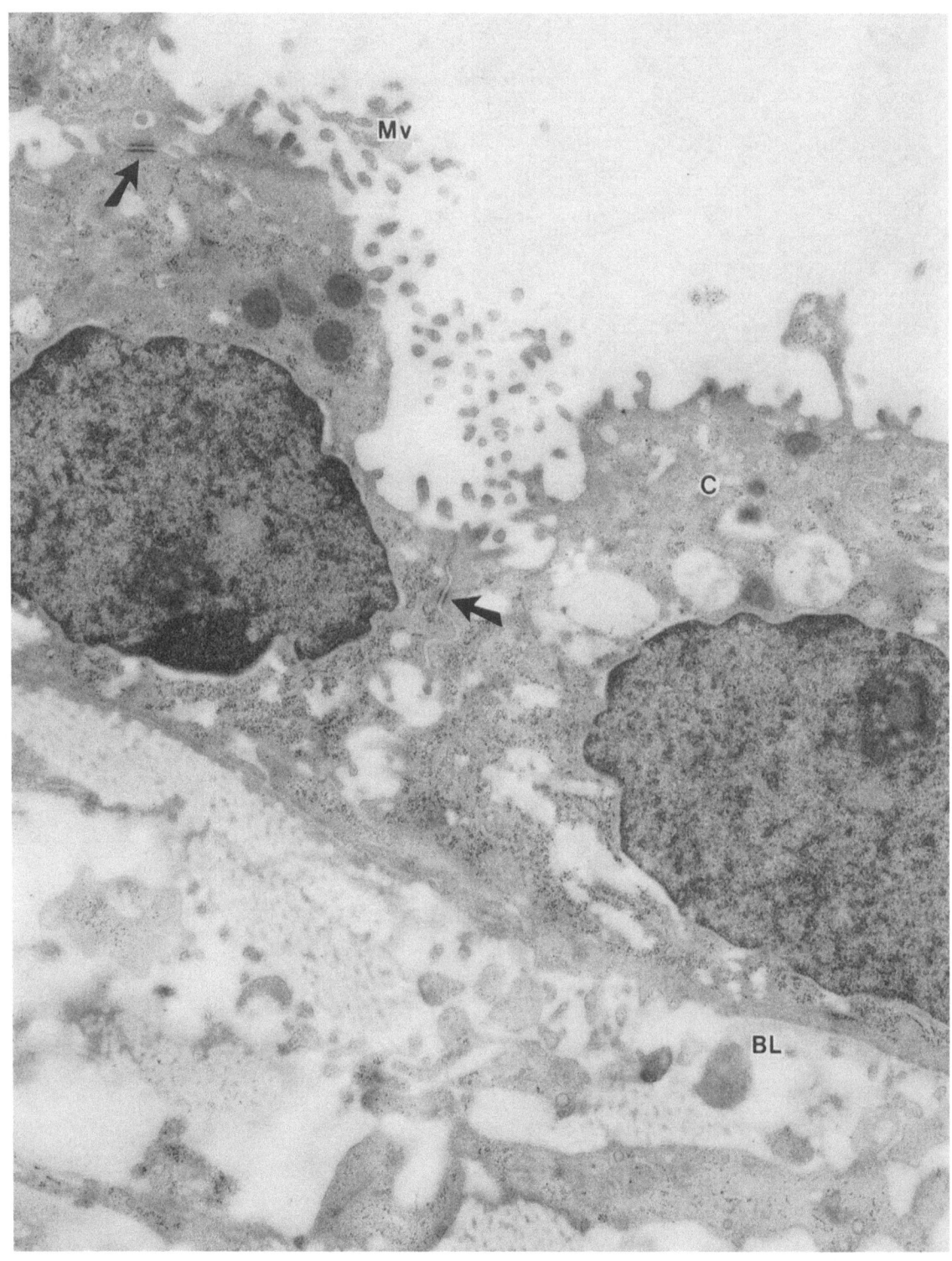

Fig. 17.4. Pineal *teratoma* (the same case as in Fig. 17.1). Desmosomes (*arrows*), microvilli (*Mv*), and a basal lamina (*BL*) are observed. *C* cuboidal cell. × 16 000

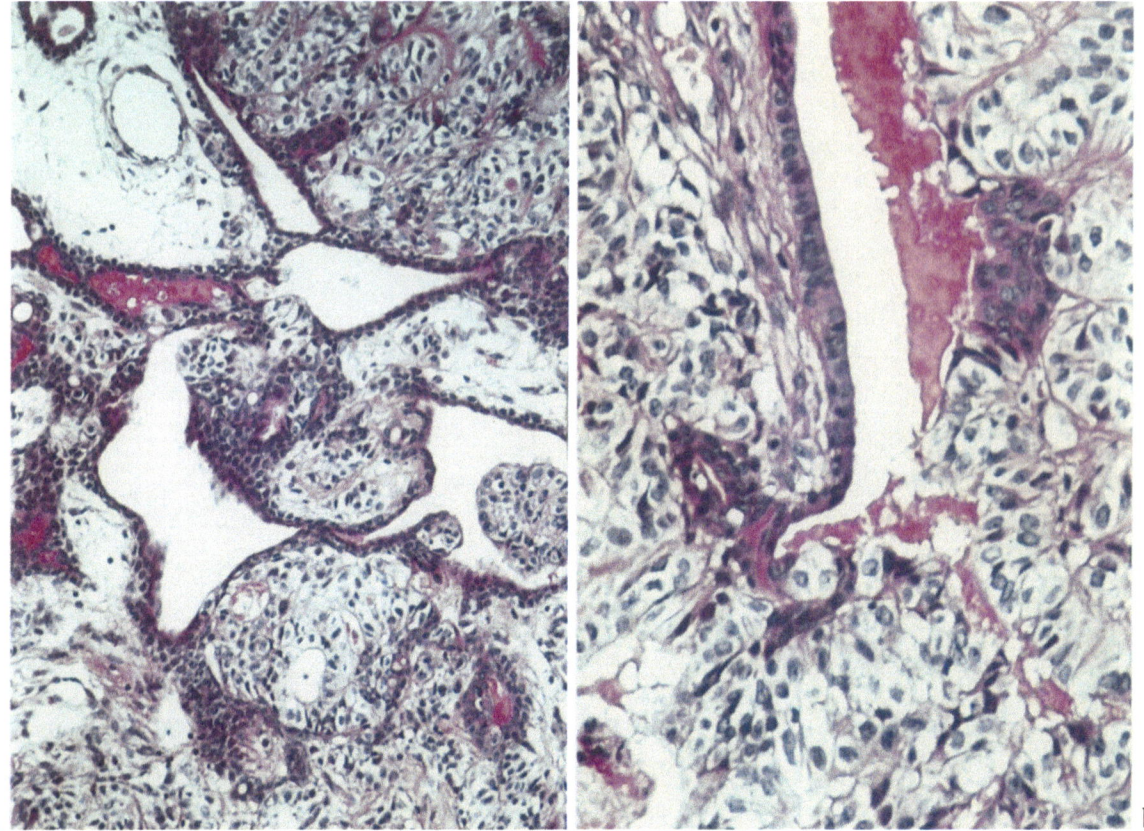

a   b

Fig. 17.5a, b. *Teratoid tumor* of the left temporo-occipital region in an 8-year-old girl. The tumor is composed of partly stratified epithelial cells and polygonal cells with clear cytoplasm. H and E; **a** × 90, **b** × 180

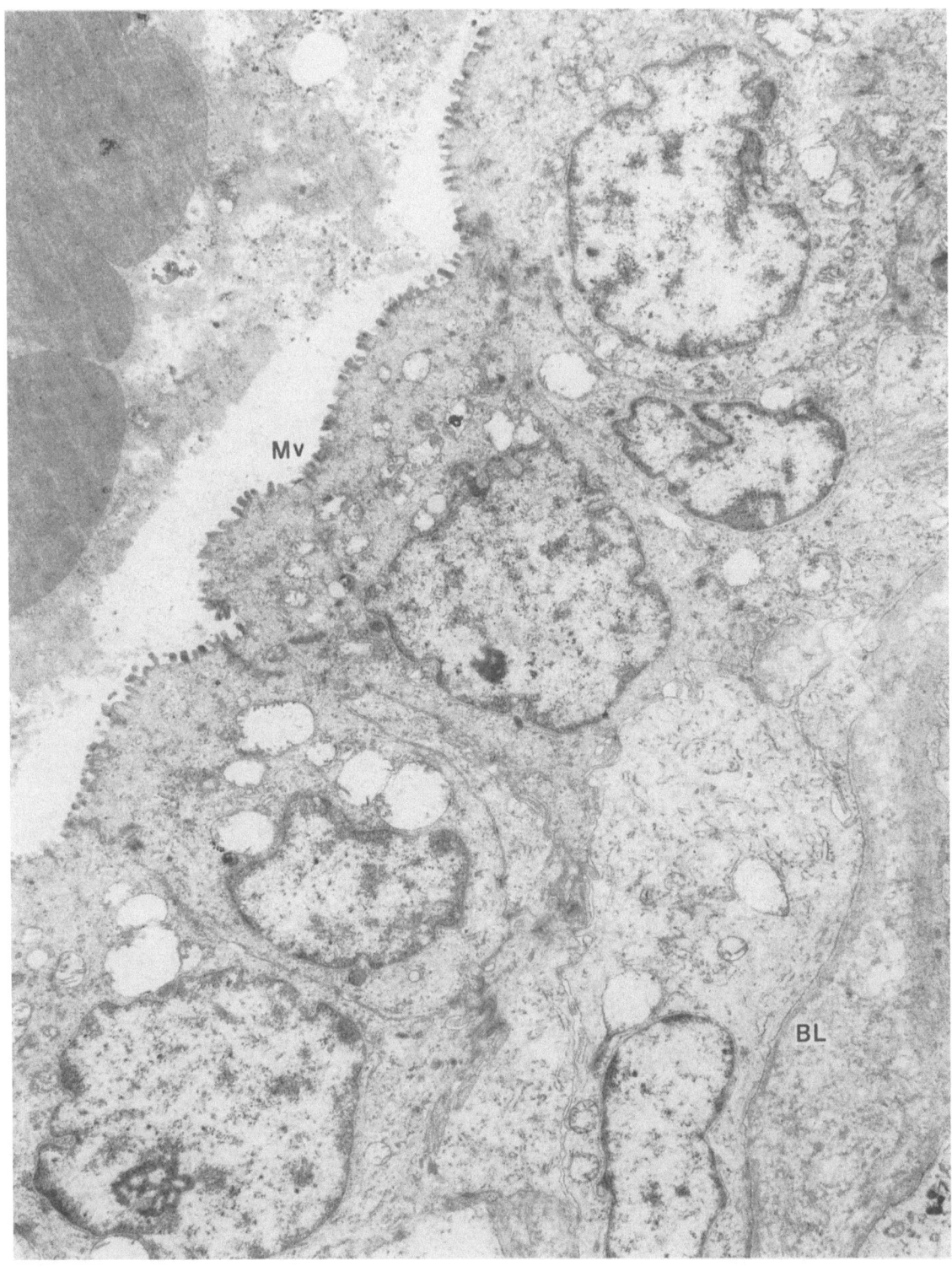

Fig. 17.6. *Teratoid tumor* (the same case as in Fig. 17.5). The epithelial cells forming a single cell layer show numerous microvilli (*Mv*). *BL* basal lamina. × 5700

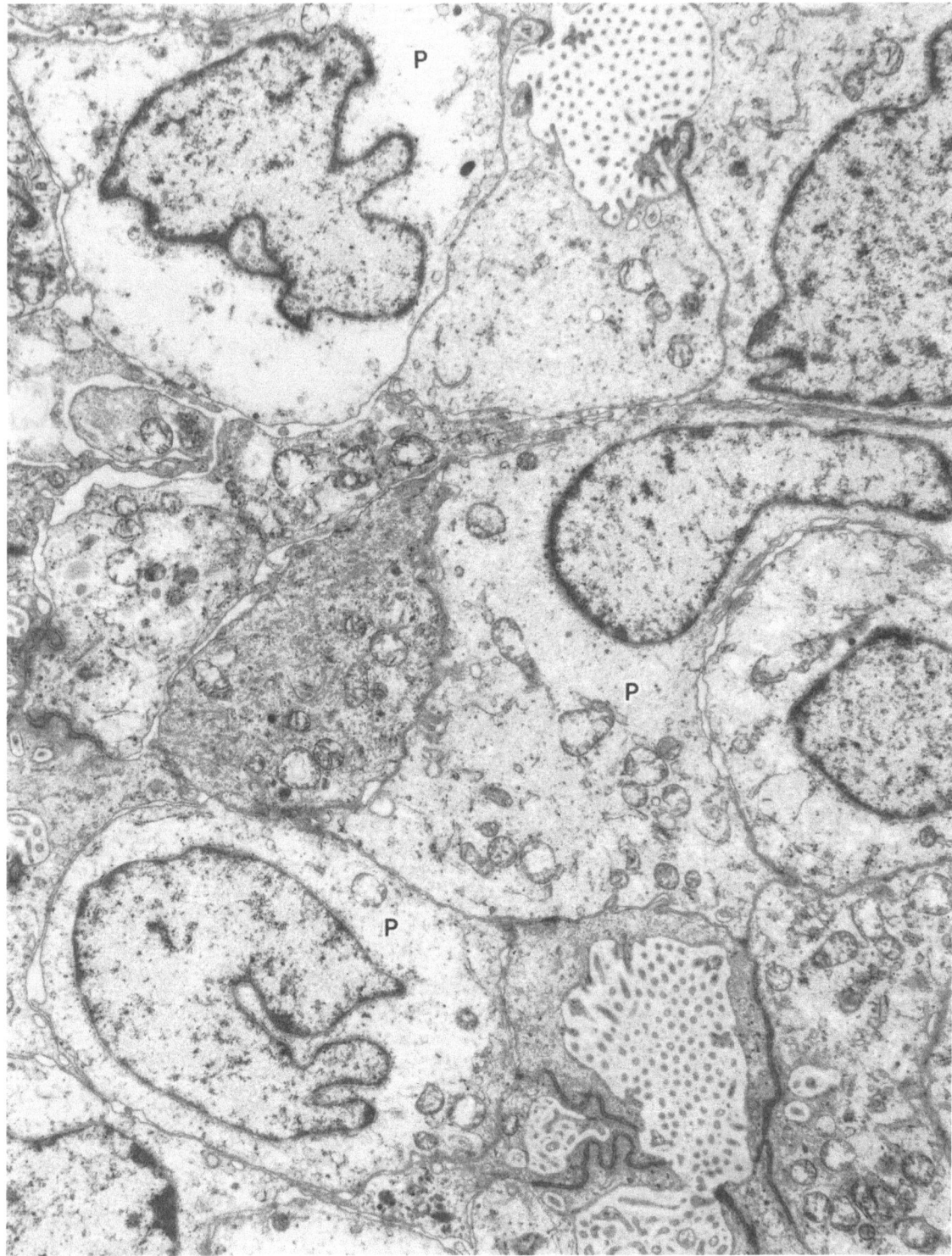

Fig. 17.7. *Teratoid tumor* (the same case as in Fig. 17.5). Polygonal cells (*P*) with clear cytoplasm have a few organelles. × 9600

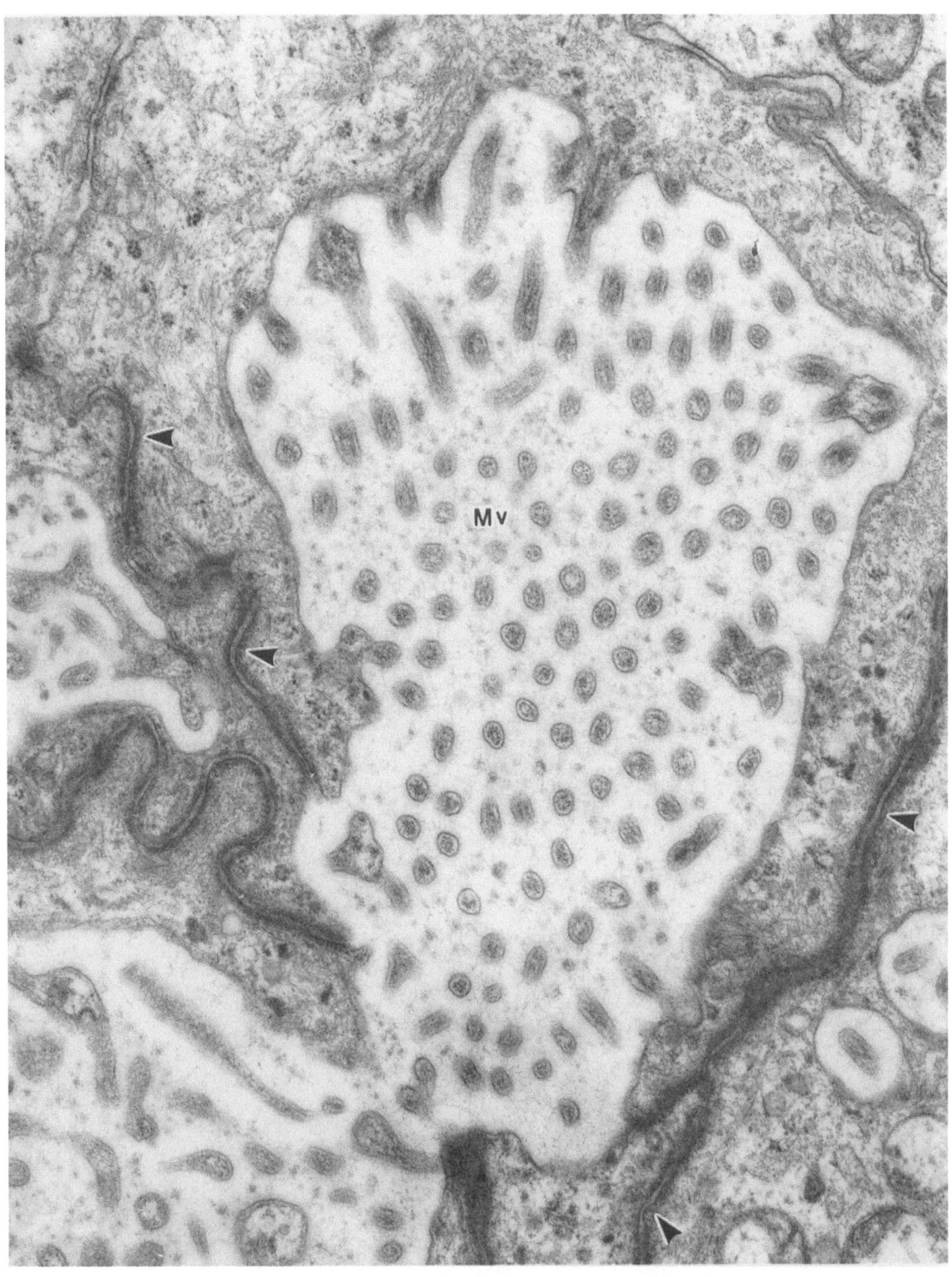

Fig. 17.8. *Teratoid tumor* (the same case as in Fig. 17.5). Higher magnification reveals details of the intercellular junctional apparatus (*arrowheads*) and transversely sectioned microvilli (*Mv*). × 35 000

18. Schwannoma

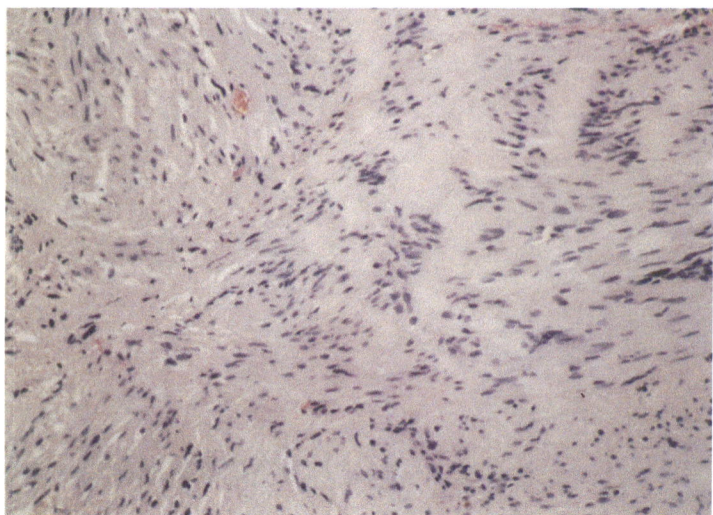

Fig. 18.1. Acoustic *schwannoma* in a 45-year-old woman. The tumor is formed of bundles of cells with elongated nuclei (Antoni's type A). Linear orientation of the nuclei and a fibrillary background characterize this tumor. H and E, × 80

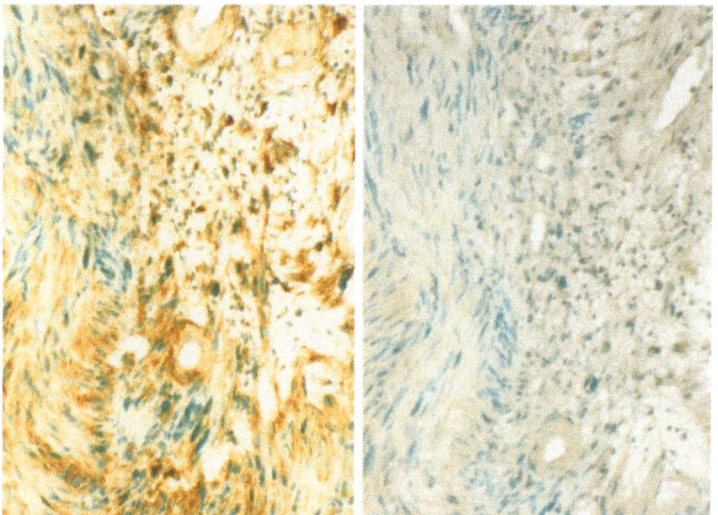

Fig. 18.2a, b. *Schwannoma* (the same case as in Fig. 18.1). Immunohistochemical examination shows positive staining for the β-subunit (**a**) but not for the α-subunit (**b**) of S-100 protein, indicating the existence of S-100b in this tumor. Peroxidase antiperoxidase method counterstained with methyl green, × 80

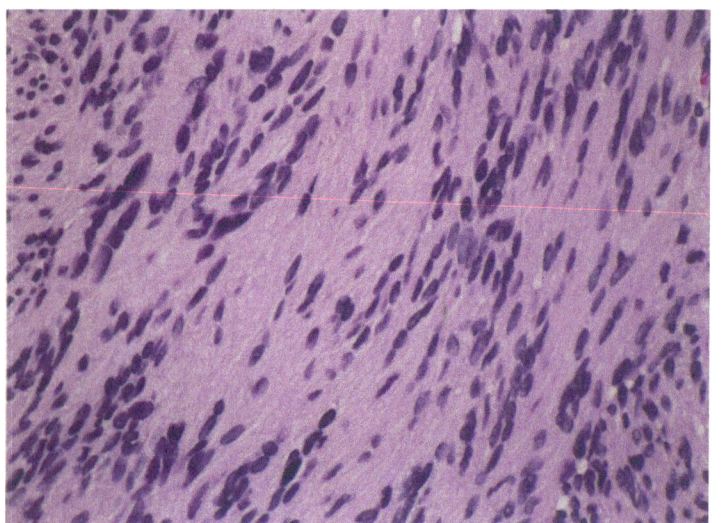

Fig. 18.3. Acoustic *schwannoma* in a 58-year-old woman. The tumor shows a parallel arrangement of elongated cells varying in nuclear size. H and E, × 160

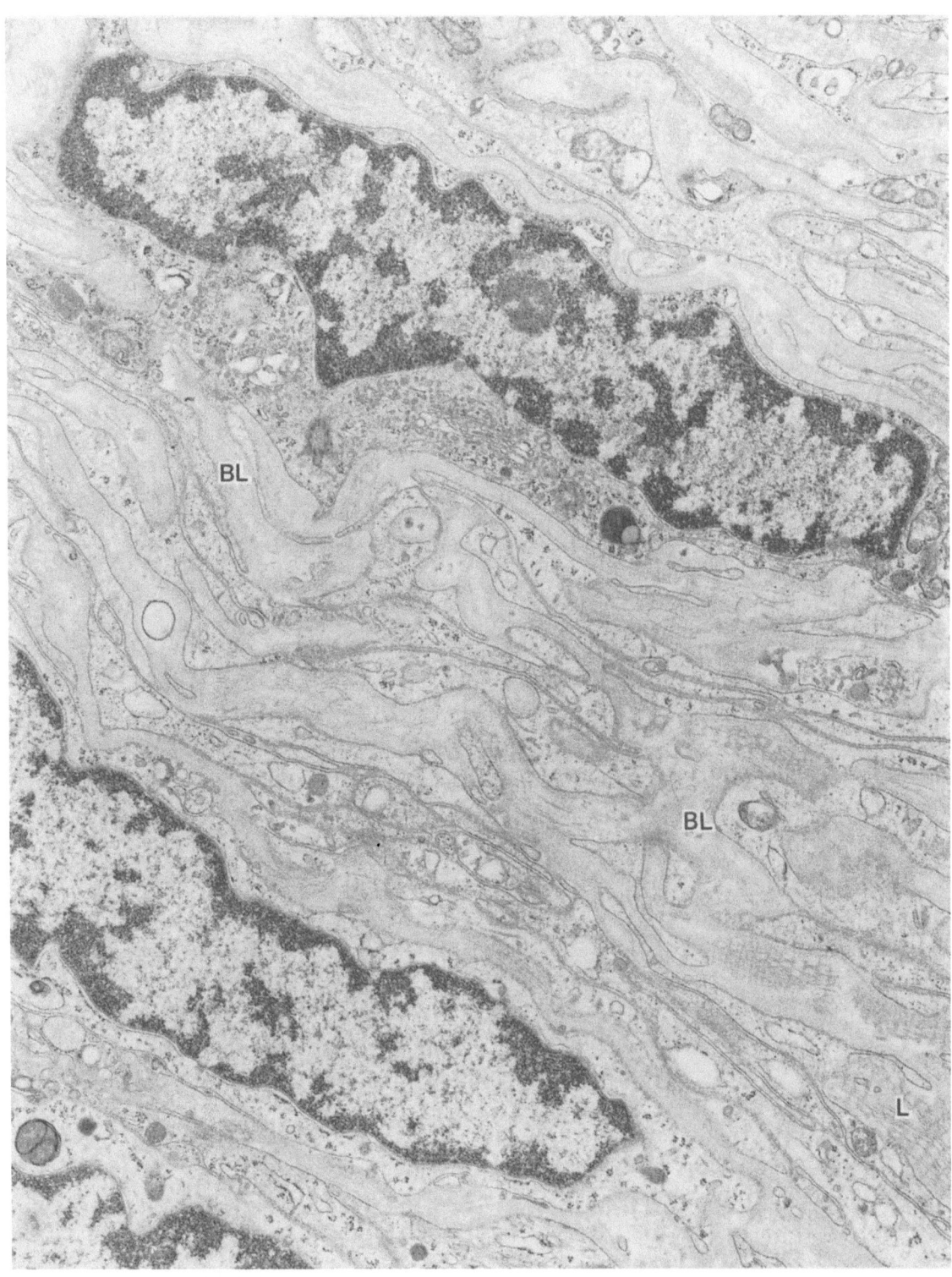

Fig. 18.4. *Schwannoma* (the same case as in Fig. 18.1). In the area of Antoni's type A, the tumor cells have elongated nuclei and narrow perikarya. The folded cytoplasmic processes are separated by basal laminae (*BL*). Long-spacing collagen fibers (Luse body) with striations, 120–150 nm apart, are also discernible. *L* Luse body. × 17 000

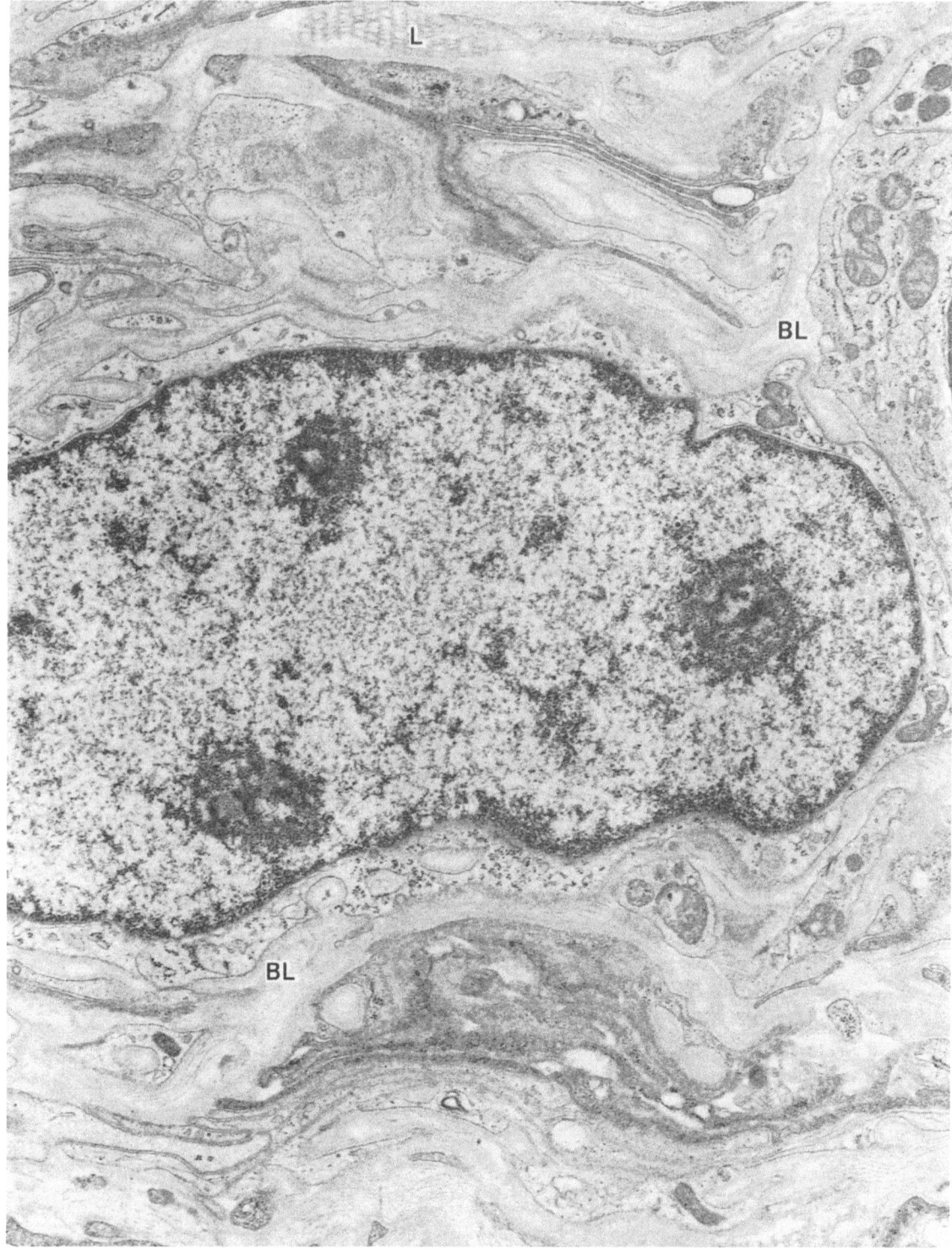

Fig. 18.5. *Schwannoma* (the same case as in Fig. 18.1). The narrow perikaryon of a schwannoma cell is completely invested with basal laminae (*BL*), which distinguish the Schwann cell from the fibroblast. A Luse body (*L*) is also seen in the extracellular matrix. × 17 000

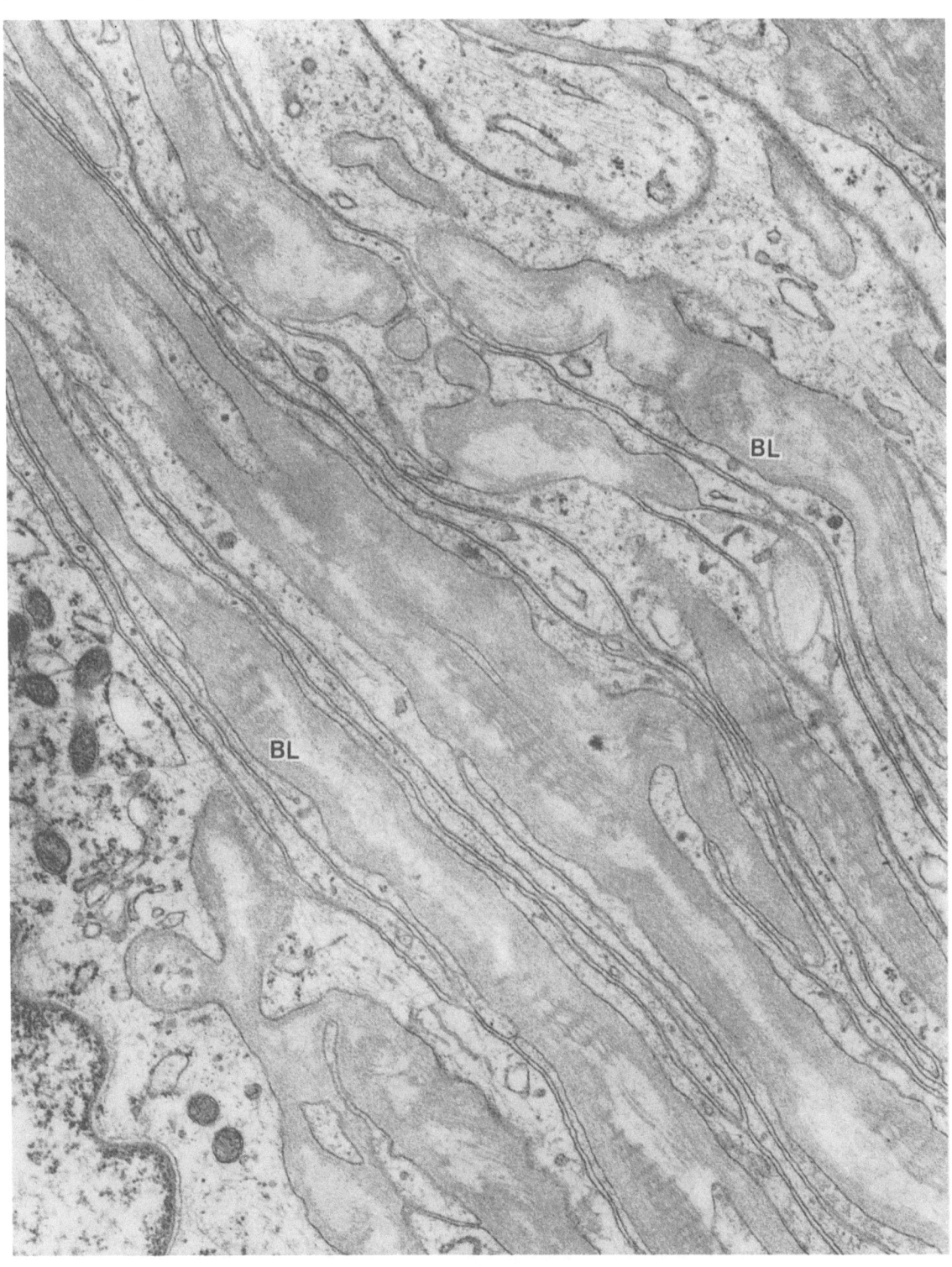

Fig. 18.6. *Schwannoma* (the same case as in Fig. 18.1). Basal laminae (*BL*) separate the parallel layers of folded cytoplasmic processes of schwannoma cells. × 27 000

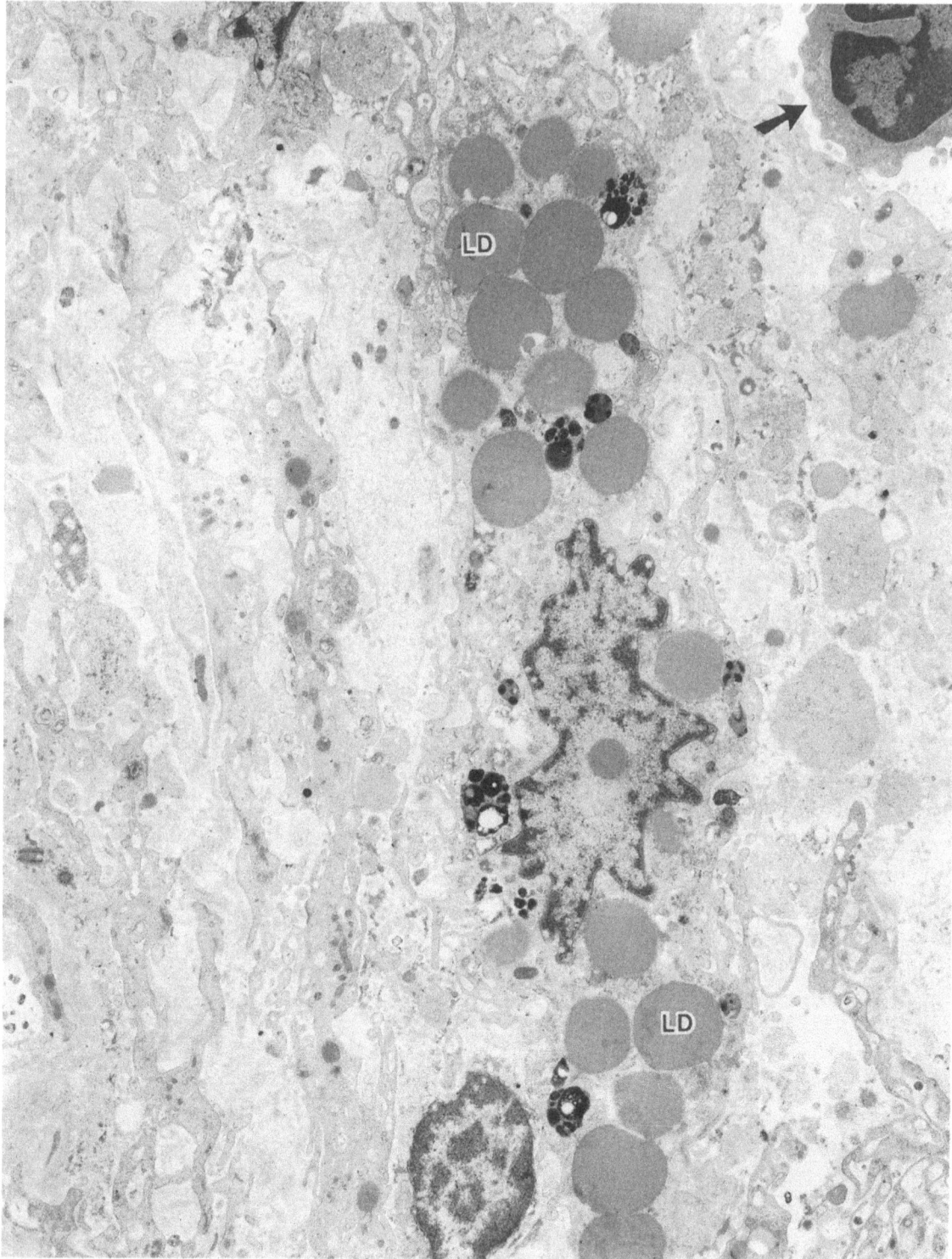

Fig. 18.7. *Schwannoma* (the same case as in Fig. 18.1). In the area of Antoni's type B, a tumor cell with an irregularly shaped nucleus bears many lipid droplets (*LD*) in the cytoplasm. A lymphocyte (*arrow*) infiltrating the tumor is also observed. × 10 000

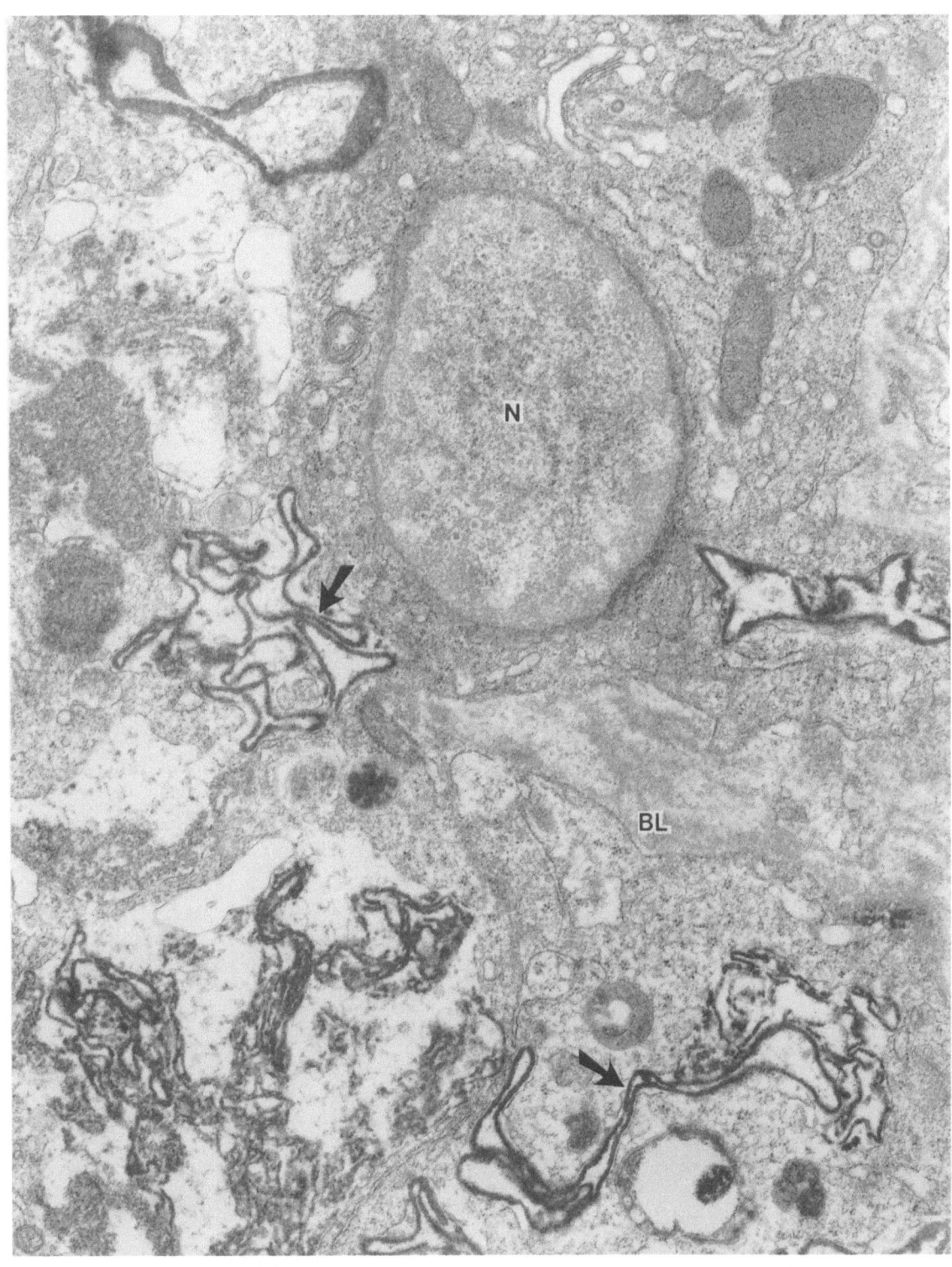

Fig. 18.8. *Schwannoma* (the same case as in Fig. 18.3). Osmiophilic membranous structures (*arrows*) are sometimes encountered in the cytoplasm of tumor cells. *N* nucleus, *BL* basal lamina. × 18 000

19. Pituitary Adenoma and Oncocytoma

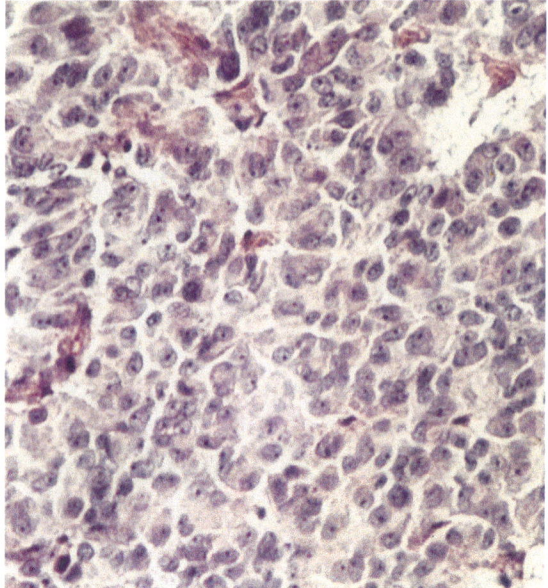

Fig. 19.1. *Pituitary adenoma* (chromophobe type, diffuse pattern) in a 30-year-old woman. H and E, × 180

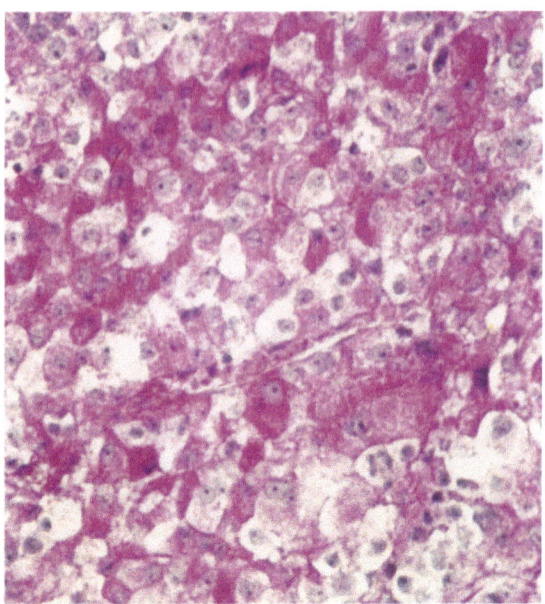

Fig. 19.2. *Pituitary adenoma* (acidophil type, diffuse pattern) in a 41-year-old man. H and E, × 180

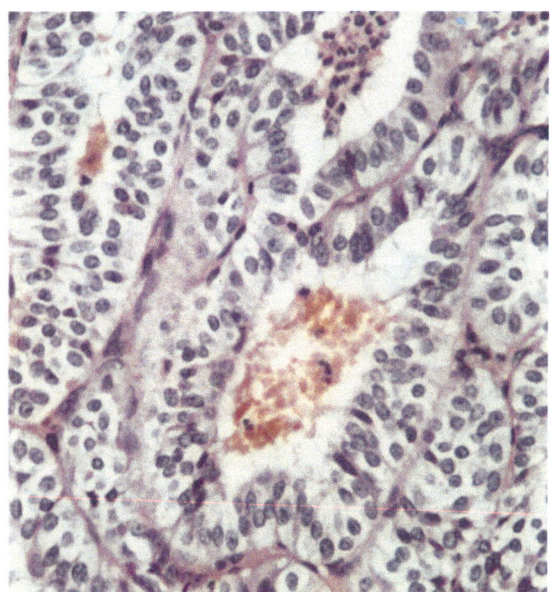

Fig. 19.3. *Pituitary adenoma* (chromophobe type, sinusoid pattern) in a 32-year-old man. H and E, × 180

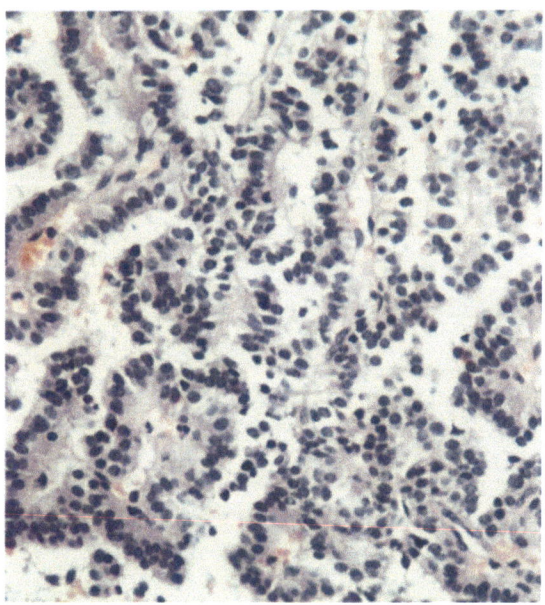

Fig. 19.4. *Pituitary adenoma* (chomophobe type, papillary pattern) in a 34-year-old woman. H and E, × 120

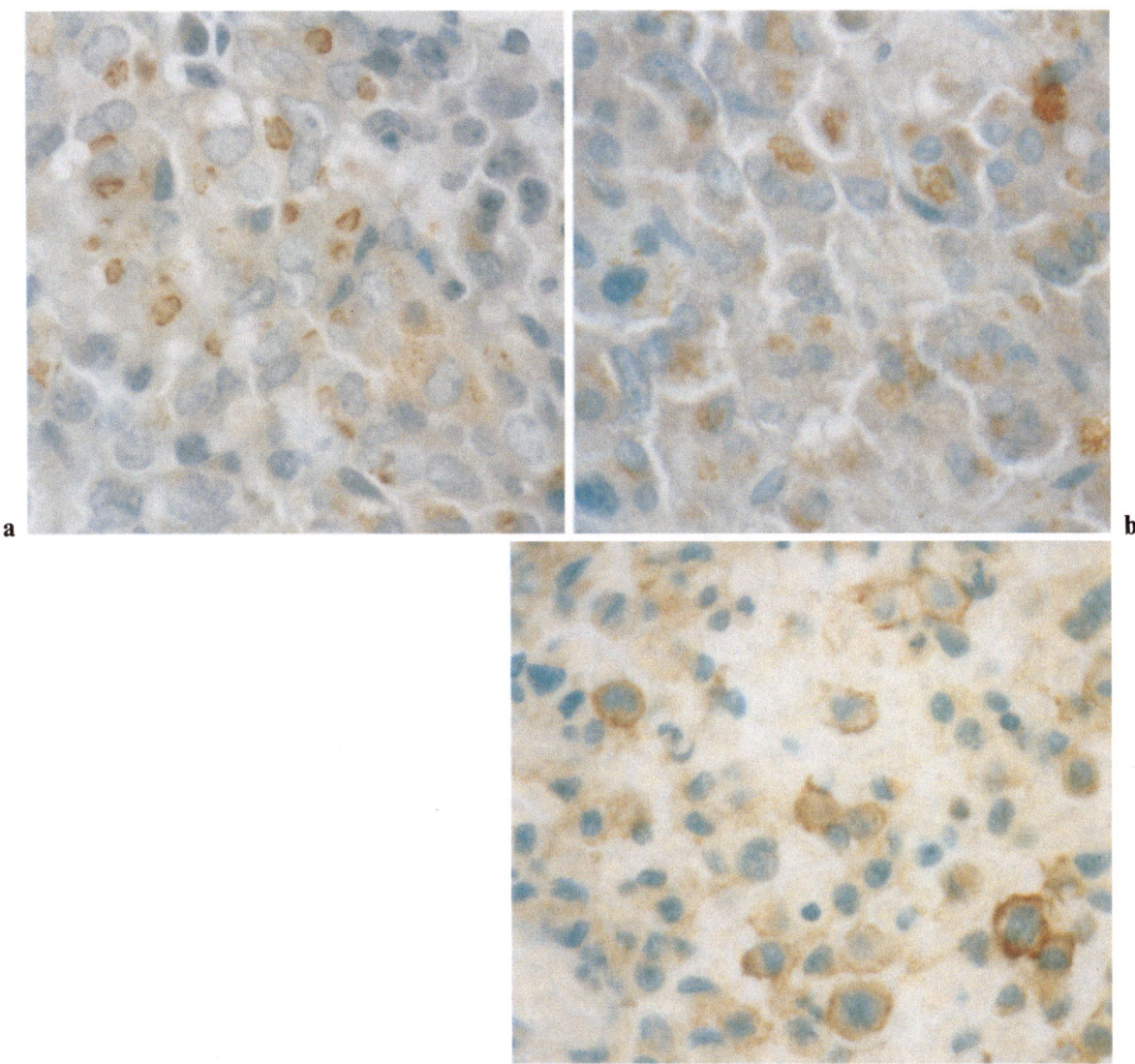

a

b

Fig. 19.5a–c. *Pituitary adenomas* stained immunohistochemically for prolactin (**a**), growth hormone (**b**), and adrenocorticotropic hormone (**c**). Traditionally, adenomas of the pituitary gland have been classified according to their tinctorial properties into three types—chromophobe, acidophil, and basophil adenomas. Recently, another division—into groups of functioning and nonfunctioning adenomas, based on the presence or absence of immunoreactive pituitary peptides (hormones), has been employed. Therefore, the immunoperoxidase method is of great importance in establishing the diagnosis of pituitary adenomas. Indirect immunoperoxidase method counterstained with methyl green, × 360

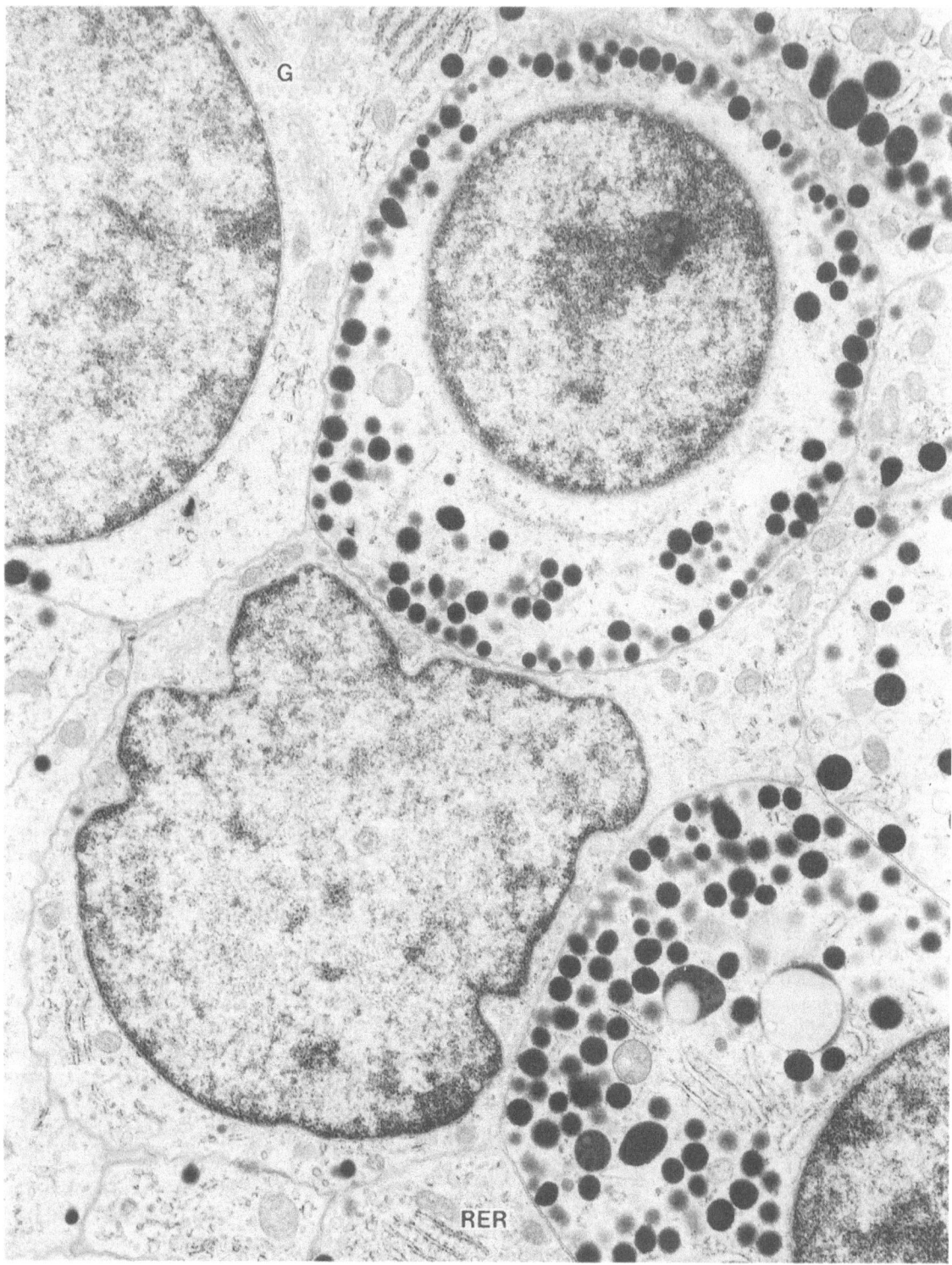

Fig. 19.6. *Prolactin cell adenoma* (the same case as in Fig. 19.1). Densely granulated round cells with a round nucleus and sparsely granulated polyhedral cells with an irregular nucleus are seen. The secretory granules are round or oval and measure 150–500 nm in diameter (average 200–300 nm). Note the well-developed lamellar rough endoplasmic reticulum (*RER*) and Golgi apparatus (*G*). × 13 500

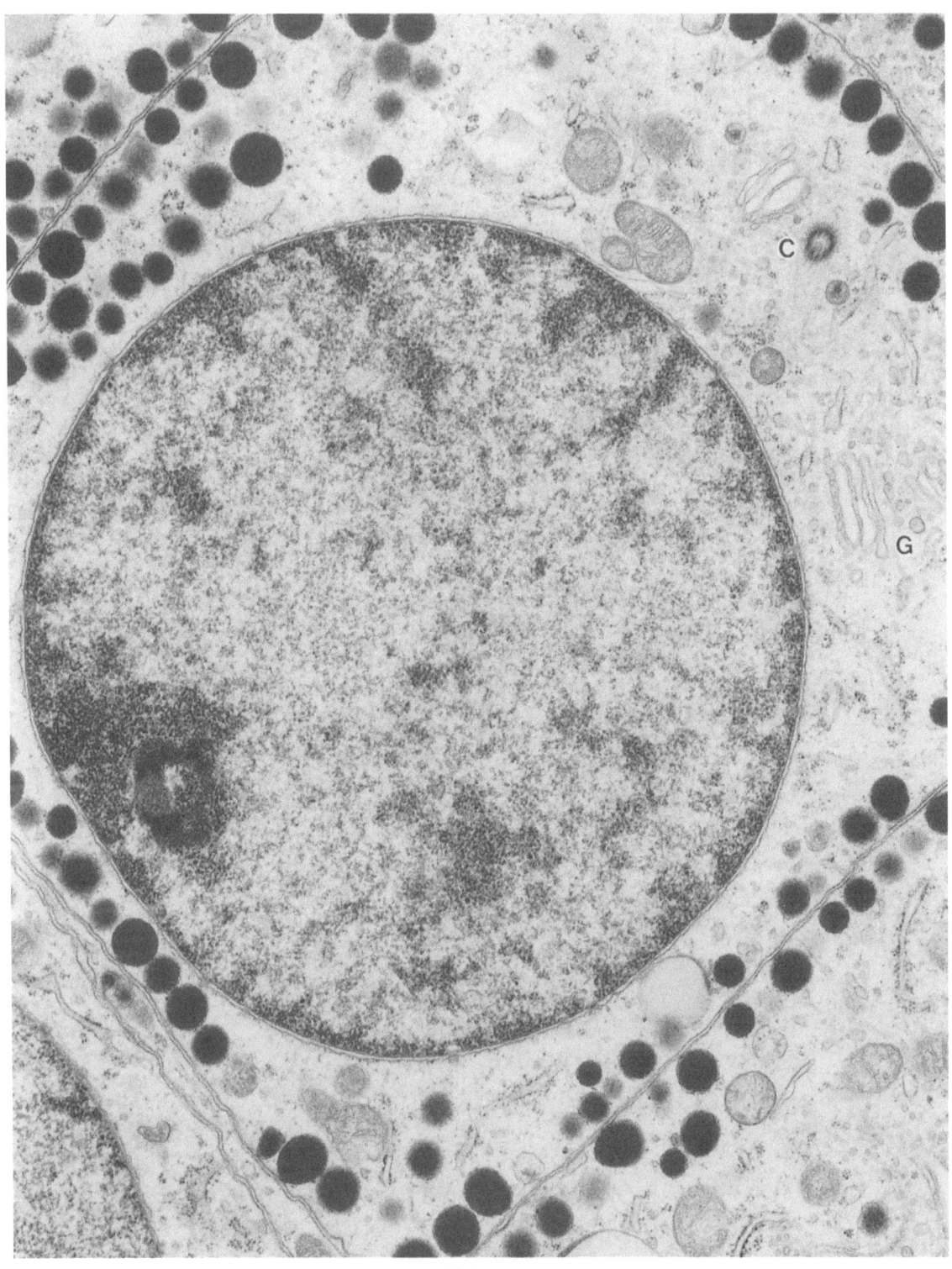

Fig. 19.7. *Prolactin cell adenoma* (the same case as in Fig. 19.1). Many of the secretory granules, 200–400 nm in diameter, are distributed along the cell membrances. *C* centriole, *G* Golgi apparatus. × 21 000

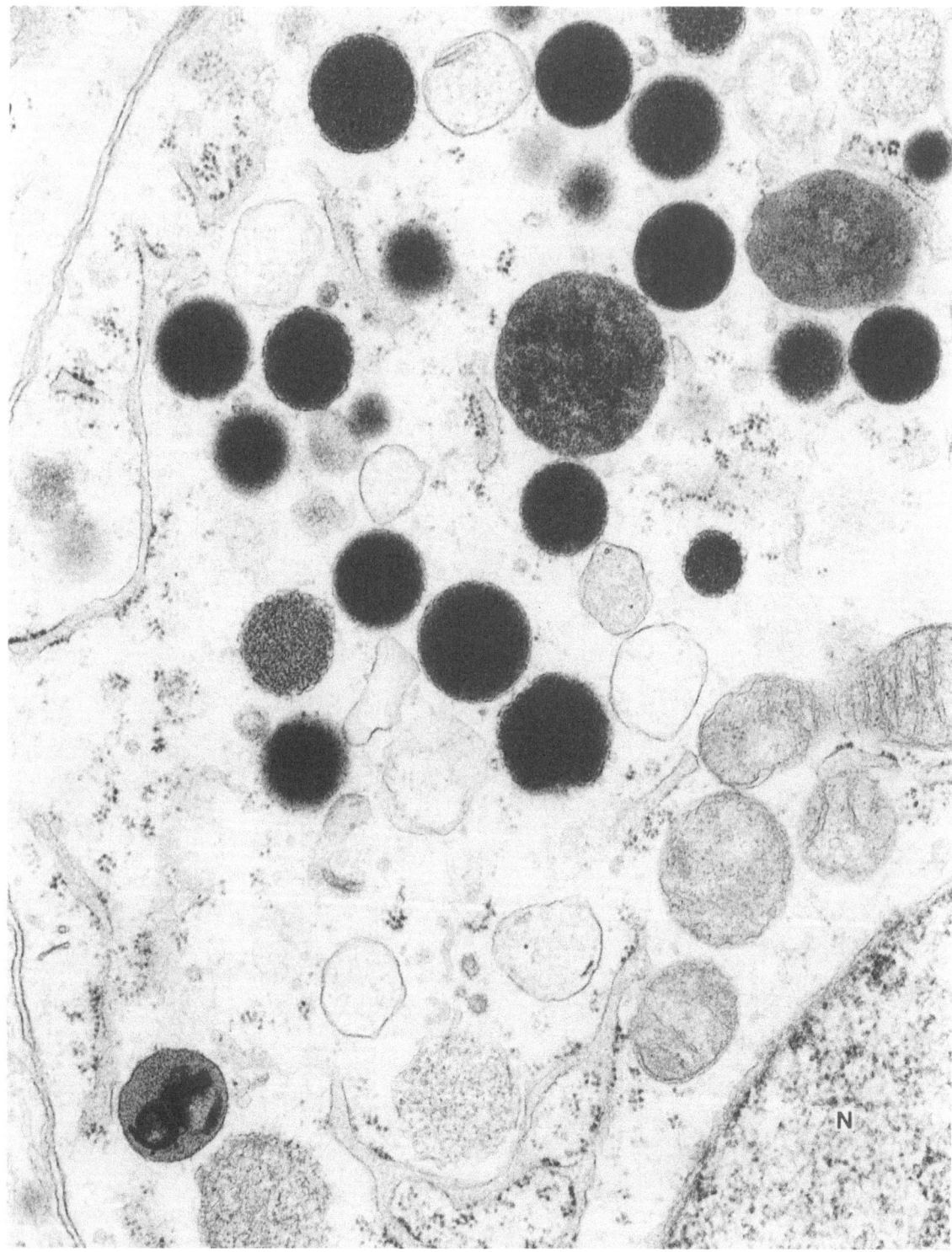

Fig. 19.8. *Prolactin cell adenoma* (the same case as in Fig. 19.1). Higher magnification discloses details of the spherical secretory granules, which differ in size and electron density. *N* nucleus. × 43 000

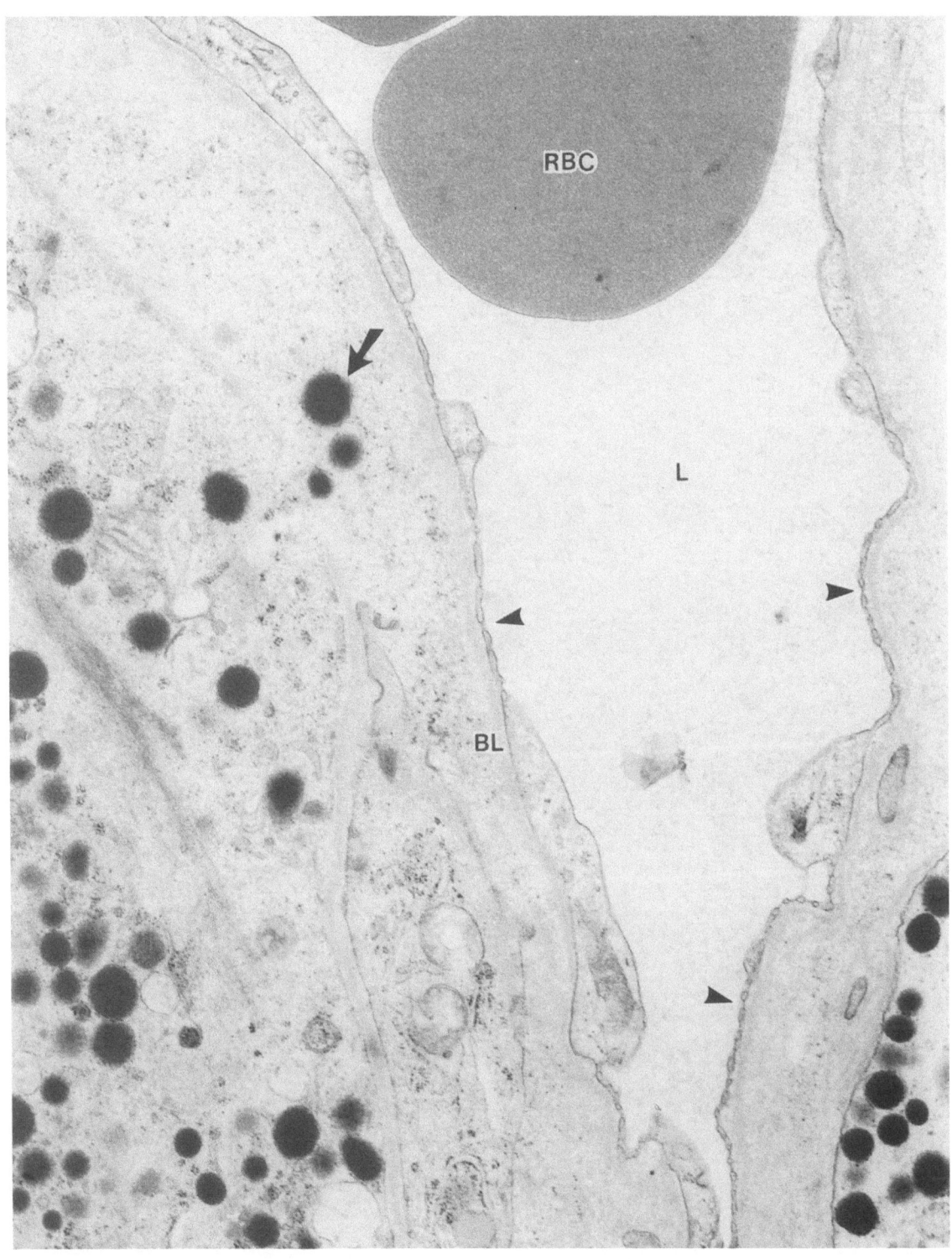

Fig. 19.9. *Prolactin cell adenoma* (the same case as in Fig. 19.1). A capillary lumen (*L*) in the adenoma is lined by endothelium with pinocytotic vesicles and numerous fenestrations (*arrowheads*). Exocytosis of the secretory granules (*arrow*) is observed, as in a normal pituitary, at the vascular pole of the cell. *BL* basal lamina, *RBC* erythrocyte. × 22 800

163

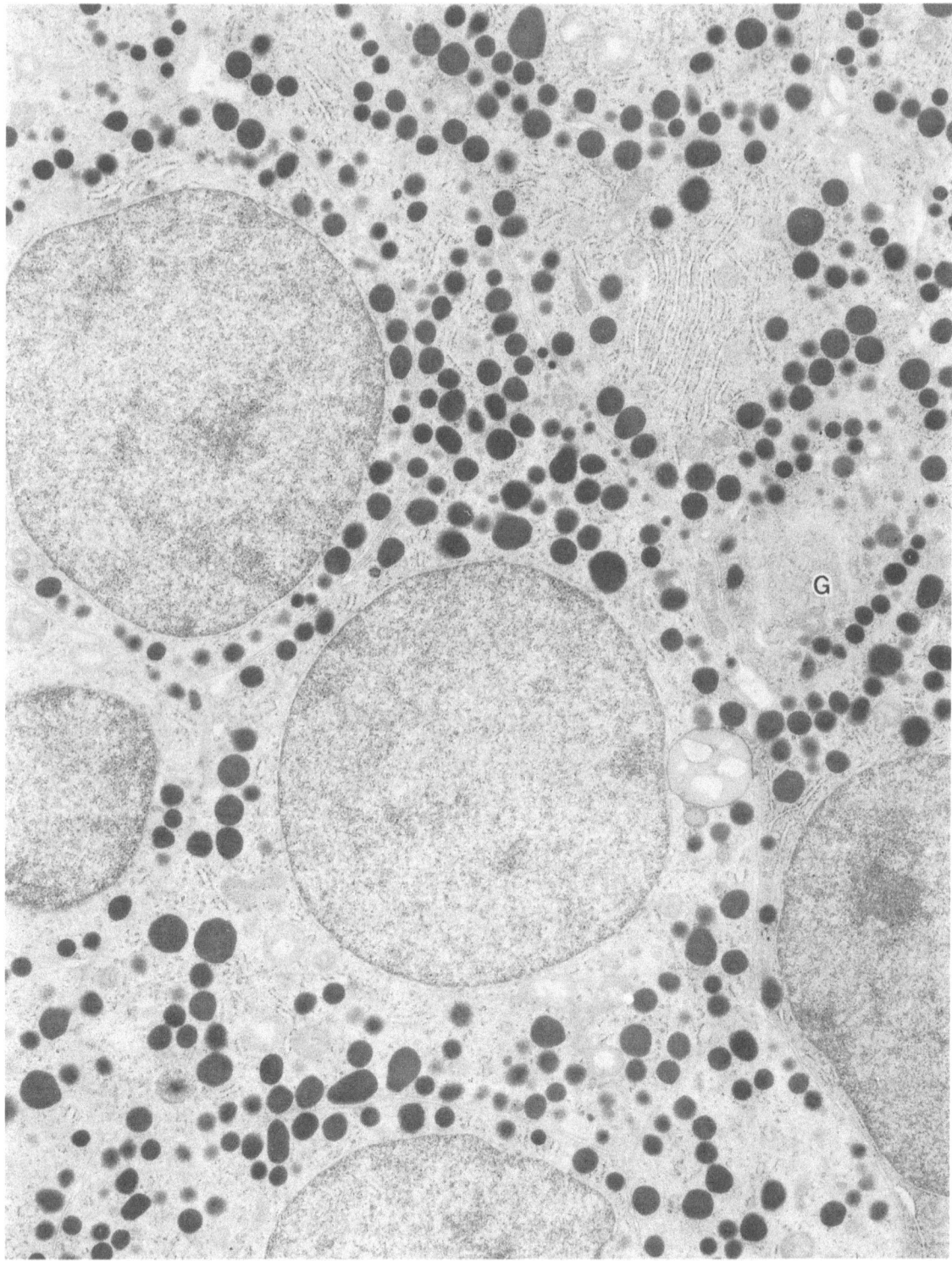

Fig. 19.10. *Growth hormone cell adenoma* (the same case as in Fig. 19.2). The adenoma cells contain many spherical, electron-dense, secretory granules, measuring 300–700 nm in diameter. The prominent Golgi apparatus (*G*) on the *right* bears some secretory granules. × 10 000

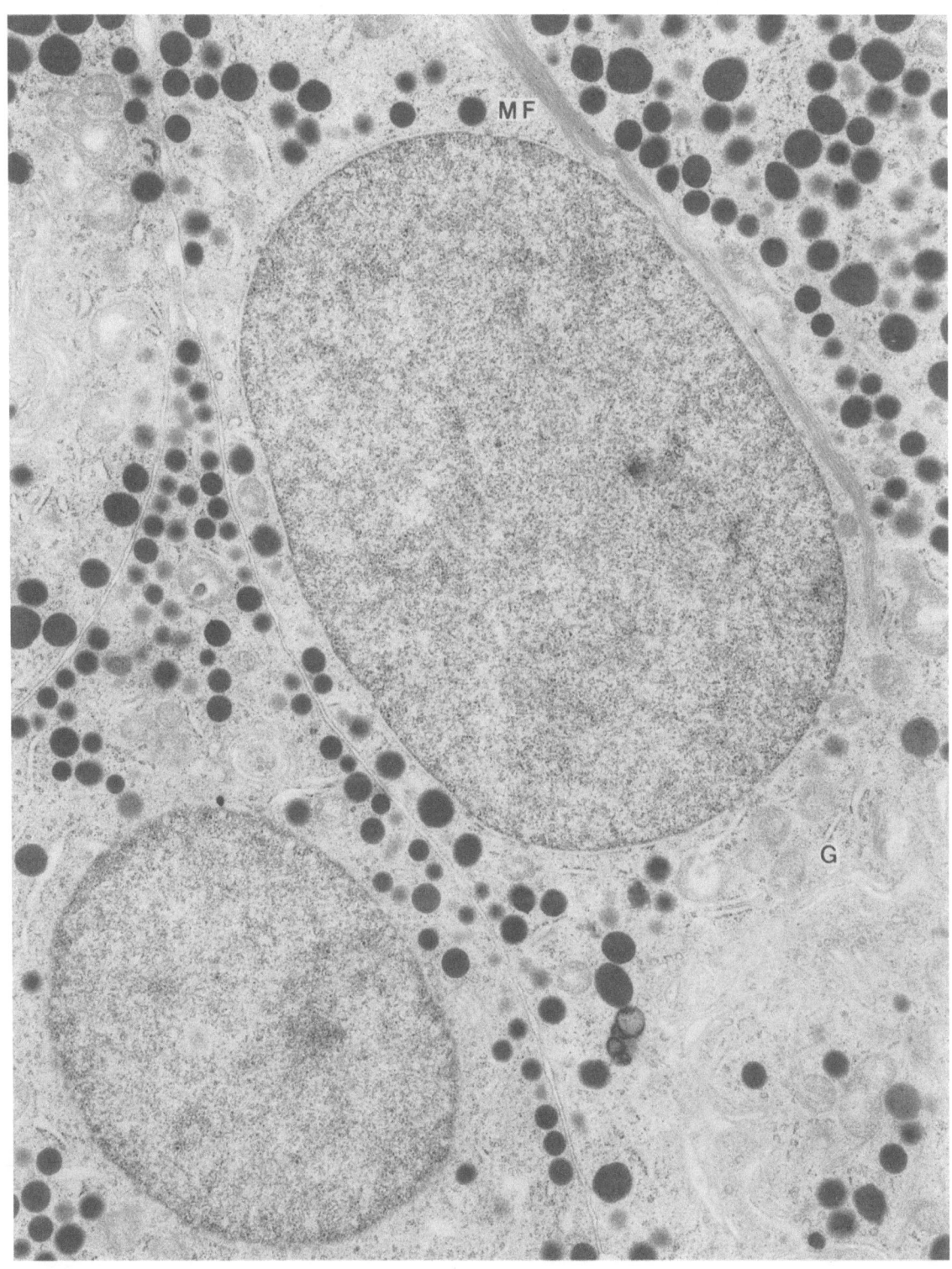

Fig. 19.11. *Growth hormone cell adenoma* (the same case as in Fig. 19.2). A bundle of microfilaments (*MF*) is sometimes seen in the well-developed cytoplasm. *G* Golgi apparatus. × 13 800

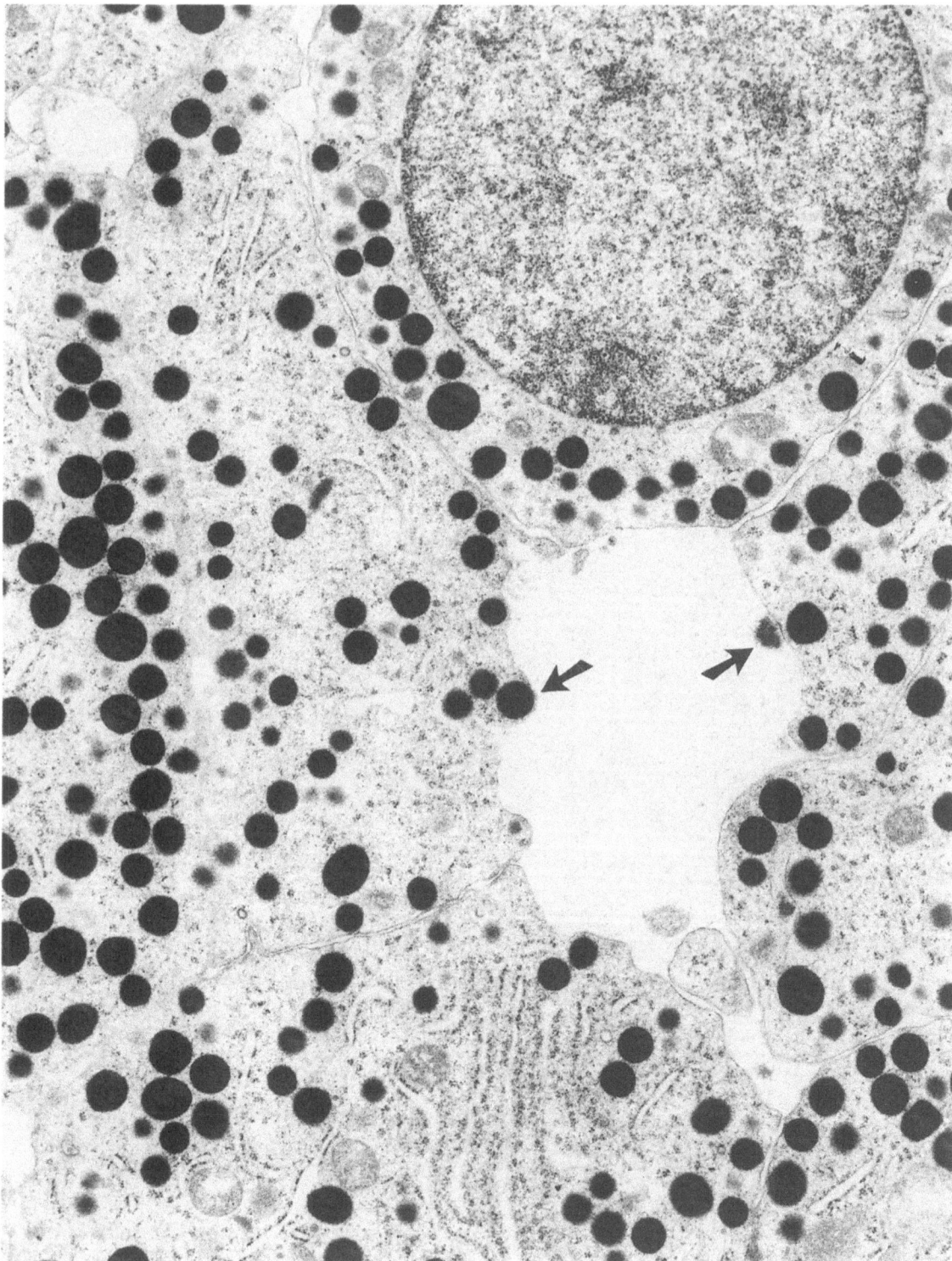

Fig. 19.12. *Growth hormone cell adenoma* (the same case as in Fig. 19.2). The densely granulated cells show excretion of secretory granules (*arrows*) into the intercellular space instead of into a capillary lumen (so-called misplaced exocytosis). × 16 400

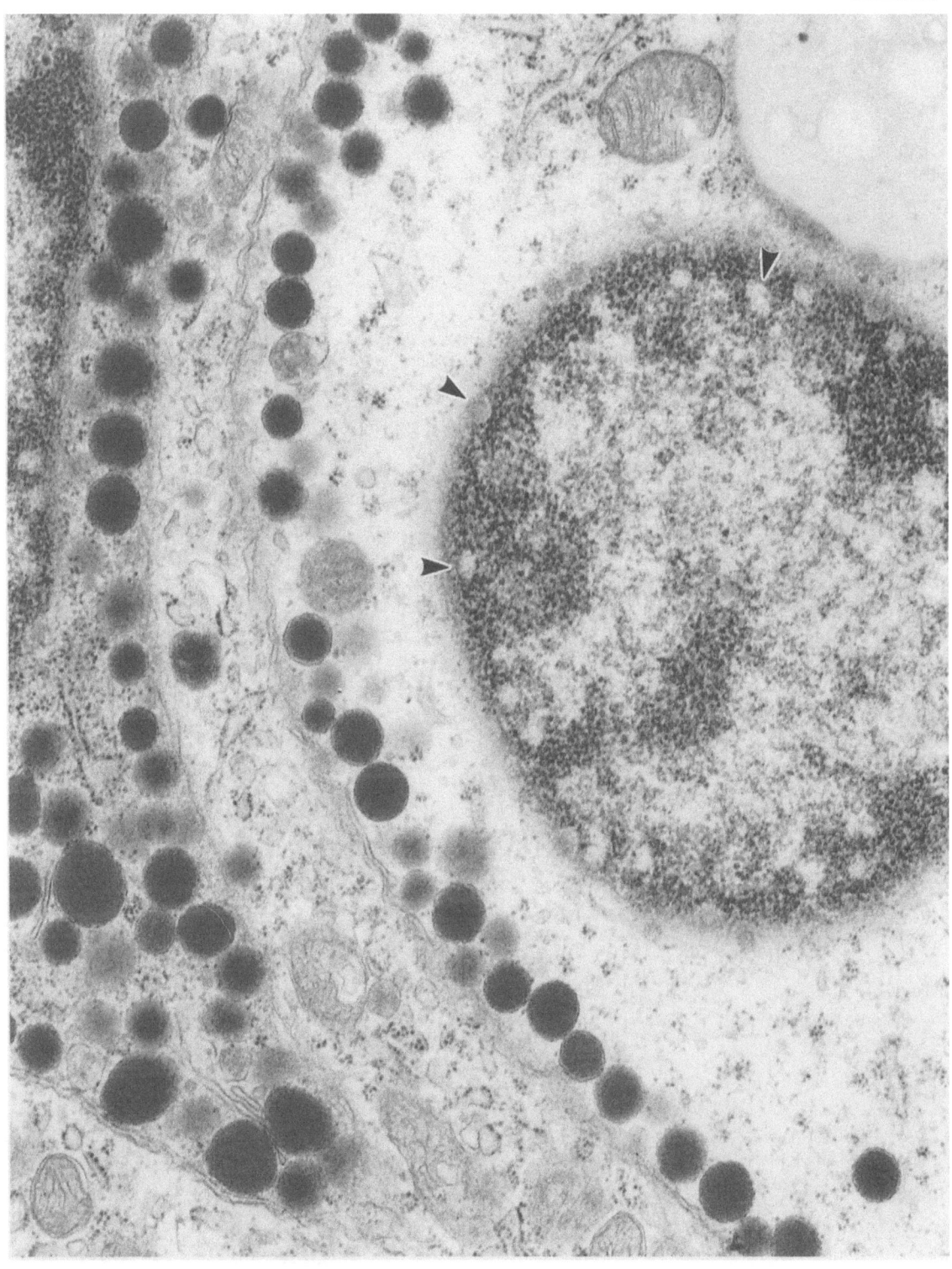

Fig. 19.13. *Growth hormone cell adenoma* (the same case as in Fig. 19.2). The secretory granules, measuring 200–300 nm in diameter, are located along the cell membranes. The tangential section of the nuclear membranes displays nuclear pores (*arrowheads*). × 35000

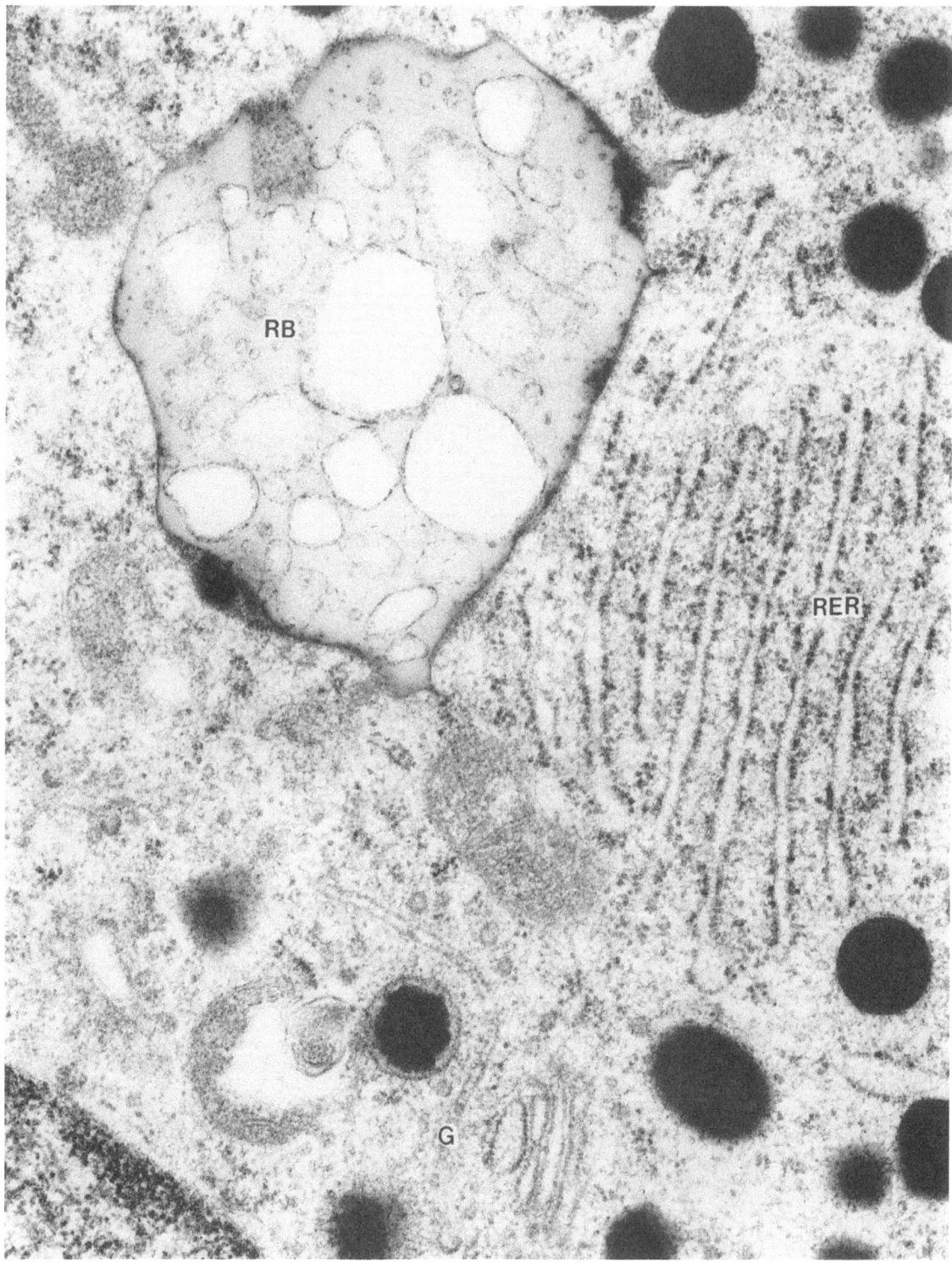

Fig. 19.14. *Growth hormone cell adenoma* (the same case as in Fig. 19.2). Higher magnification shows details of the Golgi apparatus (*G*) with developing granules, well-developed lamellar rough endoplasmic reticulum (*RER*), and the residual body (*RB*) of a lysosome. × 24 500

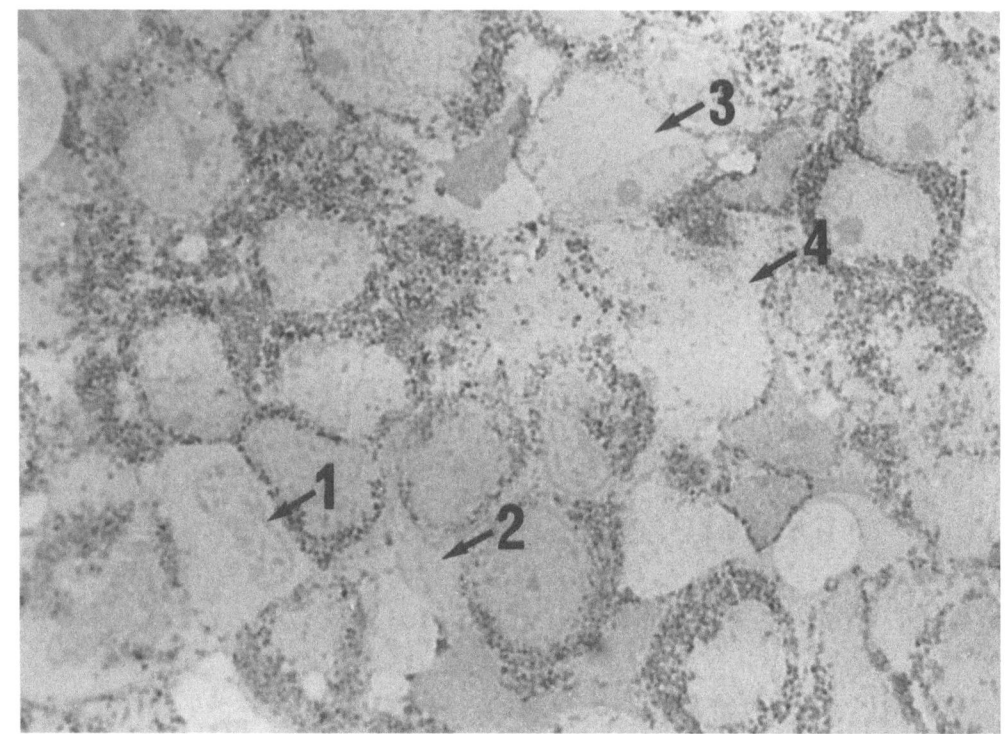

19.15

19.16

Figs. 19.15, 19.16. *Mixed growth hormone cell-prolactin cell adenoma* in a 40-year-old woman. Serial thin sections (1 μm thick, embedded in Epon-Araldite) stained immunohistochemically for growth hormone (Fig. 19.15) and prolactin (Fig. 19.16) reveal that most cells are positive for growth hormone; however, the cells numbered *1, 2, 3,* and *4* are positive for prolactin. Peroxidase antiperoxidase method without counterstain, × 1700

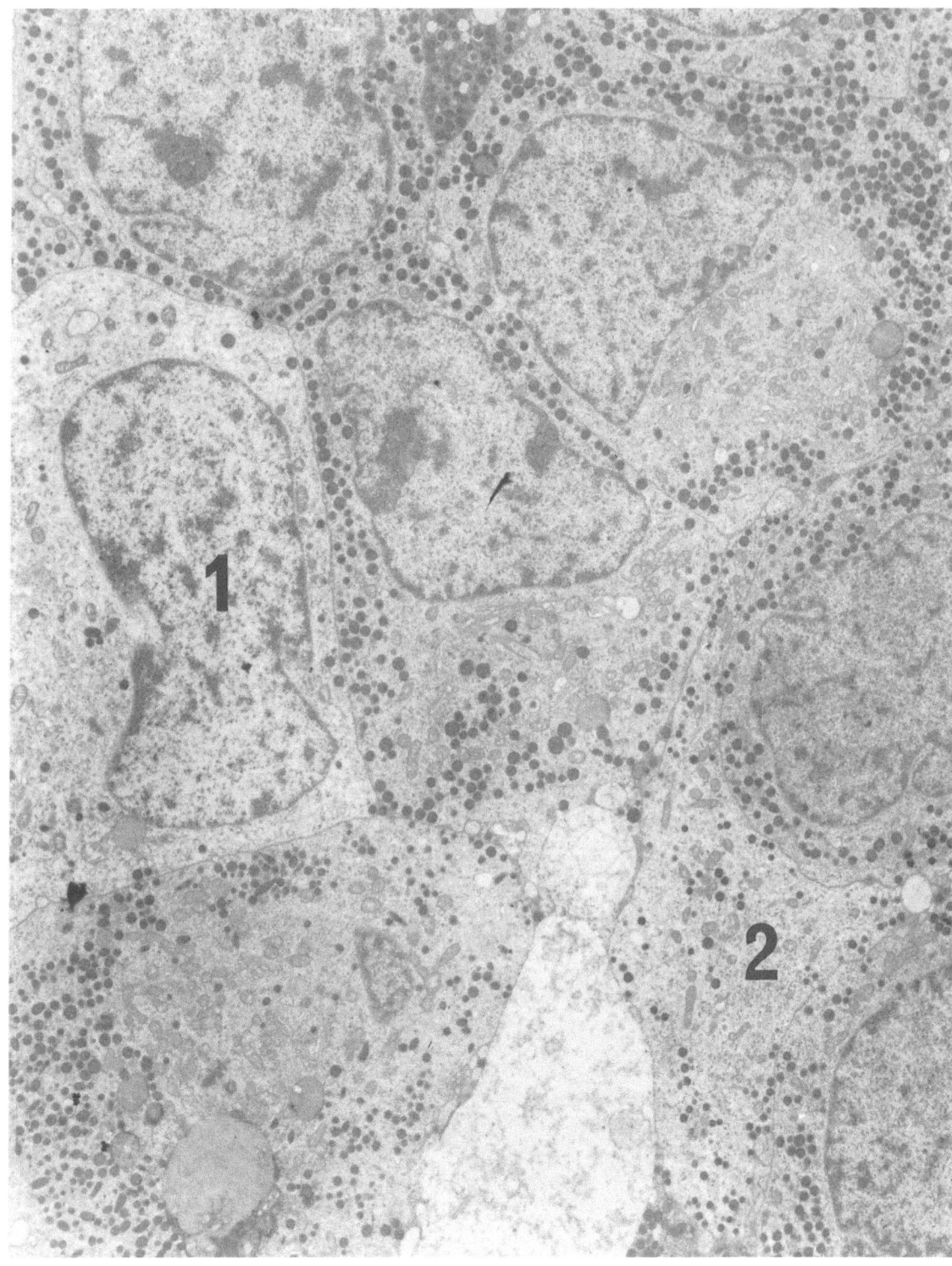

19.17

Figs. 19.17, 19.18. *Mixed growth hormone cell-prolactin cell adenoma* (the same case as in Figs. 19.15, 19.16). Electron micrographs of the serial sections comparable with those in Figs. 19.15 and 19.16 show densely and sparsely granulated cells. The cells that are positive for growth hormone are morphologically indistinguishable from those positive for prolactin cells (numbered *1*, *2*, *3*, and *4*). × 6200

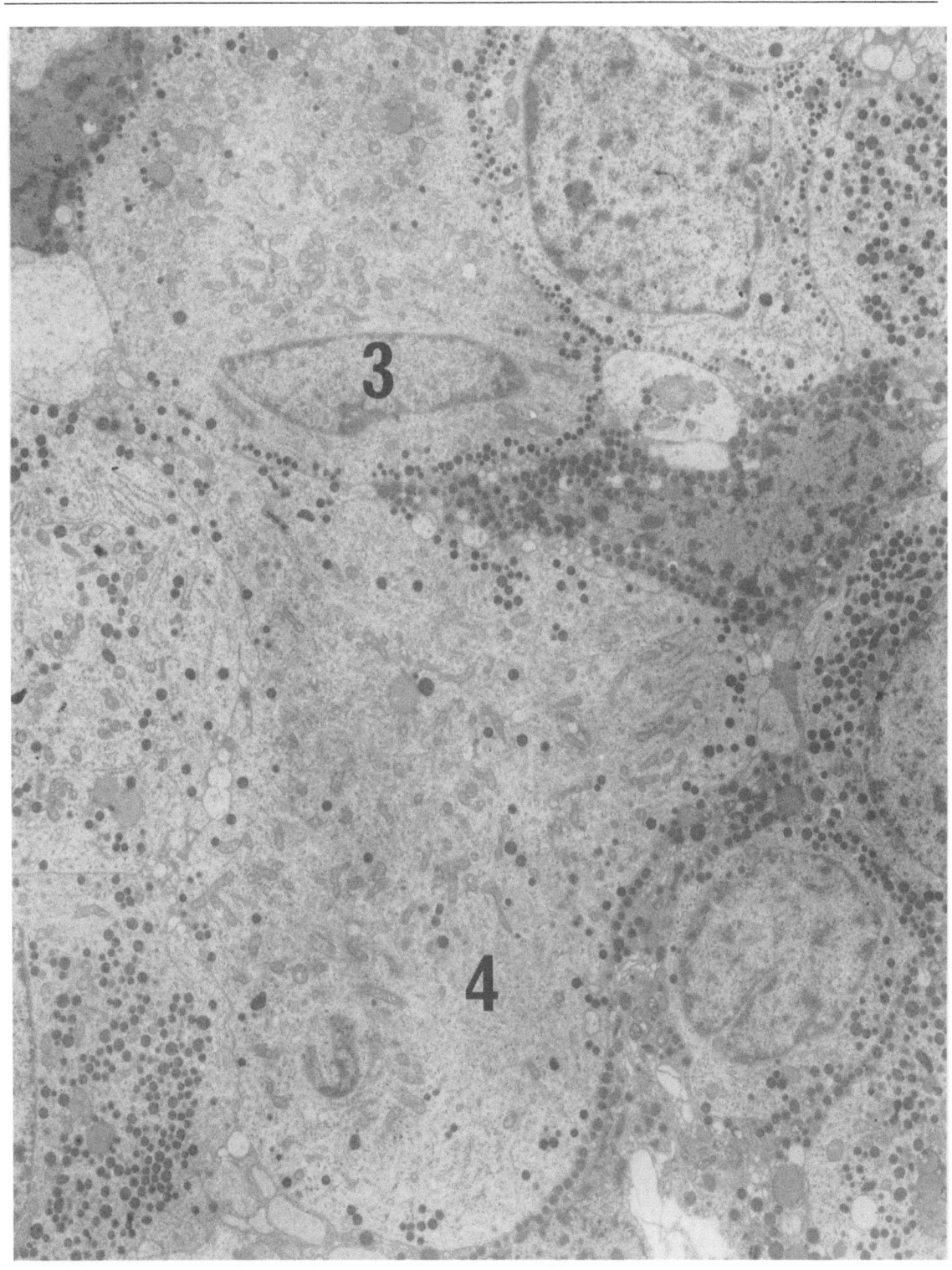

19.18

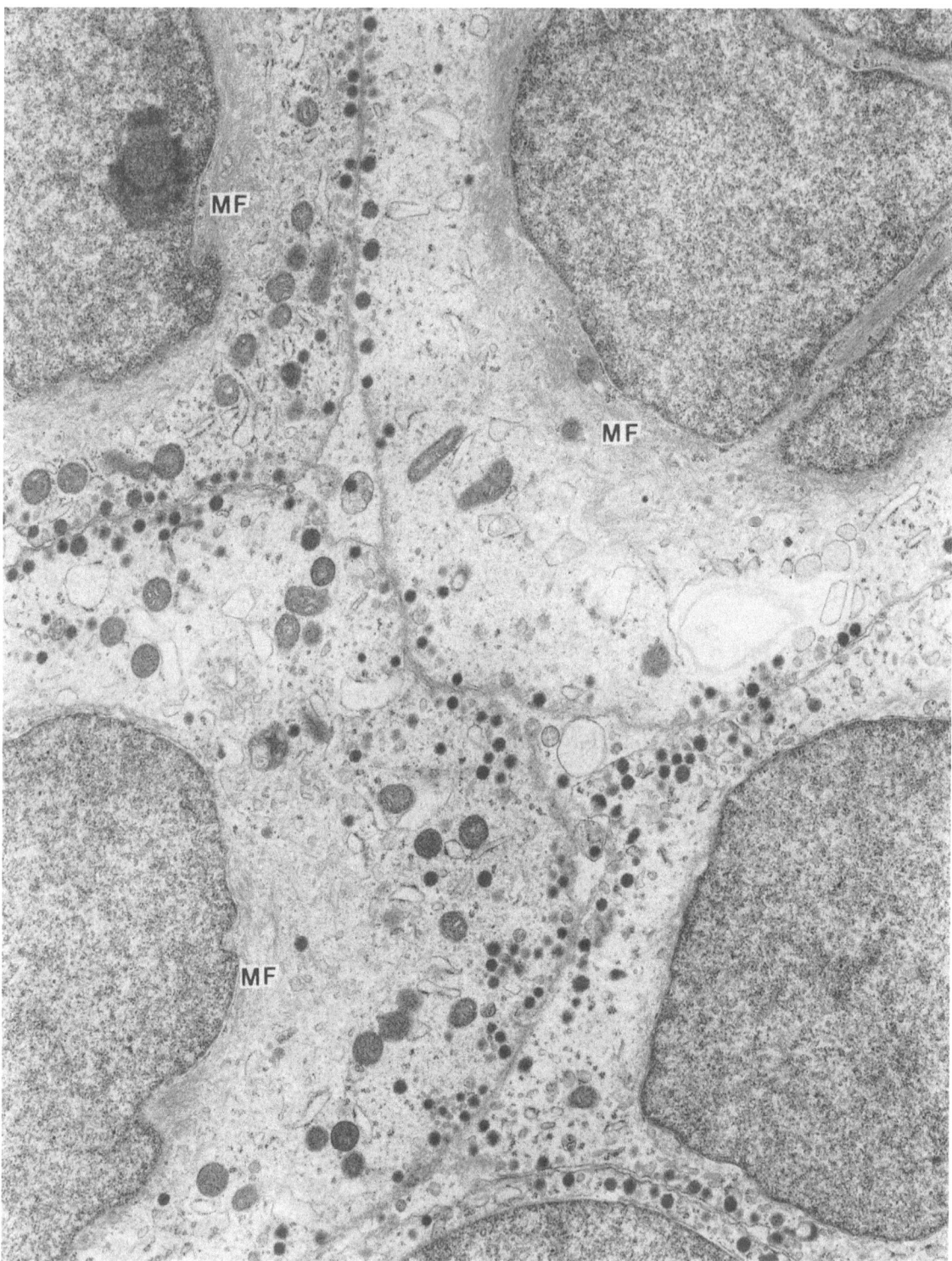

Fig. 19.19. *Corticotroph cell adenoma* of a 52-year-old woman. The secretory granules are essentially spherical and measure 150–250 nm in diameter. Note the abundant microfilaments (*MF*) around the nuclei. × 13 600

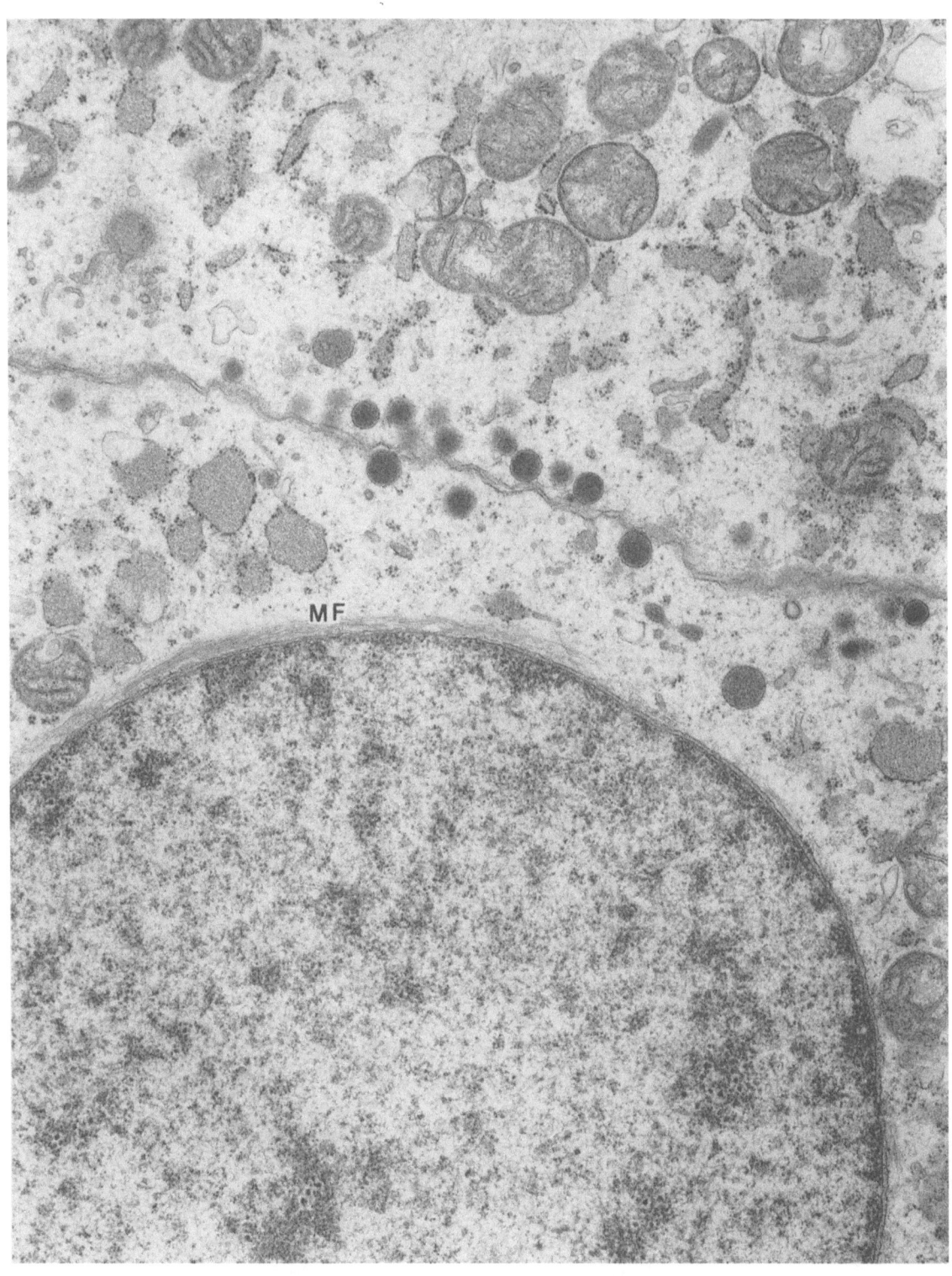

Fig. 19.20. *Corticotroph cell adenoma* (the same case as in Fig. 19.19). Secretory granules lie along the cell membranes, and perinuclear microfilaments (*MF*) are seen. × 26 000

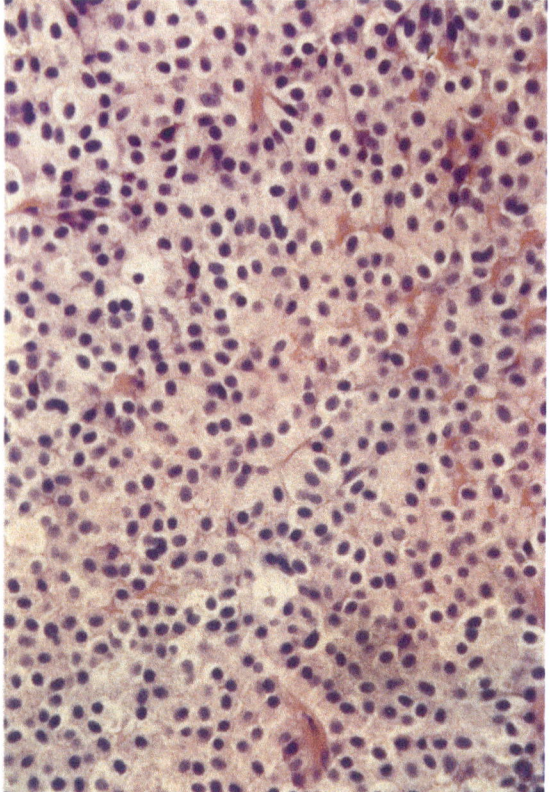

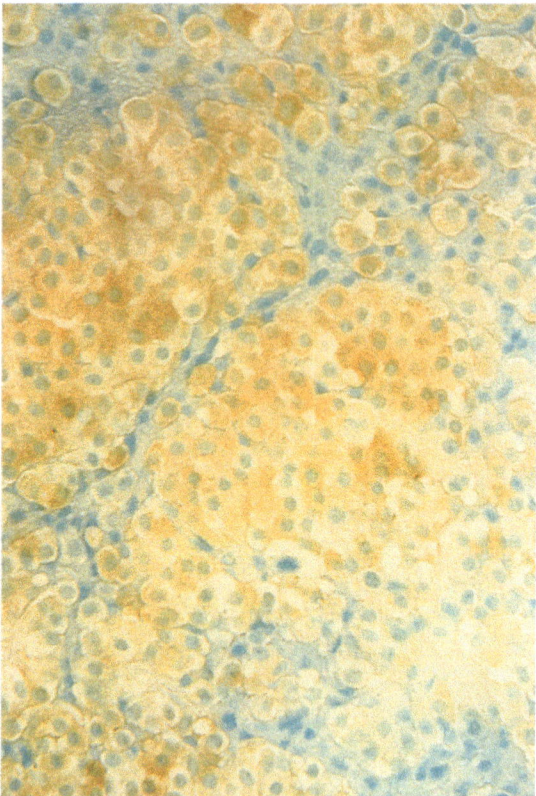

Fig. 19.21. *Pituitary oncocytoma* in a 55-year-old man with high levels of serum luteinizing hormone (LH) and follicle-stimulating hormone (FSH). The tumor consists of chromophobe cells with well-developed cytoplasm. H and E, × 120

Fig. 19.22. *Pituitary oncocytoma* (the same case as in Fig. 19.21). A weak but unequivocally positive staining for luteinizing hormone (LH) is localized in the cytoplasm of the tumor cells. Peroxidase antiperoxidase method counterstained with methyl green, × 120

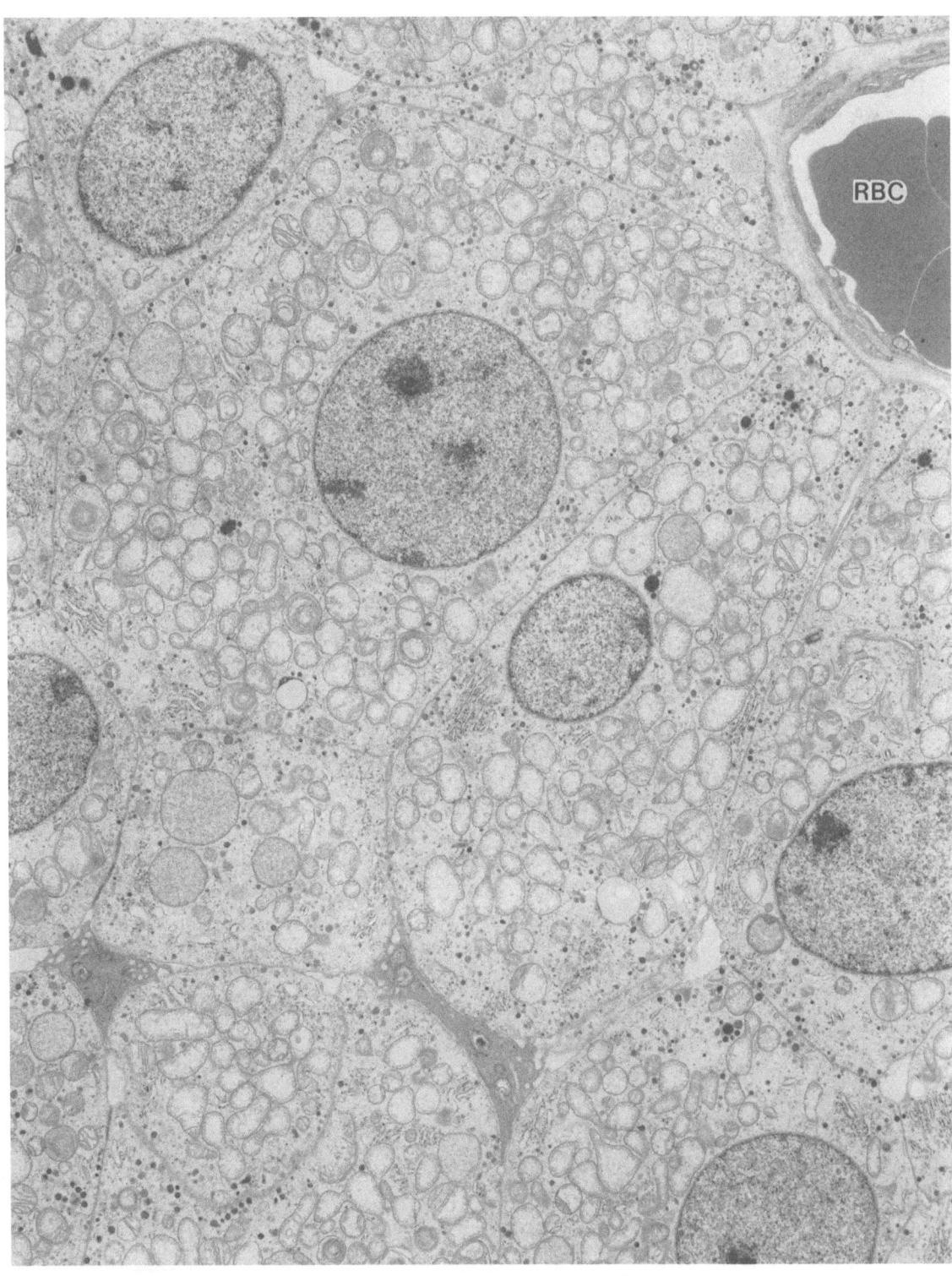

Fig. 19.23. *Pituitary oncocytoma* (the same case as in Fig. 19.21). At a lower magnification, the oncocytic cells display numerous mitochondria, obliterating other cytoplasmic organelles. Sparse secretory granules and intercellular junctional apparatus are also discernible. *RBC* erythrocyte. × 5500

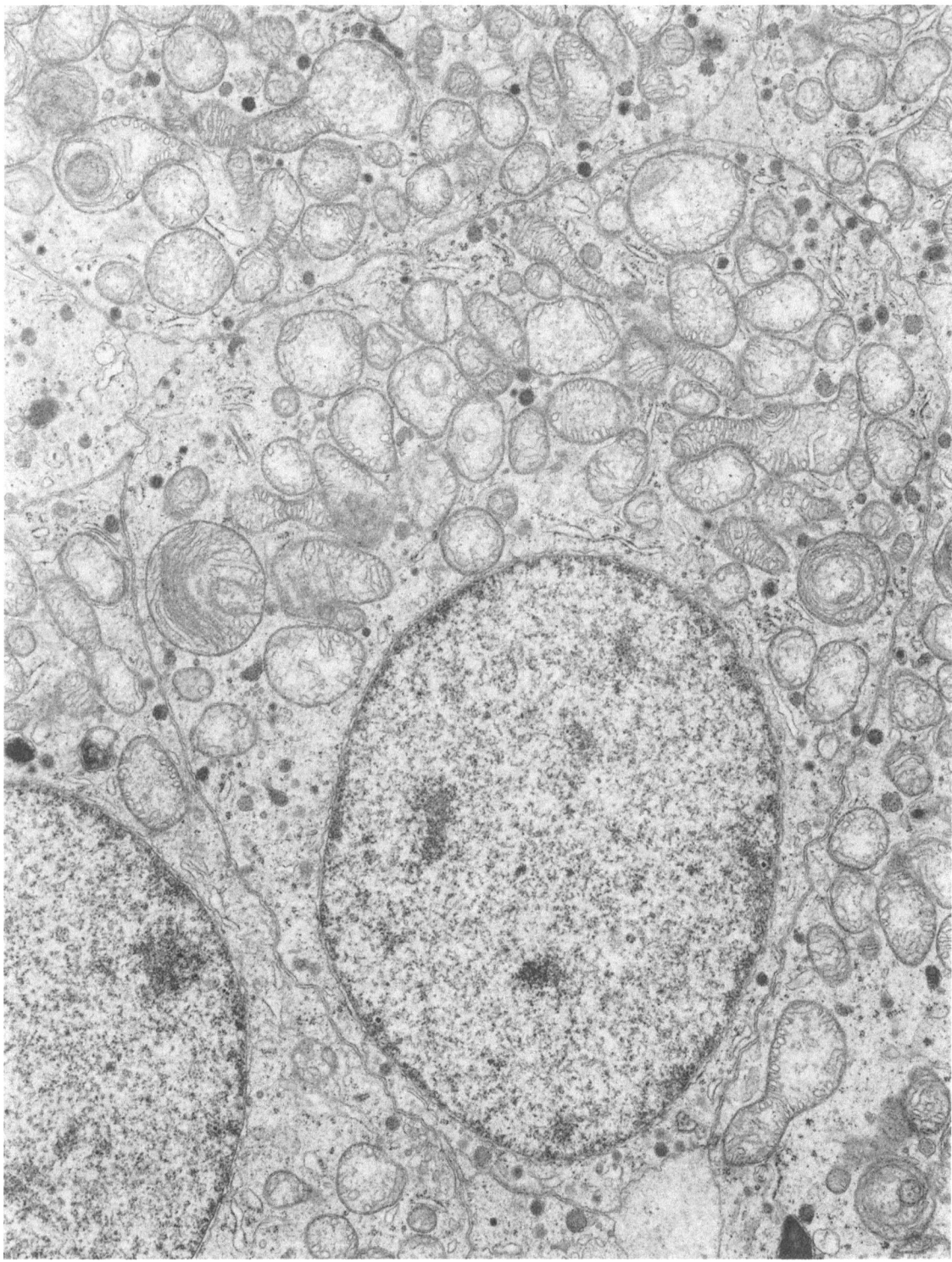

Fig. 19.24. *Pituitary oncocytoma* (the same case as in Fig. 19.21). An oncocytic cell with a round nucleus contains many pleomorphic mitochondria and sparse secretory granules measuring 150–200 nm in diameter. × 13 600

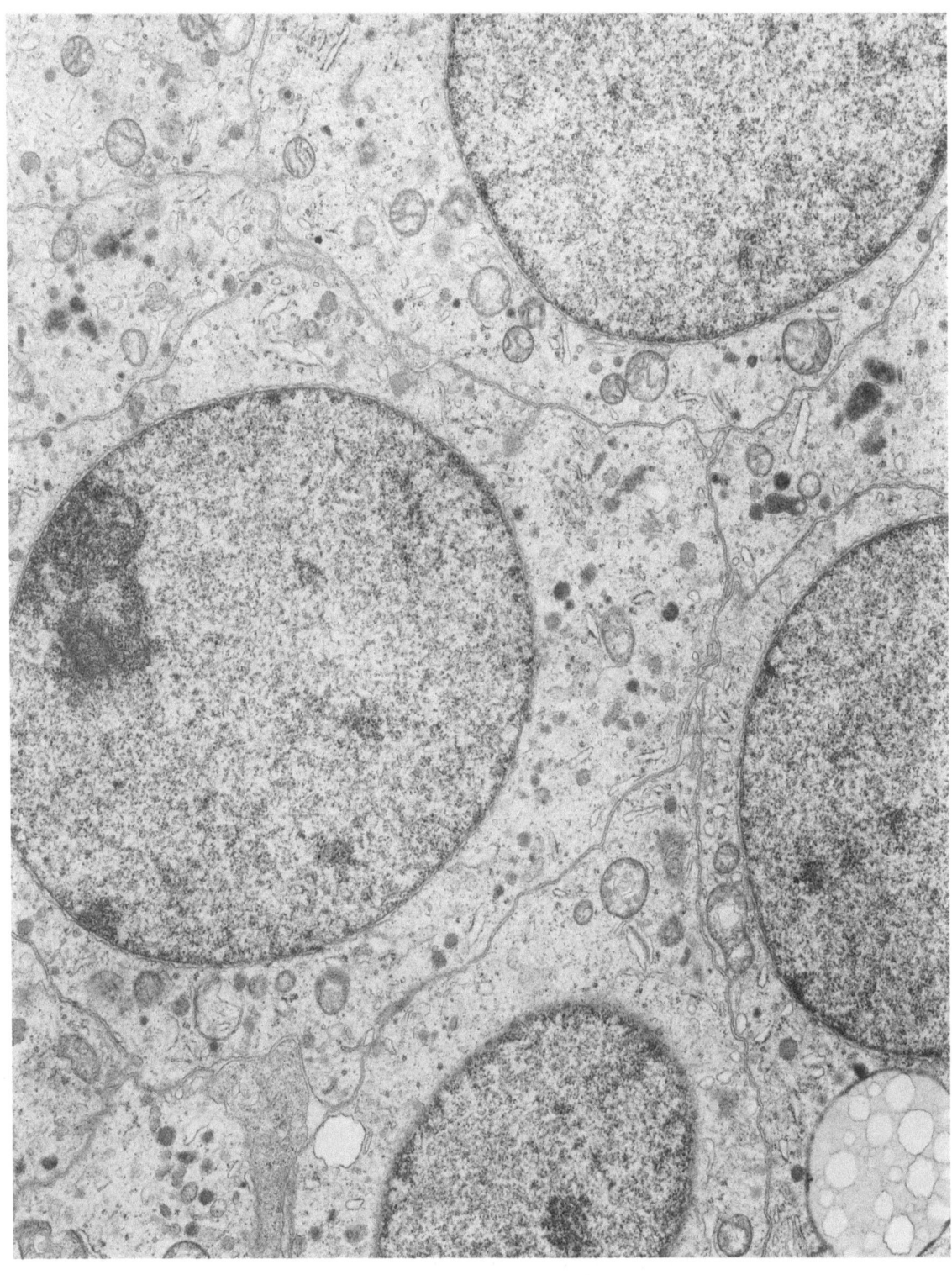

Fig. 19.25. *Pituitary oncocytoma* (the same case as in Fig. 19.21). In some parts of the tumor, the cells with sparse secretory granules do not have many mitochondria. × 17 000

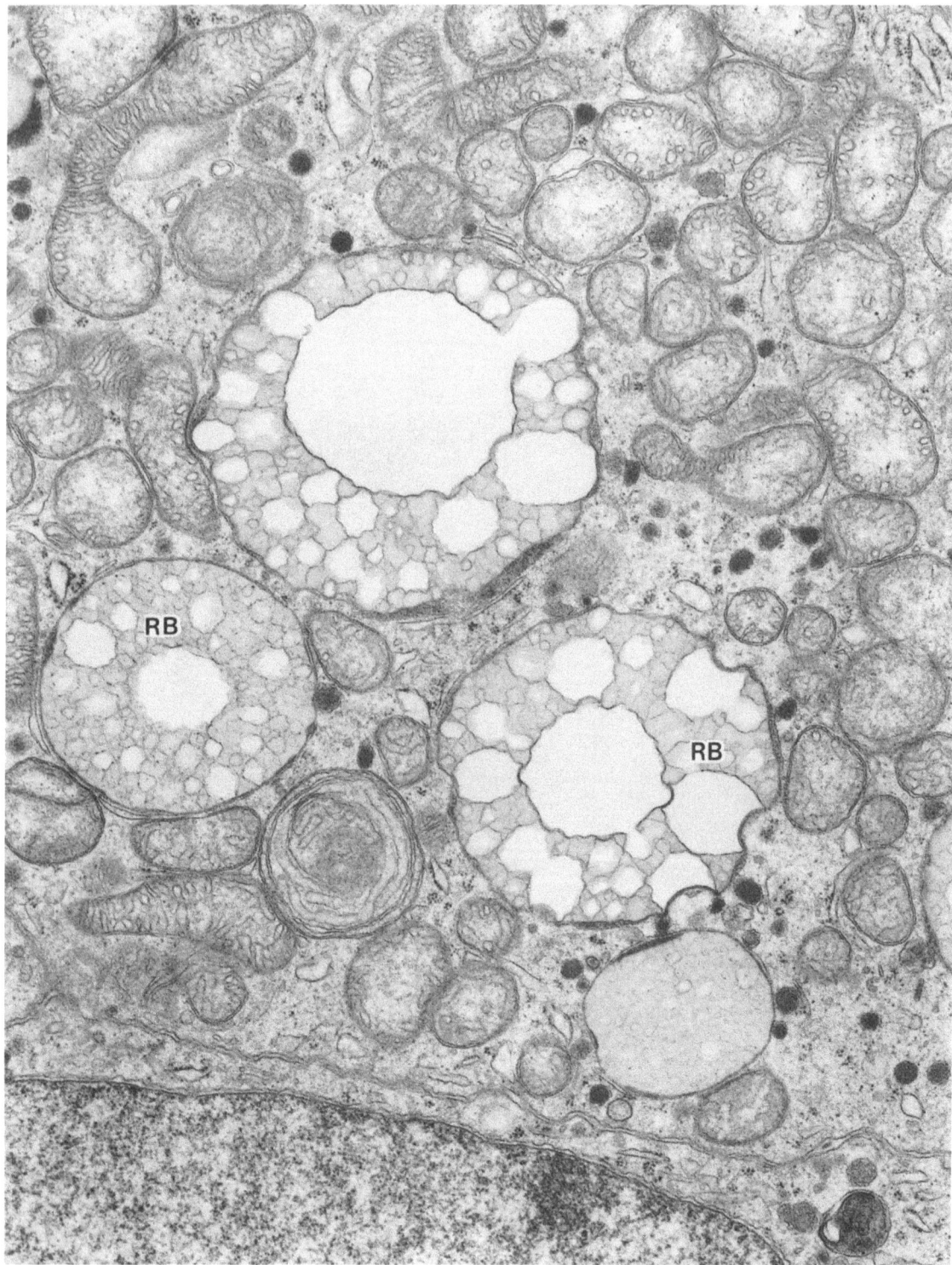

Fig. 19.26. *Pituitary oncocytoma* (the same case as in Fig. 19.21). Higher magnification reveals densely packed pleomorphic mitochondria with tubular, vesicular, or lamellar cristae. Residual bodies (*RB*) of lysosomes are often encountered. × 22 000

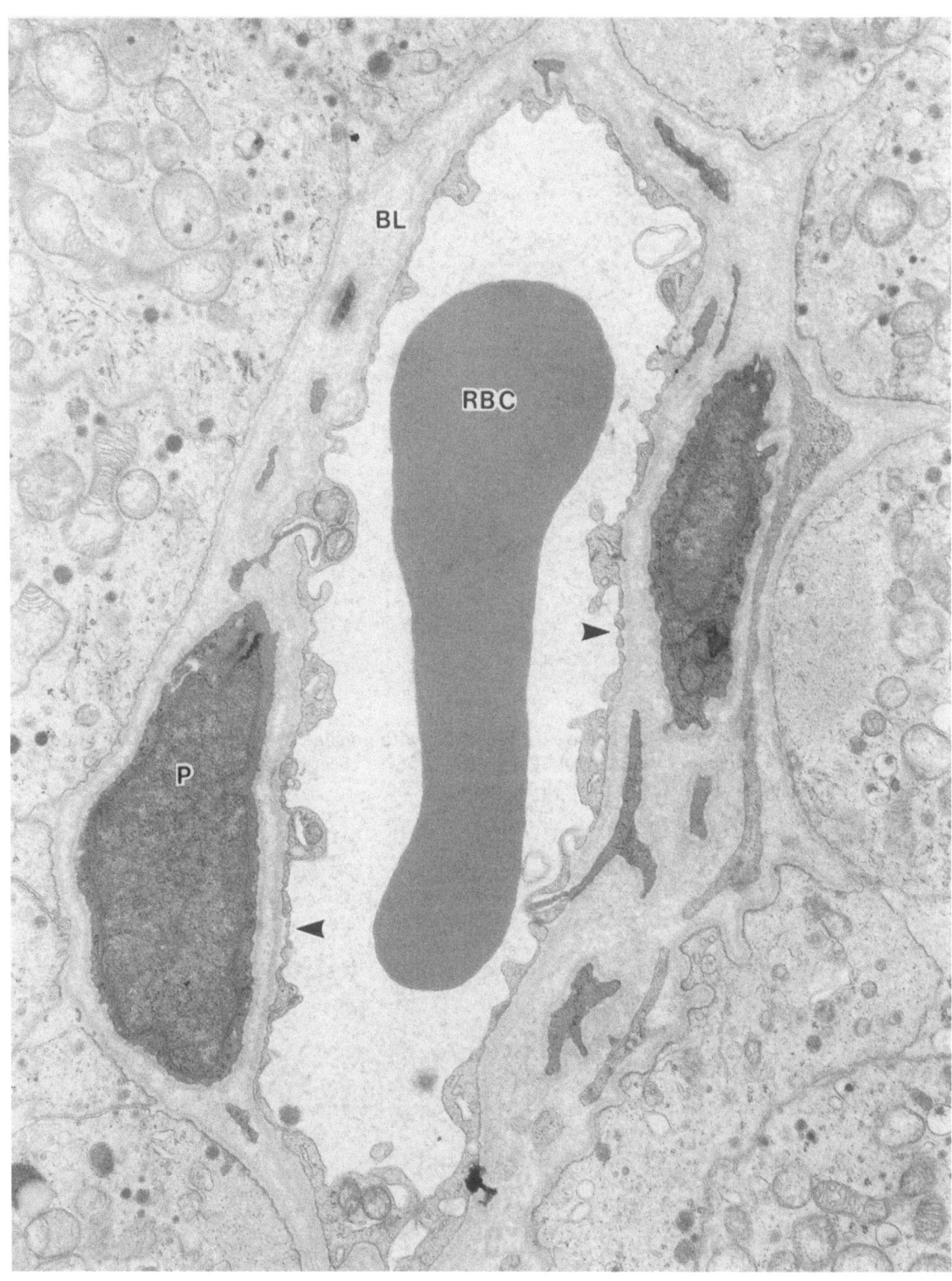

Fig. 19.27. *Pituitary oncocytoma* (the same case as in Fig. 19.21). Endothelial fenestrations (*arrowheads*) are clearly observed in a capillary of an oncocytoma. *RBC* erythrocyte, *BL* basal lamina, *P* pericyte. × 13 600

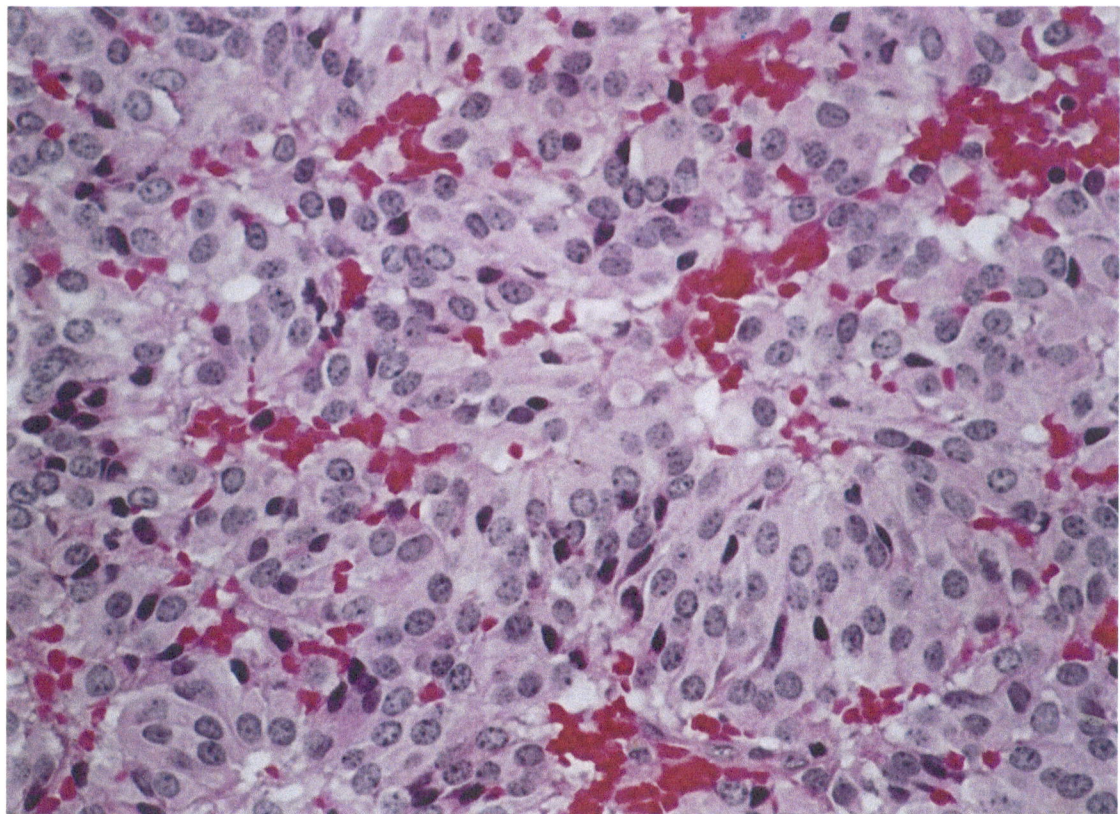

Fig. 19.28. *Pituitary oncocytoma* in a 49-year-old woman with no clinical, biochemical, or immunohisto-chemical evidence of hormone production. The tumor shows a sheet of chromophobe cells which have round to oval nuclei with prominent nucleoli. H and E, × 250

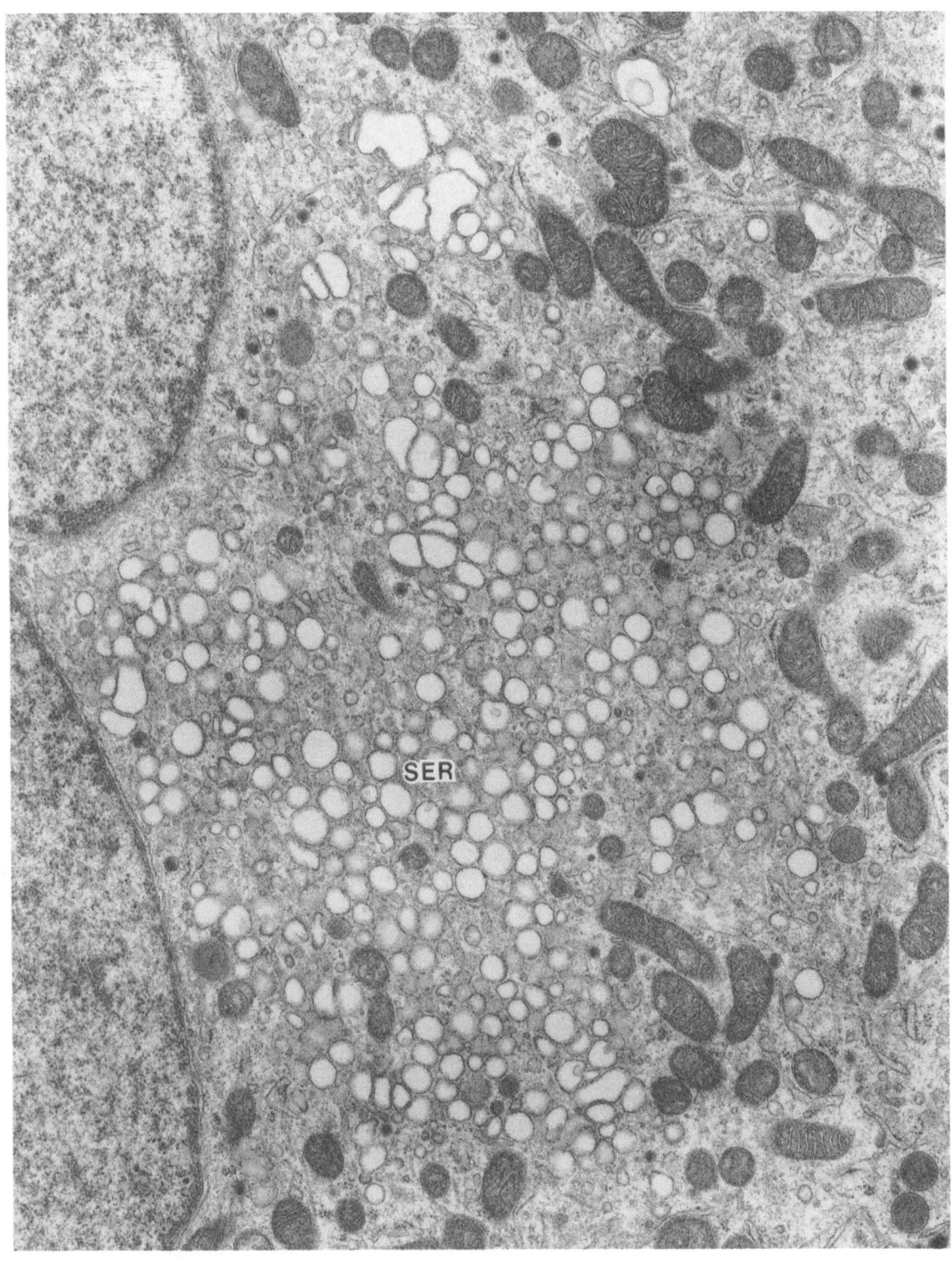

Fig. 19.29. *Pituitary oncocytoma* (the same case as in Fig. 19.28). The cytoplasm of an oncocytic cell contains extensive dilated smooth endoplasmic reticulum (*SER*) and mitochondria. × 22 000

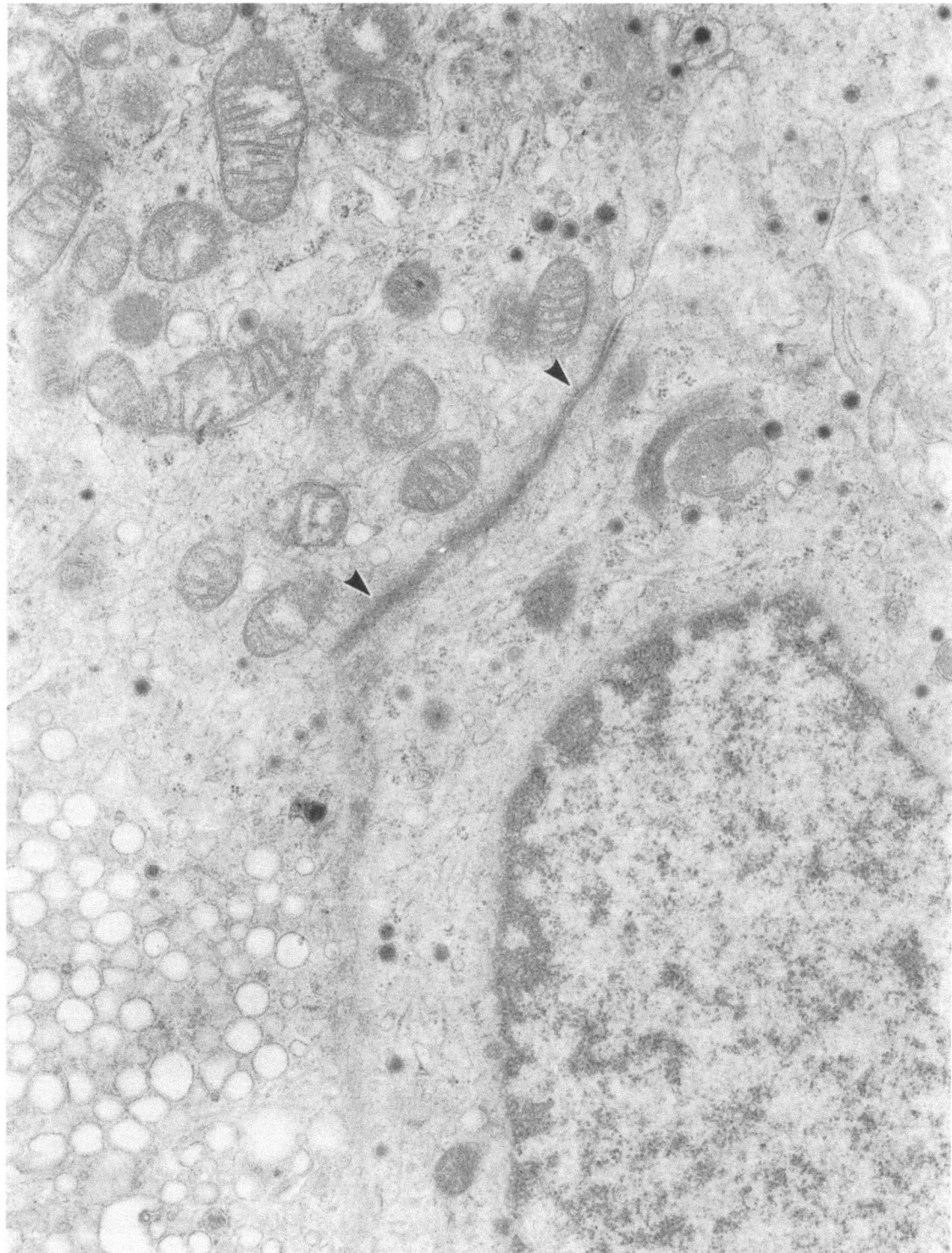

Fig. 19.30. *Pituitary oncocytoma* (the same case as in Fig. 19.28). Dilated smooth endoplasmic reticulum, sparse secretory granules of 120–200 nm in diameter, microtubules, and intercellular junctional apparatus (*arrowheads*) are observed. × 27 000

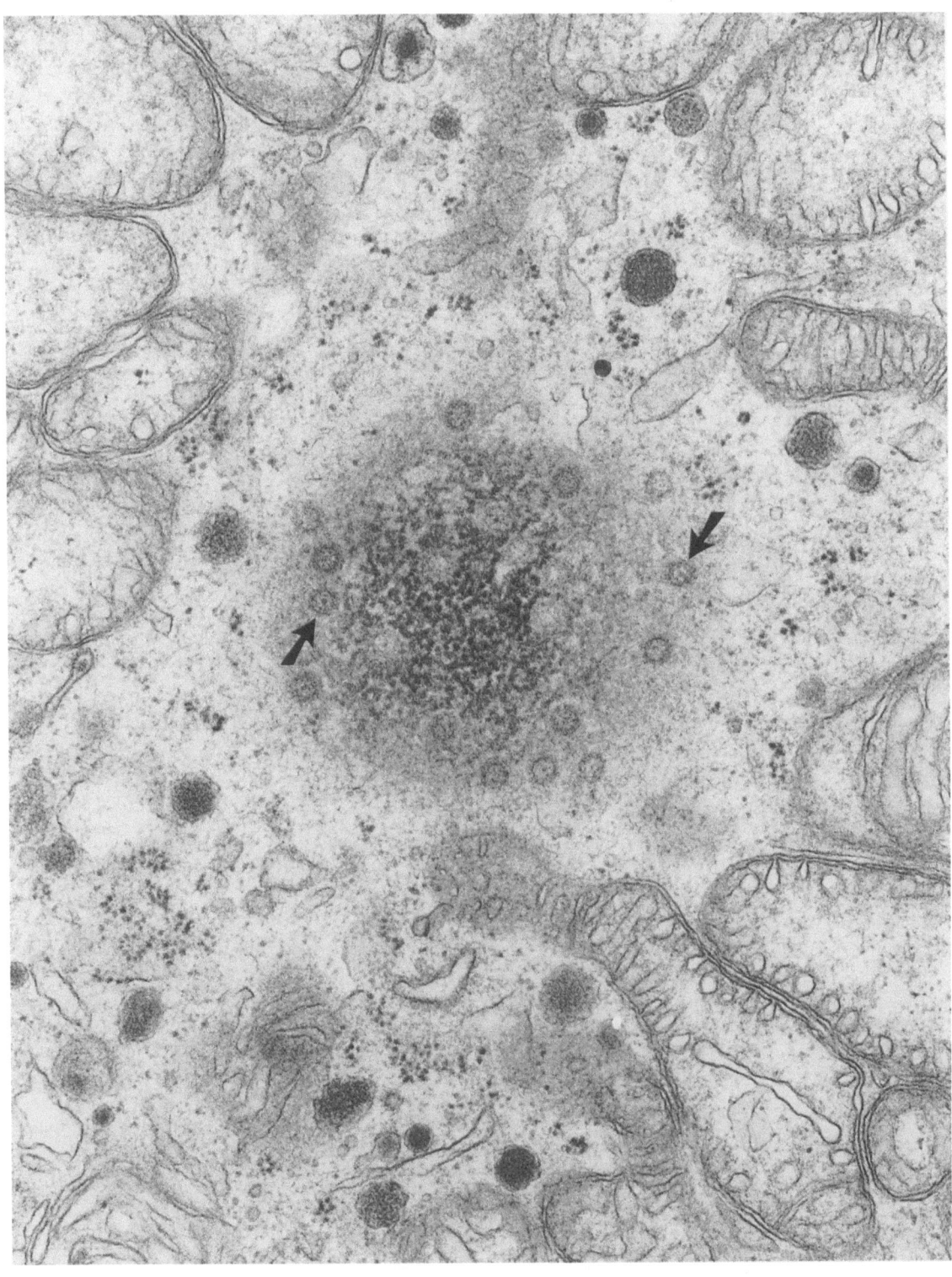

Fig. 19.31. *Pituitary oncocytoma* (the same case as in Fig. 19.28). A tangential section of the nuclear membranes of an oncocytic cell reveals details of the nuclear pores (*arrows*). × 54 000

20. Meningioma

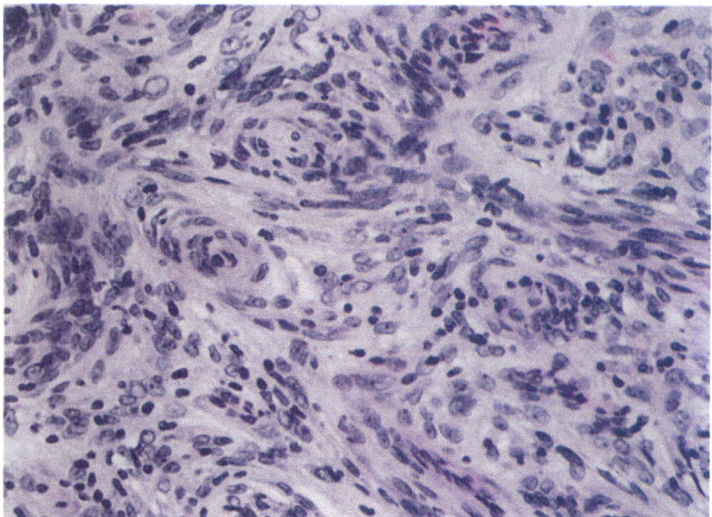

Fig. 20.1. Tuberculum sellae *meningioma* in a 48-year-old woman. Whorl formation of elongated cells, interwoven fascicles, and nuclear vacuolations mark the fibroblastic meningioma. H and E, × 160

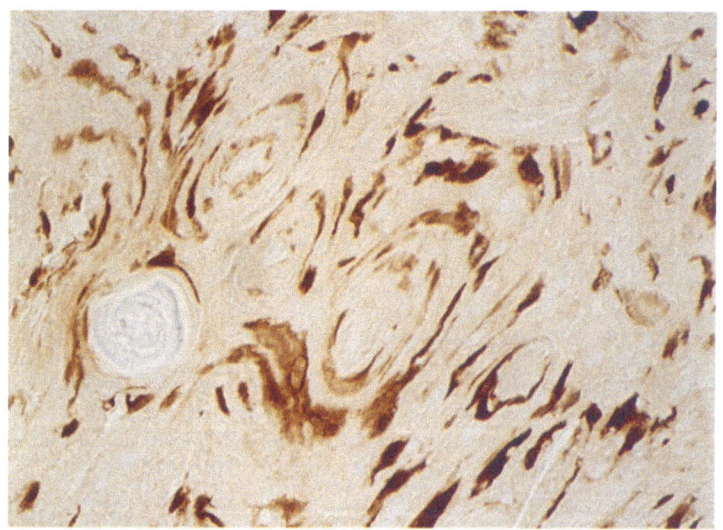

Fig. 20.2. *Meningioma* (the same case as in Fig. 20.1). Definite meningioma, as shown here, reveals a positive reaction for S-100 protein, suggesting that the histogenesis of this meningioma is different from that of others. Indirect immunoperoxidase method without counterstain, × 160

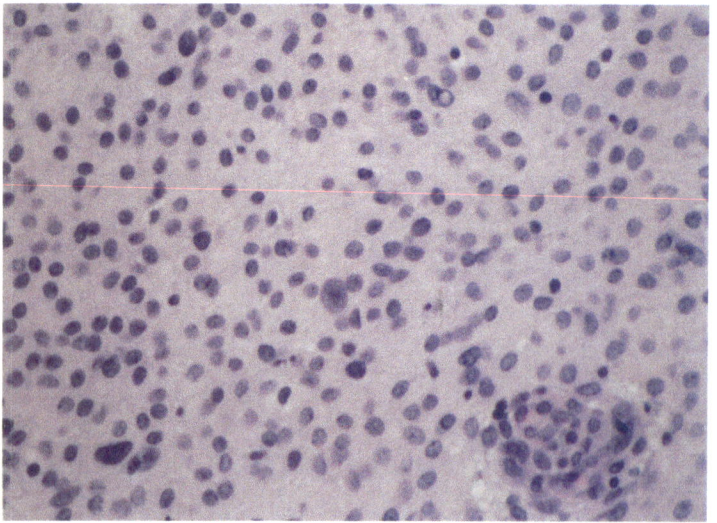

Fig. 20.3. Parasagittal *meningioma* in a 55-year-old man. Tumor cells with indistinct borders and oval, often vacuolated nuclei characterize meningotheliomatous meningioma. H and E, × 160

Fig. 20.4. Psammoma bodies (calcospherites) in a *meningioma* lie at the centers of whorls. H and E, × 160

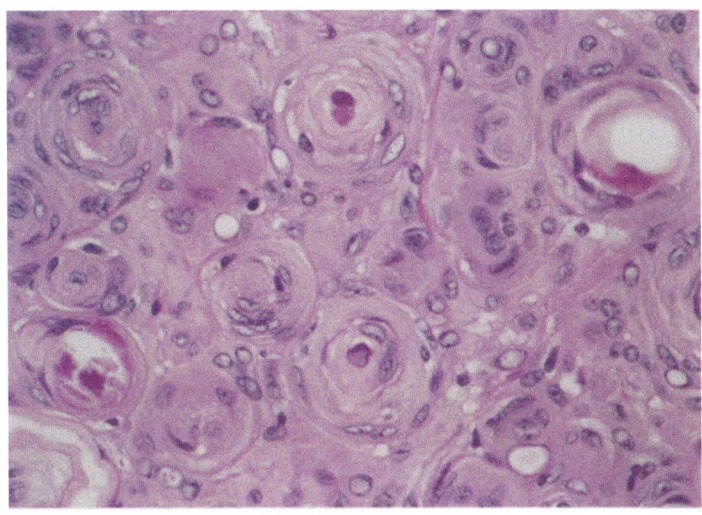

Fig. 20.5. *Fibroblastic meningioma* of the left sphenoidal ridge in a 50-year-old woman. Xanthomatous changes are sometimes seen as a conspicuous element of meningioma. H and E, × 160

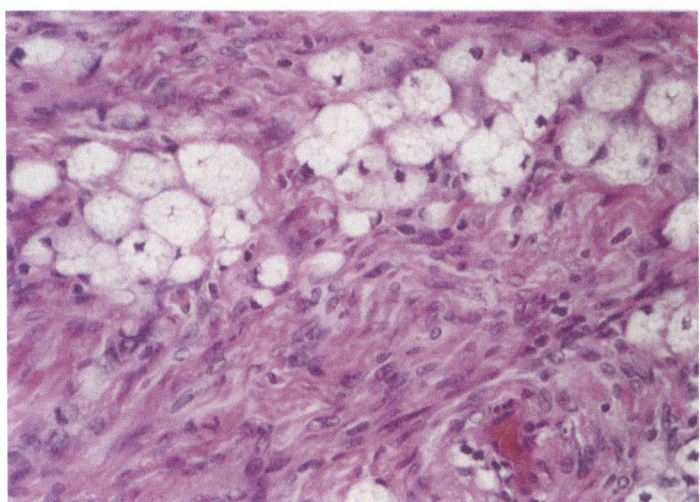

Fig. 20.6. *Meningioma* (the same case as in Fig. 20.5). Unequivocally positive staining for S-100 protein is observed in the elongated meningioma cells but not in the xanthomatous cells. Indirect immunoperoxidase method counterstained with methyl green, × 160

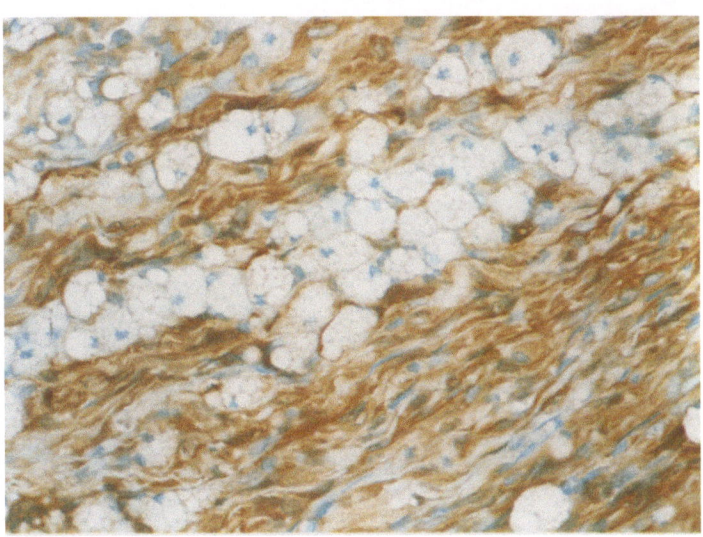

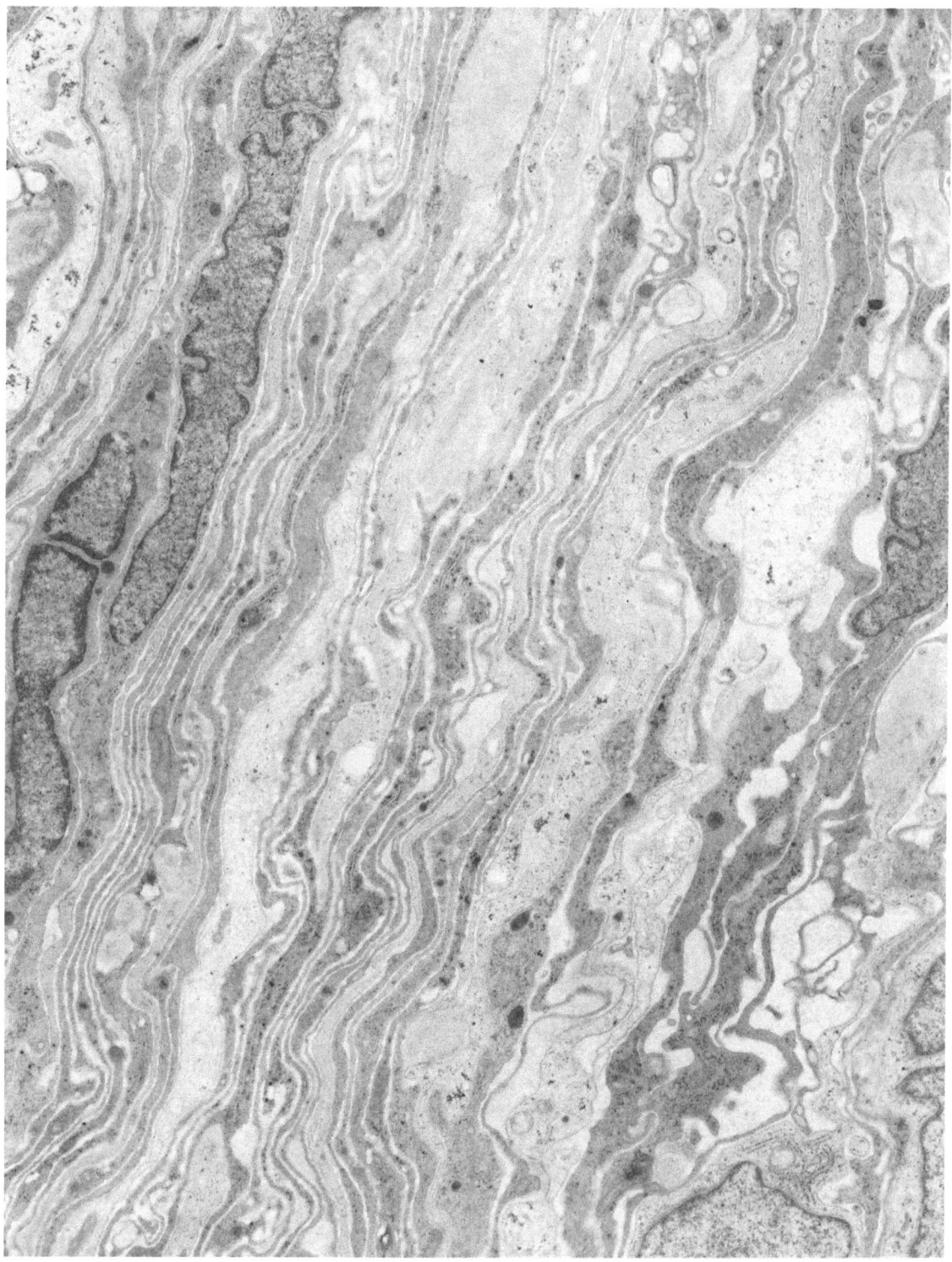

Fig. 20.7. *Meningioma* (the same case as in Fig. 20.1). Fibroblastic meningioma shows numerous parallel layers of longitudinally sectioned narrow cytoplasm. × 8000

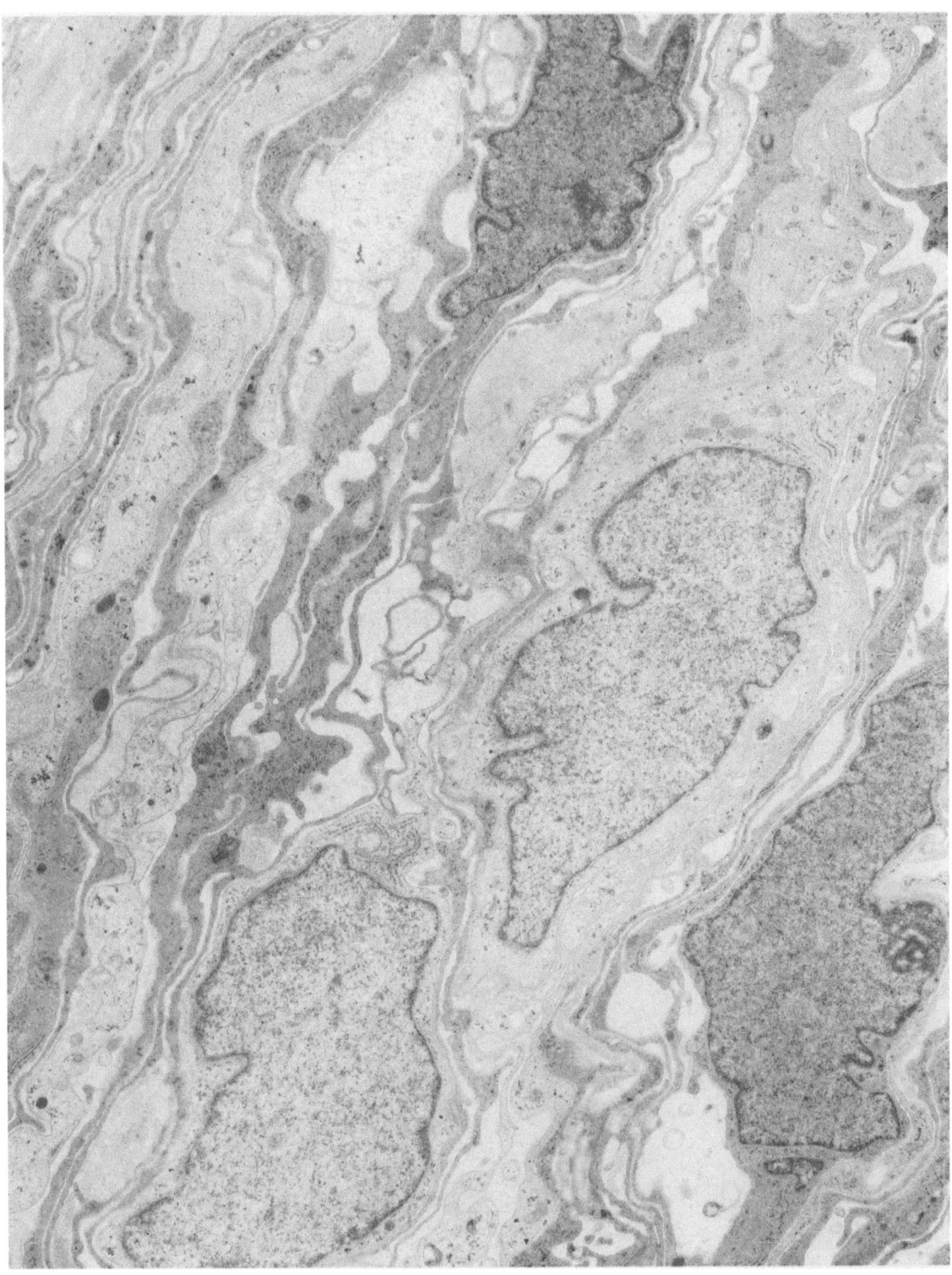

Fig. 20.8. *Meningioma* (the same case as in Fig. 20.1). The tumor is characterized by interdigitation of the narrow folded cytoplasm. The extracellular spaces are scanty and a basal lamina is not present. × 8000

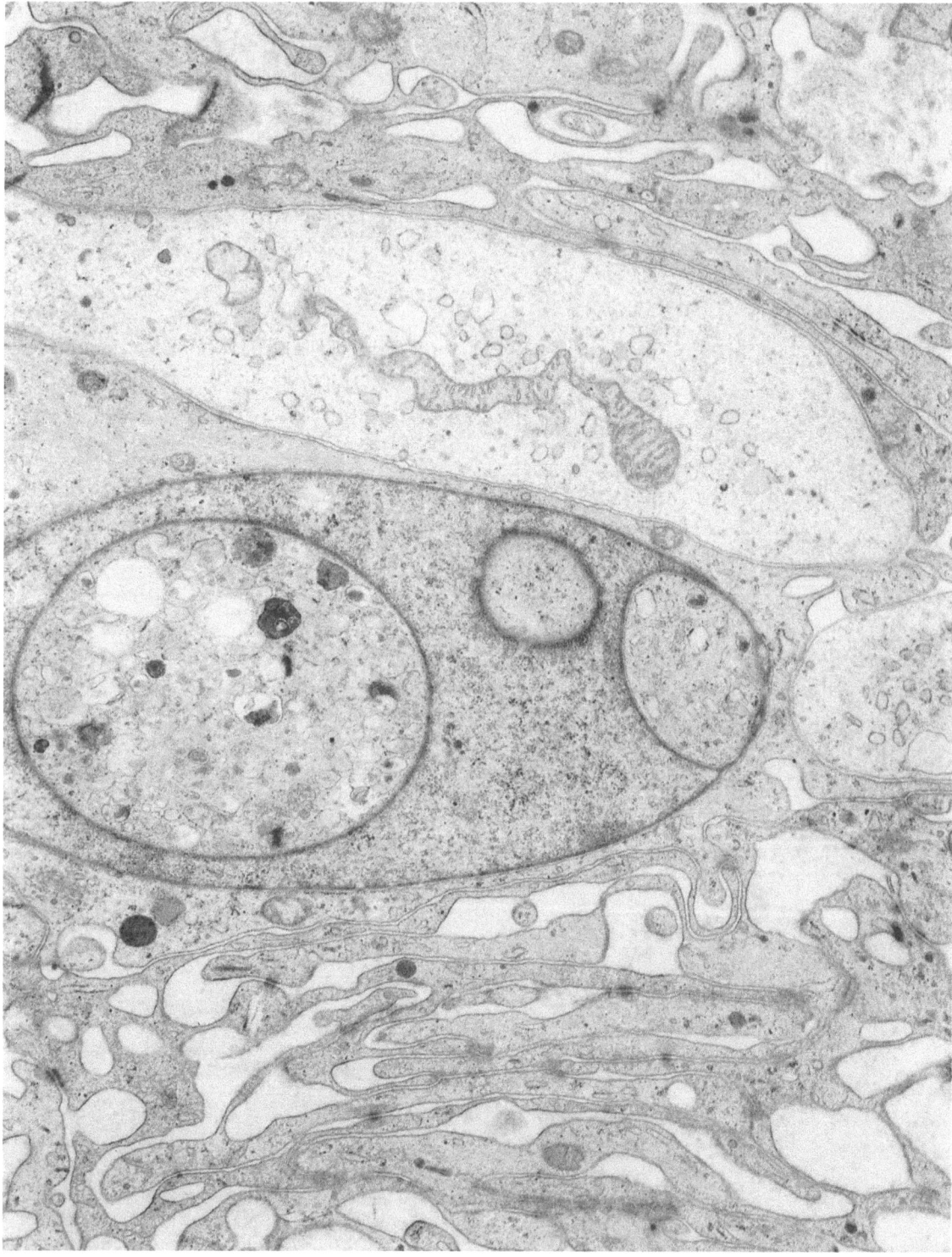

Fig. 20.9. *Meningioma* (the same case as in Fig. 20.1). There are three intranuclear pseudoinclusions, which appear as nuclear vacuolations under the light microscope. × 15 000

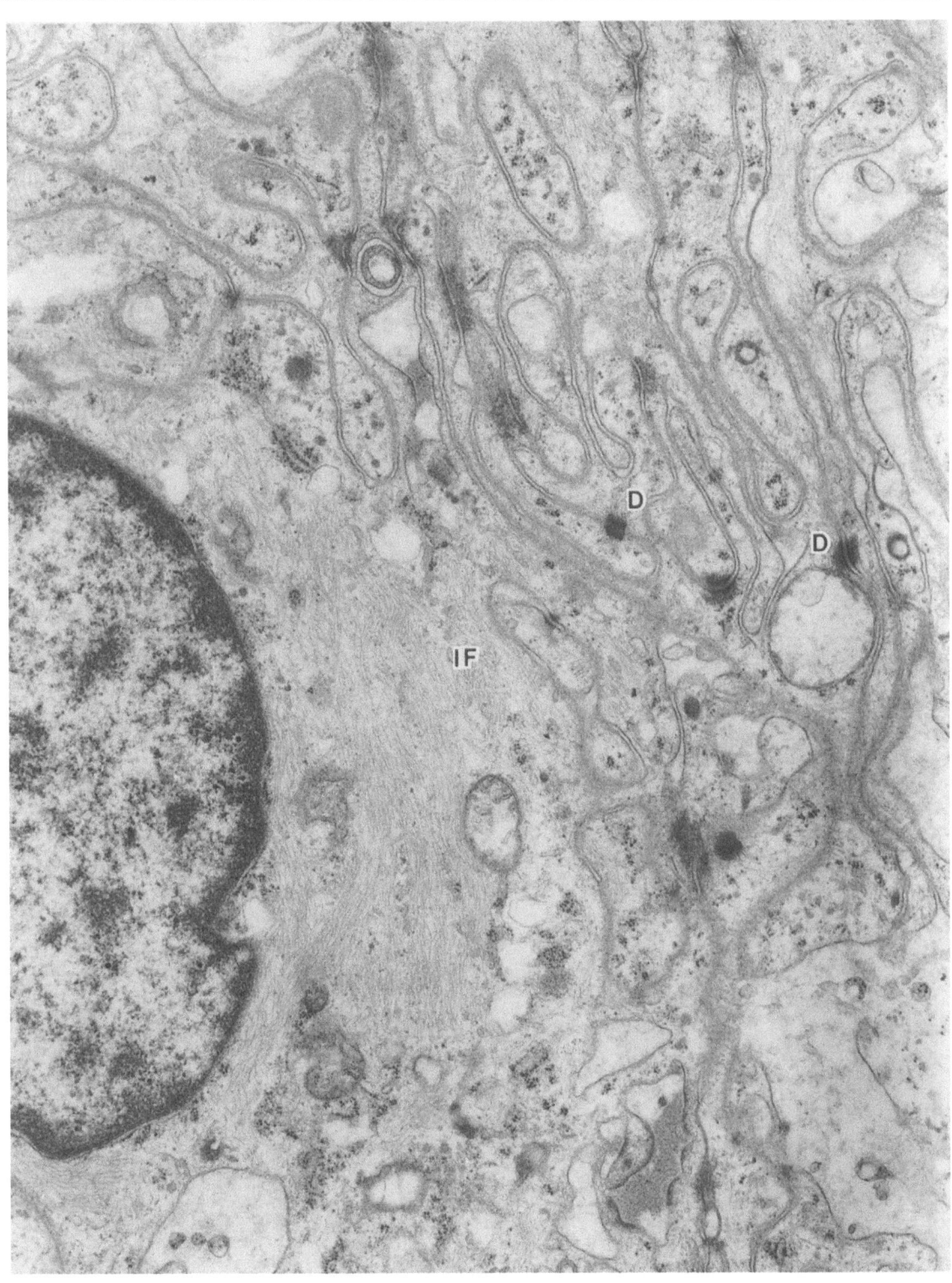

Fig. 20.10. *Meningioma* (the same case as in Fig. 20.3). The meningioma cell is characterized by intra-cytoplasmic 10-nm intermediate filaments (*IF*) and many desmosomes (*D*) between areas of narrow folded cytoplasm. × 21 000

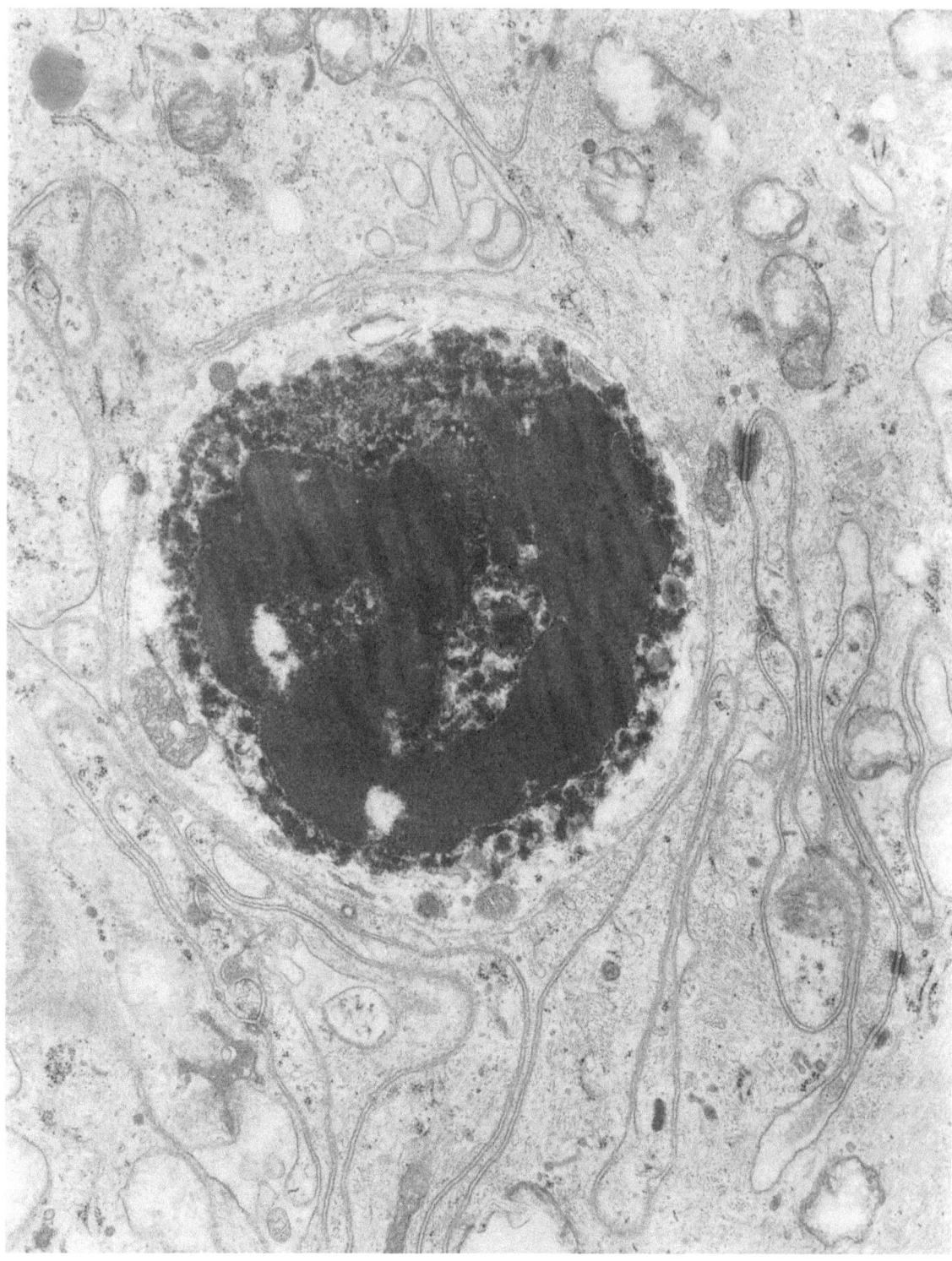

Fig. 20.11. *Meningioma* (the same case as in Fig. 20.3). Pyknosis and watery clear cytolasm indicate a degenerating meningioma cell. × 21 000

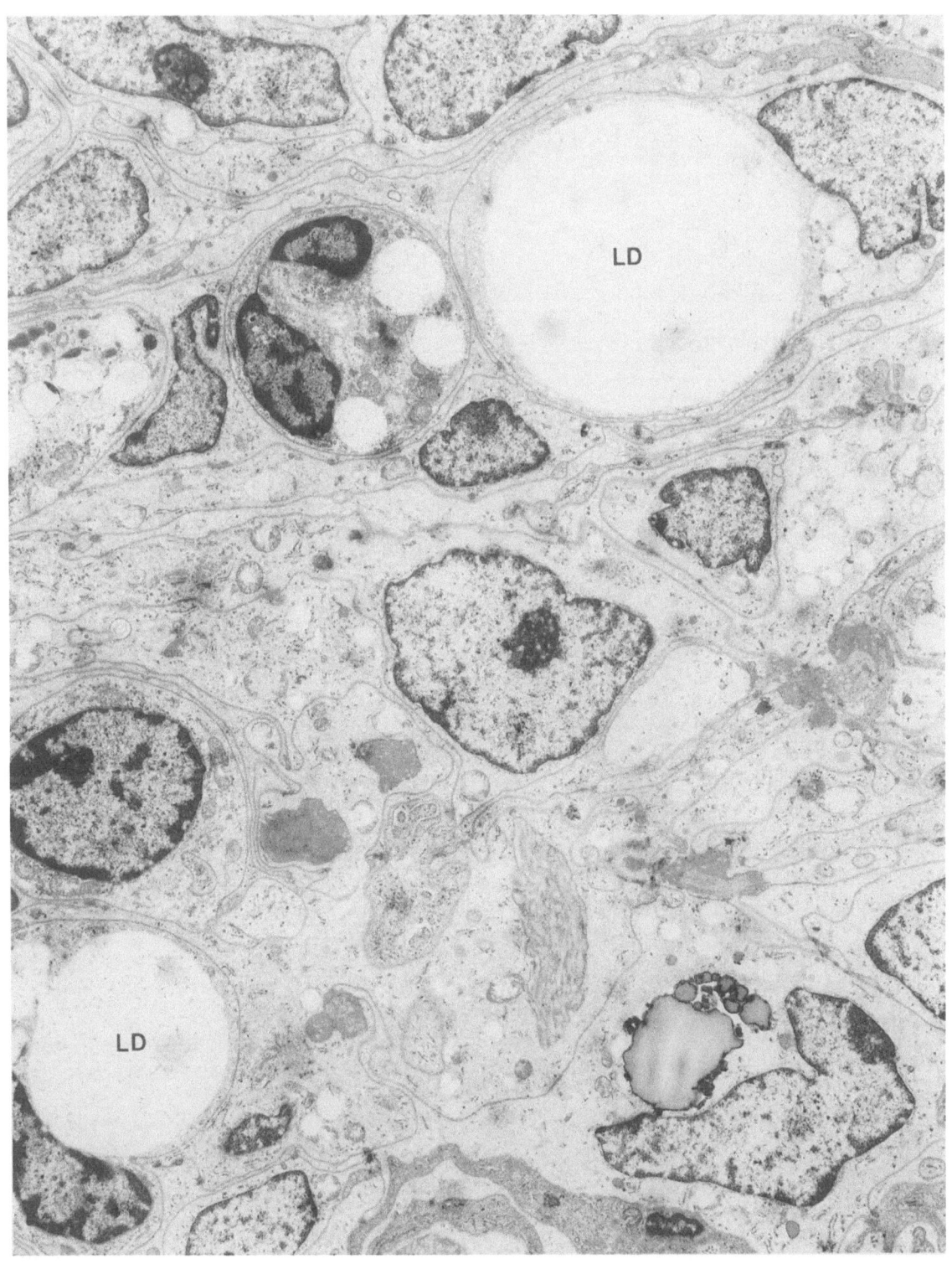

Fig. 20.12. *Meningioma* (the same case as in Fig. 20.5). Several xanthomatous cells with intracytoplasmic lipid droplets (*LD*) are interspersed in the compact sheet of cells and areas of narrow folded cytoplasm. × 6500

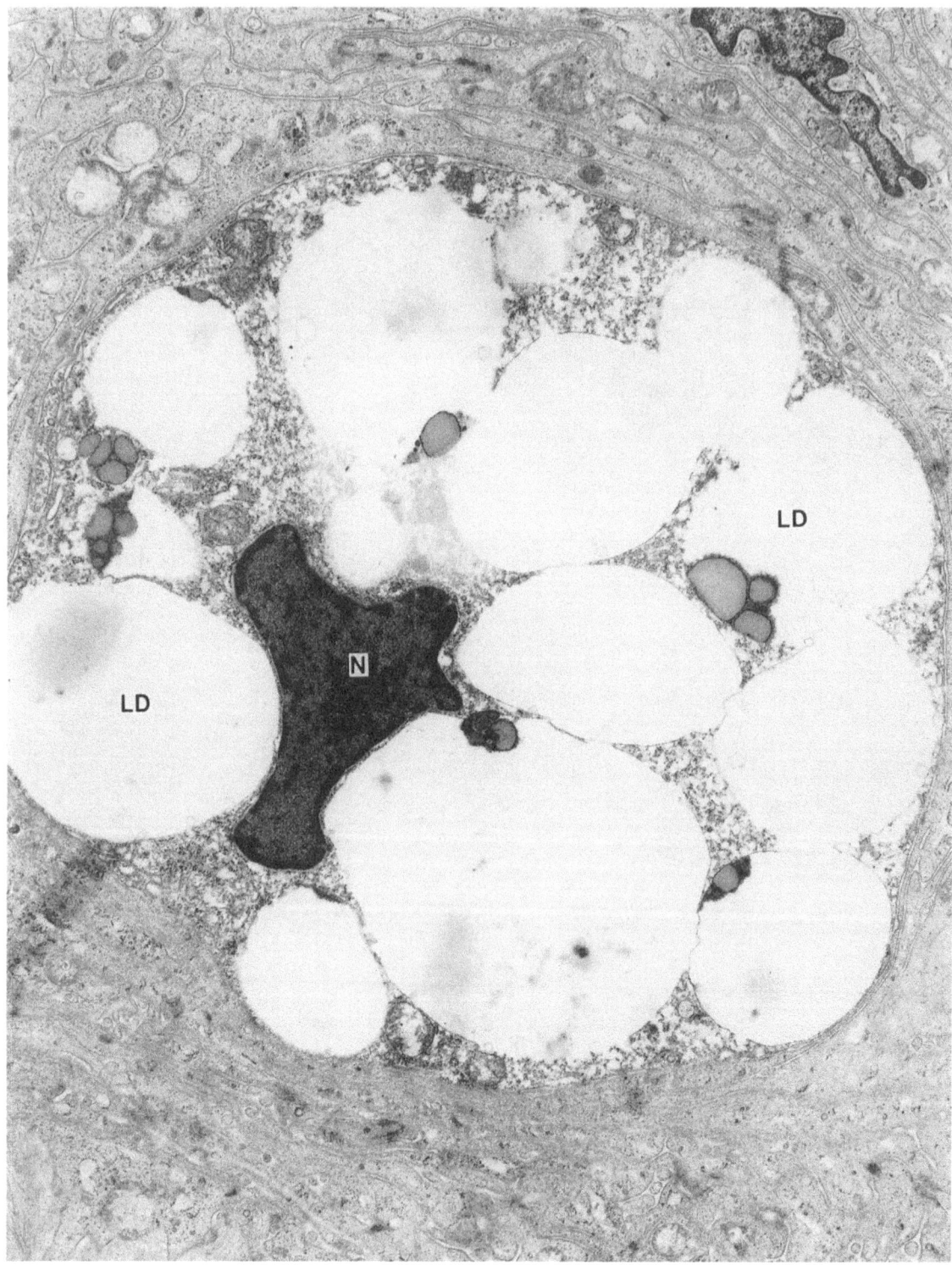

Fig. 20.13. *Meningioma* (the same case as in Fig. 20.5). Higher magnification of a xanthomatous cell shows the nucleus (*N*) distorted by intracytoplasmic lipid droplets (*LD*). × 11 000

21. Meningioangiomatosis

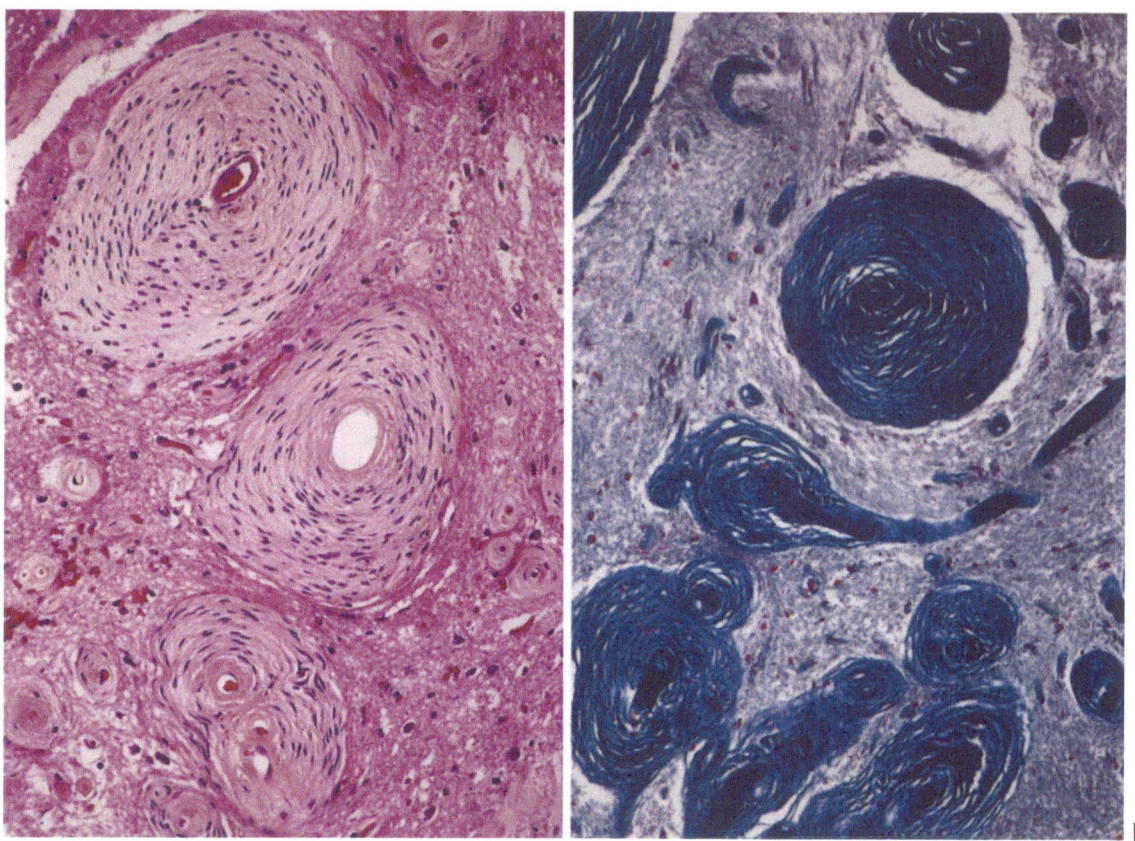

Fig. 21.1a, b, *Meningioangiomatosis* of the right parietal lobe in a 39-year-old man. Proliferated capillaries are surrounded by a concentric lamellar arrangement of spindle-shaped cells in association with intervening neural tissue. **a** H and E, × 90; **b** Azan, × 90

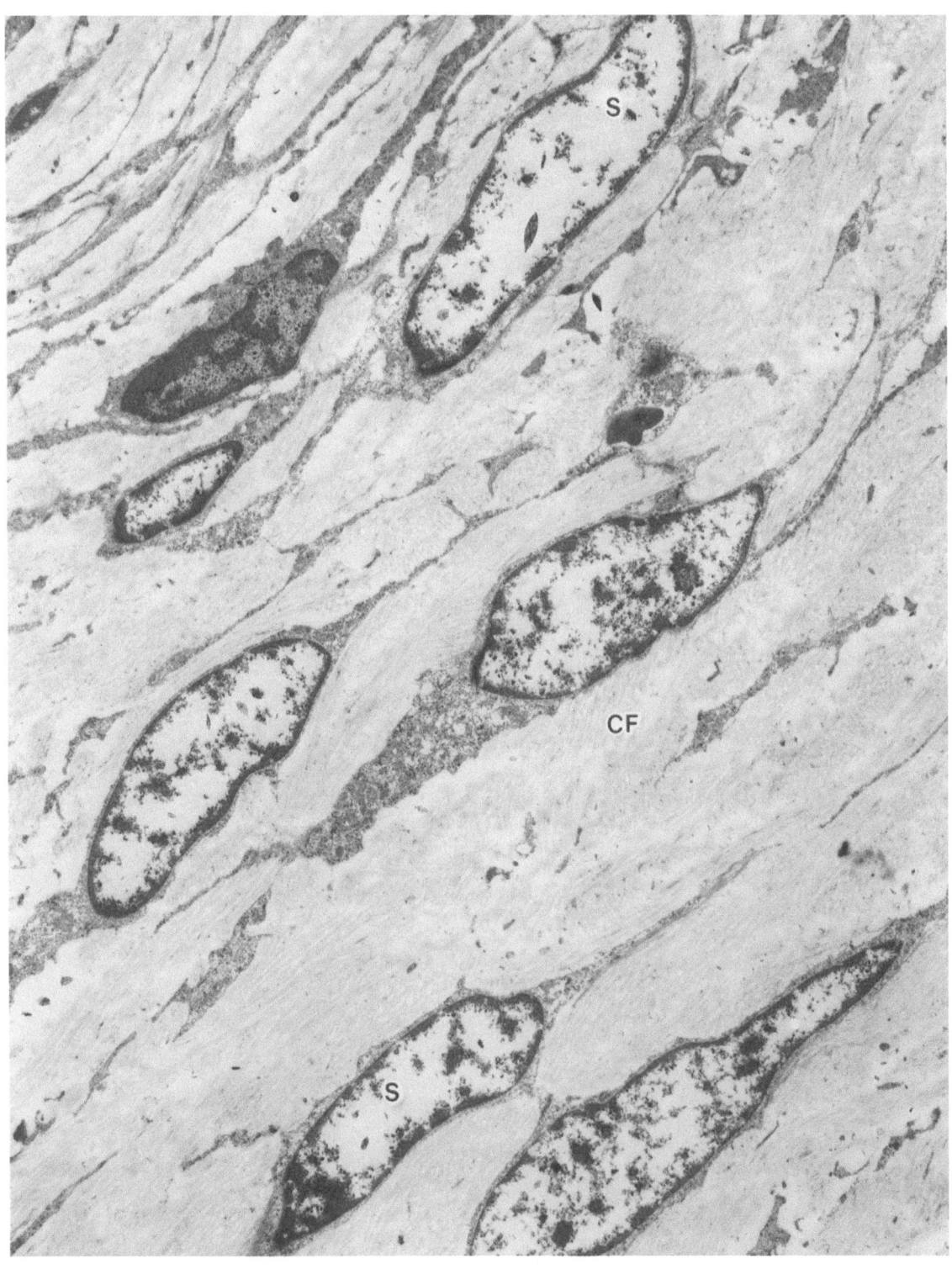

Fig. 21.2. *Meningioangiomatosis* (the same case as in Fig. 21.1). Spindle-shaped cells (*S*) of the thickened capillary wall are invested in collagen fibers (*CF*) and extend irregular cell processes. An intercellular junction is not seen. × 7000

22. Hemangioblastoma

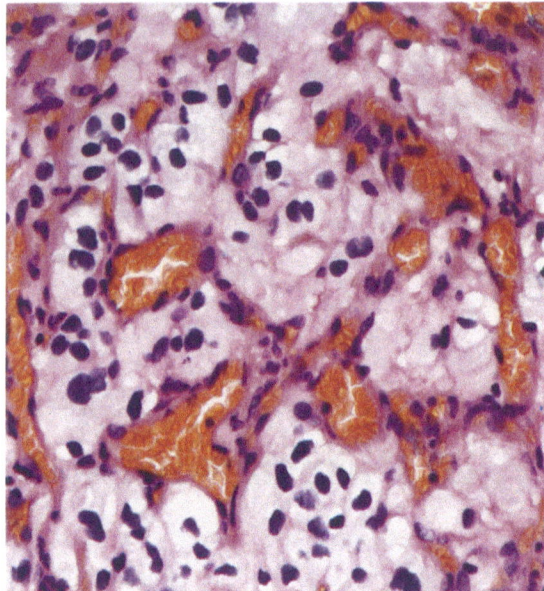

Fig. 22.1. *Hemangioblastoma* of the cerebellum in a 34-year-old woman. The tumor consists of two cellular components: One includes the endothelial cells and pericytes, and the other the foamy (lipid-containing) "stromal" cells. H and E, × 180

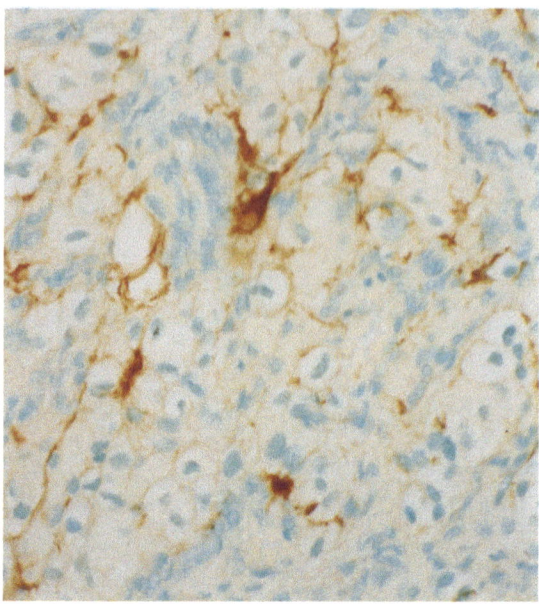

Fig. 22.2. Cerebellar *hemangioblastoma* (the same case as in Fig. 22.1). Positive staining for glial fibrillary acidic protein (GFAP) is observed exclusively in the astrocytes, which are considered to be entrapped in the tumor, but not in the "stromal" cells. Indirect immunoperoxidase method counterstained with methyl green, × 180

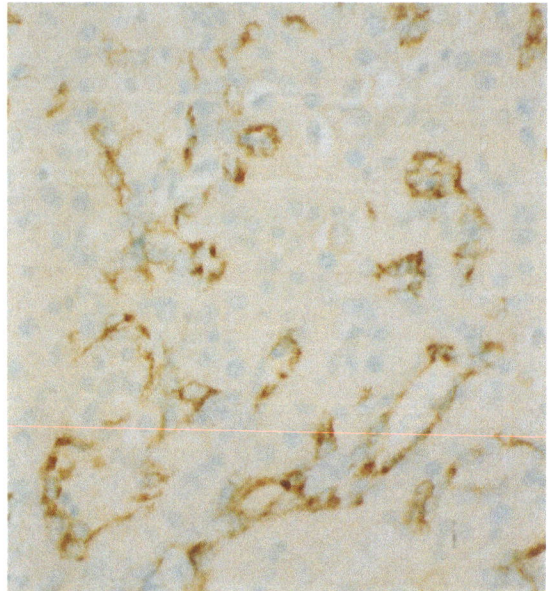

Fig. 22.3. Cerebellar *hemangioblastoma* (the same case as in Fig. 22.1). Endothelial cells of the capillary are positive for Factor VIII-related (von Willebrand) antigen. Indirect immunoperoxidase method counterstained with methyl green, × 180

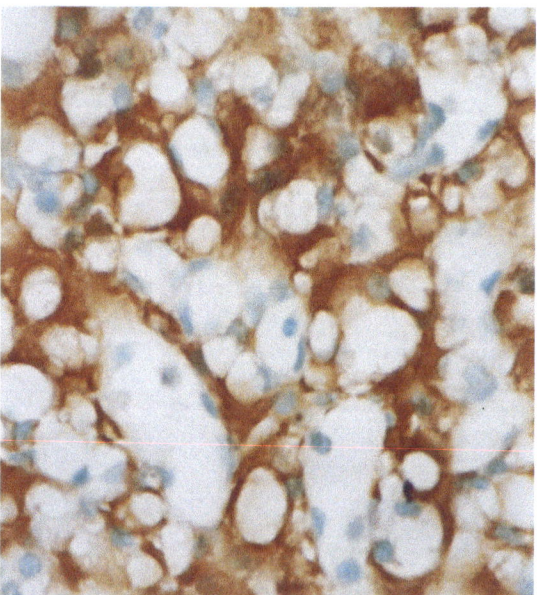

Fig. 22.4. Cerebellar *hemangioblastoma* (the same case as in Fig. 22.1). A positive reaction for S-100 protein is seen in the "stromal" cells of this tumor. Indirect immunoperoxidase method counterstained with methyl green, × 360

200

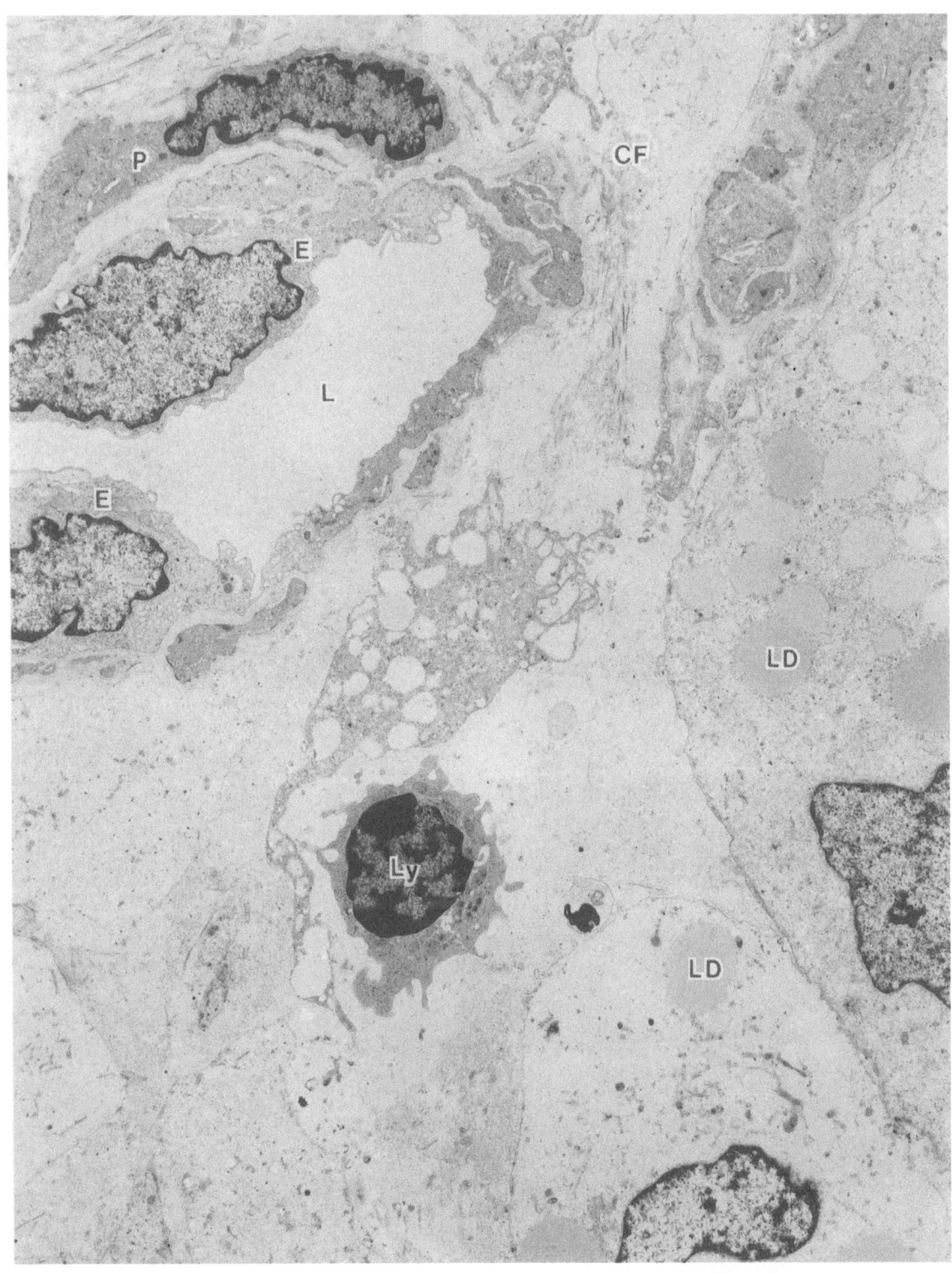

Fig. 22.5. Cerebellar *hemangioblastoma* (the same case as in Fig. 22.1). The "stromal" cells with lipid droplets (*LD*), endothelial cells (*E*), and a pericyte (*P*) are morphologically different from each other. A lymphocyte (*Ly*) and pericapillary collagen fibers (*CF*) are seen. *L* capillary lumen. × 6000

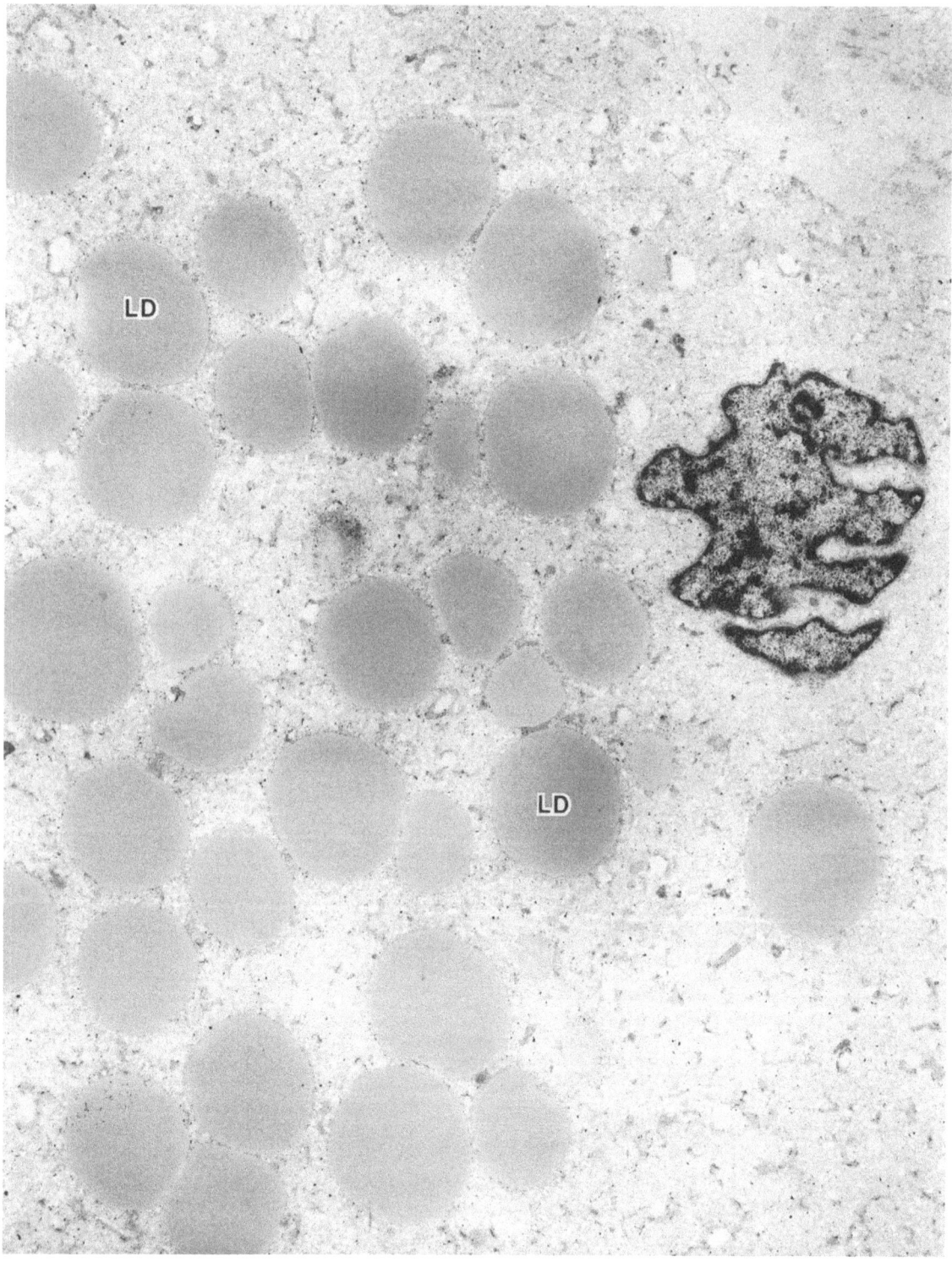

Fig. 22.6. Cerebellar *hemangioblastoma* (the same case as in Fig. 22.1). Many lipid droplets (*LD*) lie in the uniform cytoplasmic background of a "stromal" cell. × 8000

23. Hemangiopericytoma

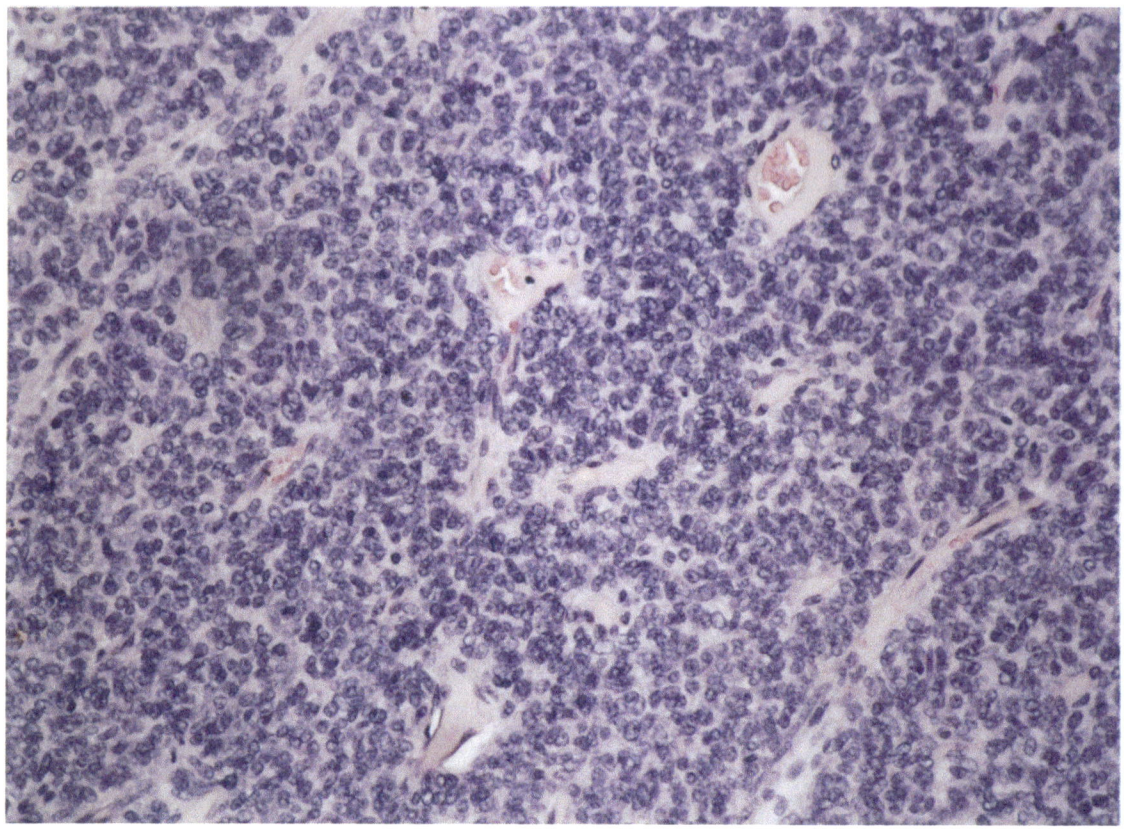

Fig. 23.1. *Hemangiopericytoma* of the right parietal region in a 40-year-old woman. The tumor is composed of round, ovoid or fusiform cells with prominent vesicular nuclei. In highly cellular parts of this tumor, as shown here, the vasculature is sometimes indistinct. H and E, × 125

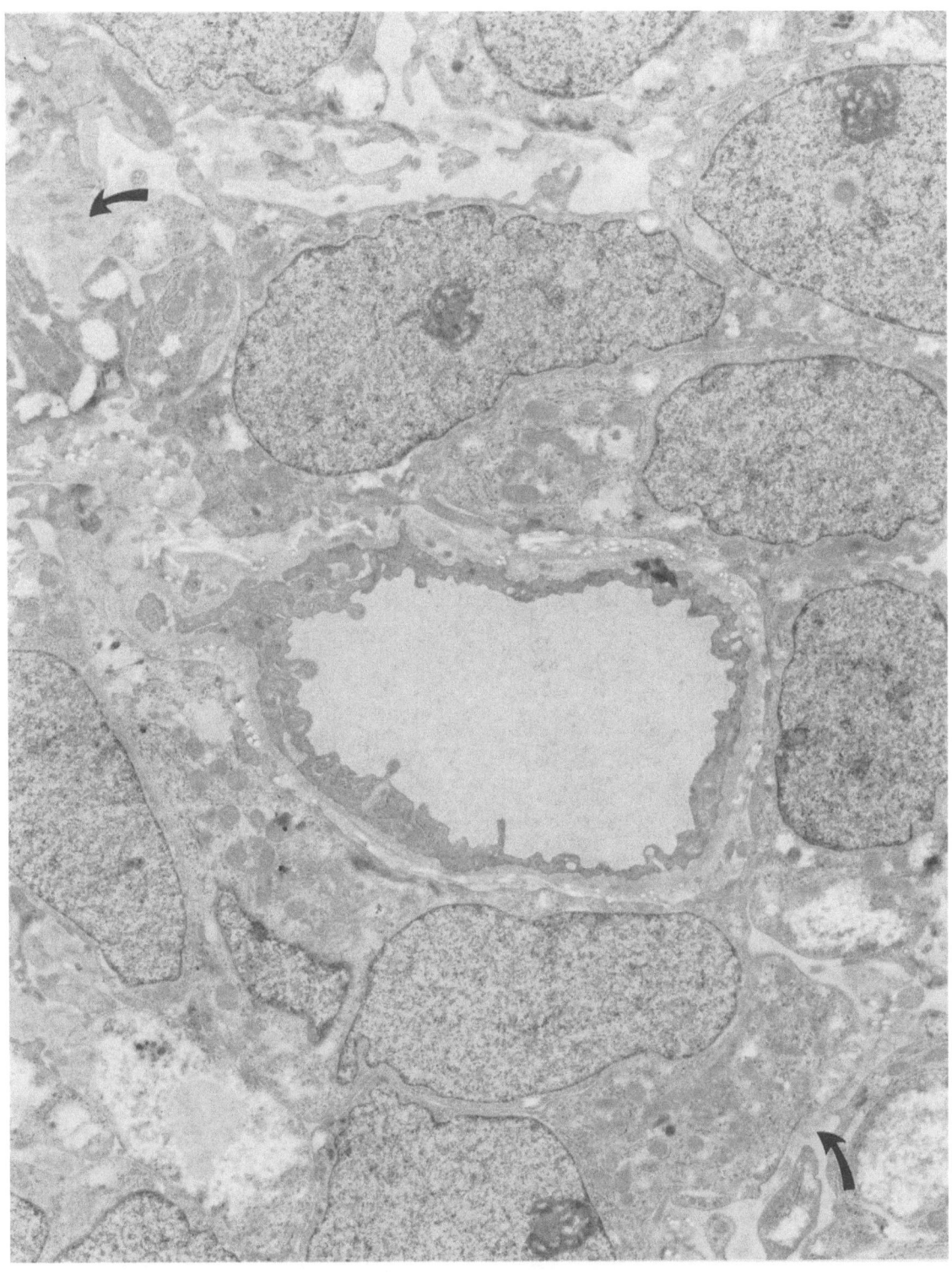

Fig. 23.2. *Hemangiopericytoma* (the same case as in Fig. 23.1). The tumor cells surround a capillary. The light-gray substance of the extracellular matrix (*arrows*) is discernible. The individual tumor cells are not invested with this substance. × 7500

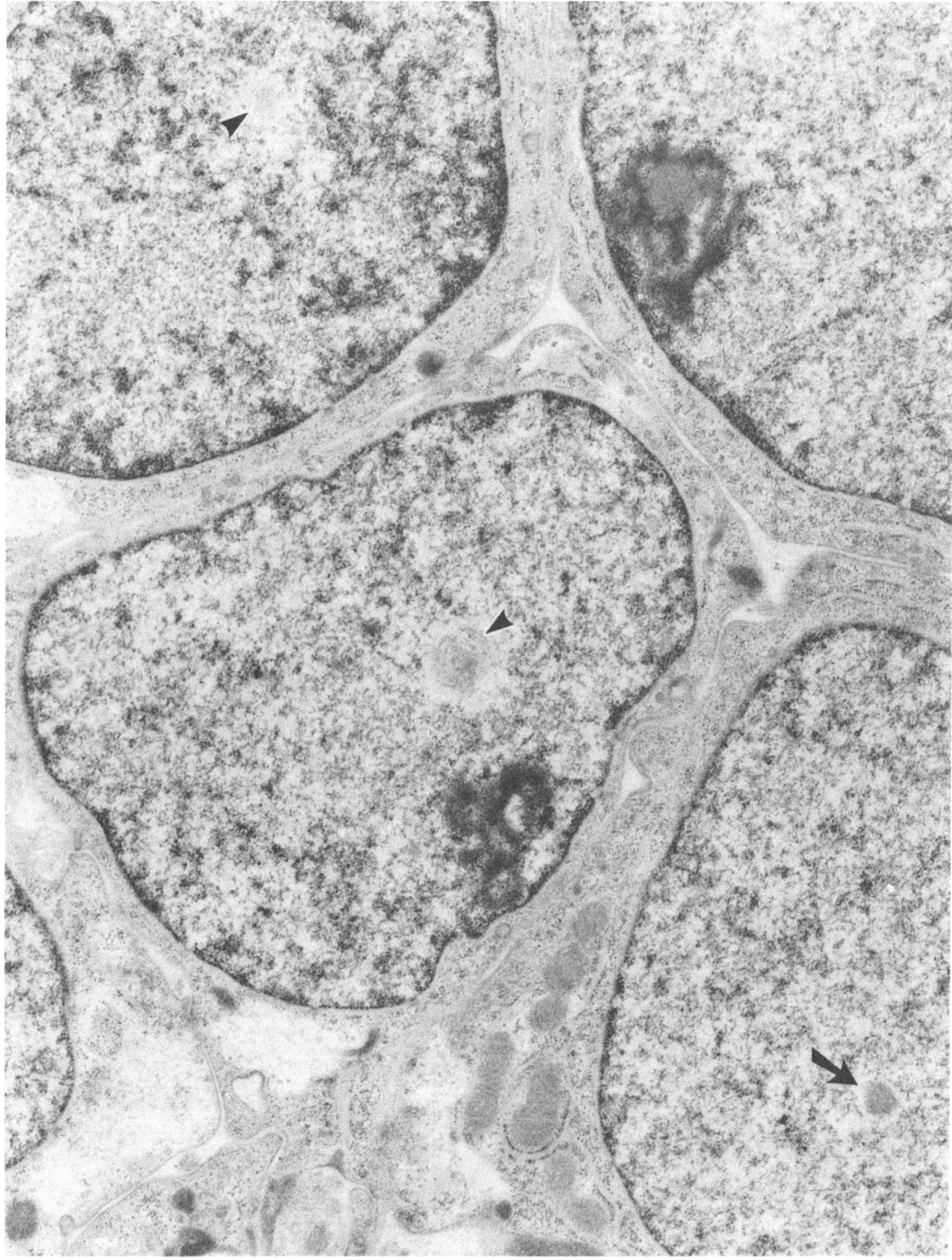

Fig. 23.3. *Hemangiopericytoma* (the same case as in Fig. 23.1). The tumor cells have little cytoplasm and round to oval nuclei with fine chromatin granules. Nuclear bodies (*arrowheads*) and a filamentous intranuclear inclusion (*arrow*) are seen. There is no junctional apparatus between the tumor cells. × 18 000

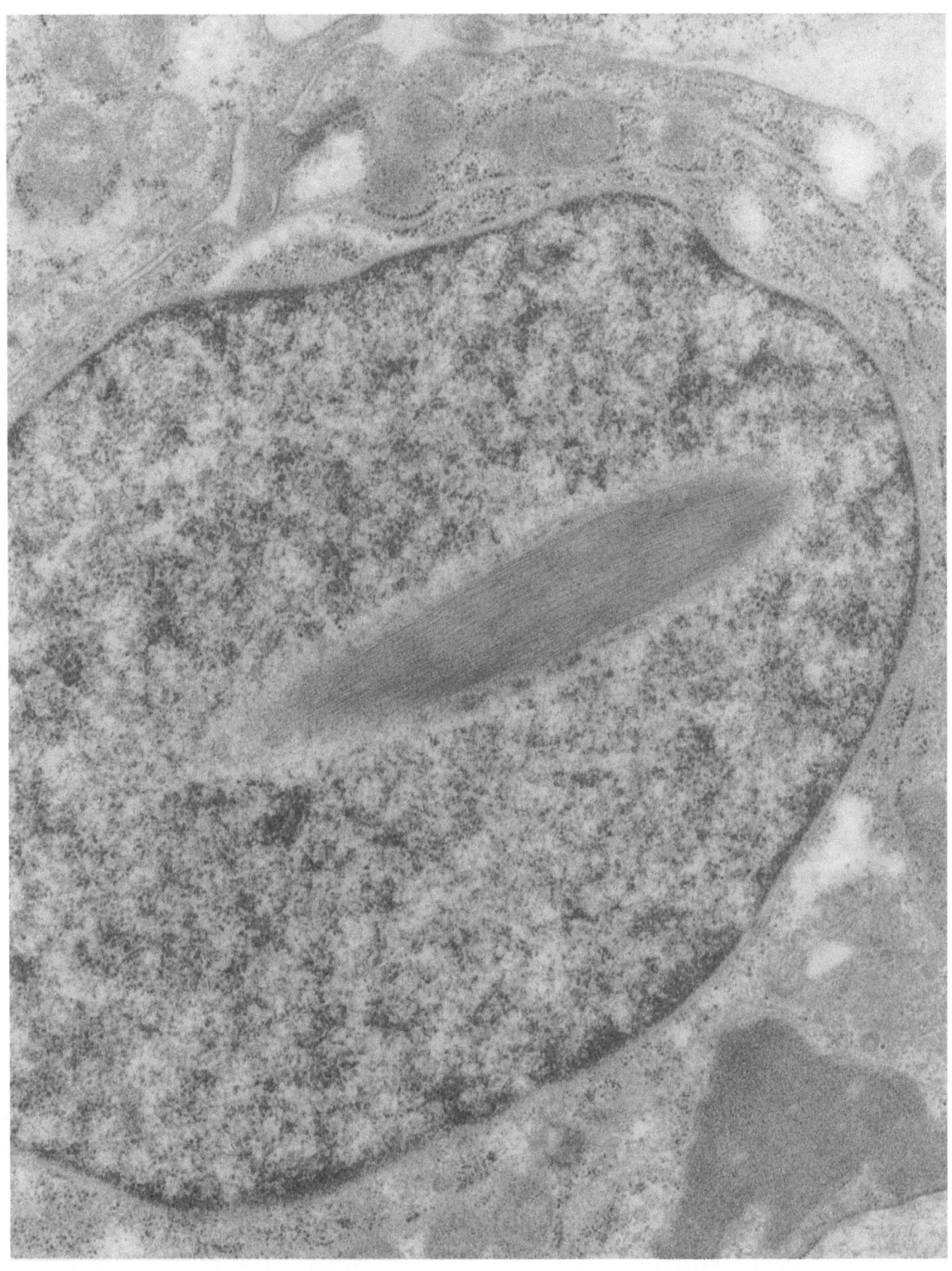

Fig. 23.4. *Hemangiopericytoma* (the same case as in Fig. 23.1). A large filamentous intranuclear inclusion is evident in a tumor cell. × 30 000

24. Melanoma

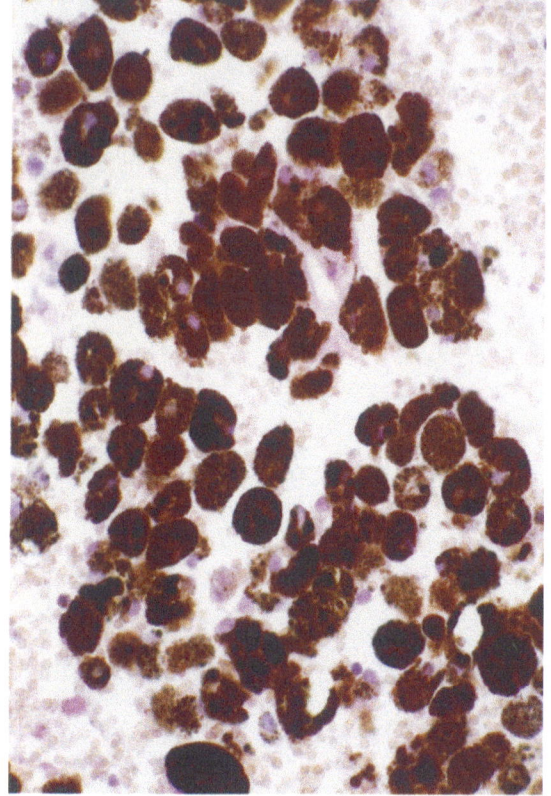

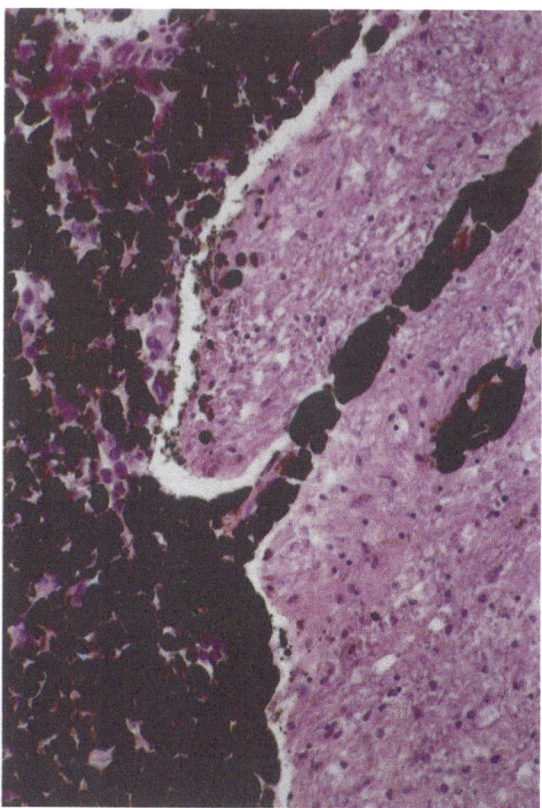

Fig. 24.1. Primary intracranial *malignant melanoma* of the right parietal region in a 35-year-old man. The tumor cells are characterized by abundant melanin. H and E, × 180

Fig. 24.2. Primary intracranial *malignant melanoma* of the pineal region in a 62-year-old woman. Malignant melanocytes easily disseminate through the subarachnoid space. H and E, × 90

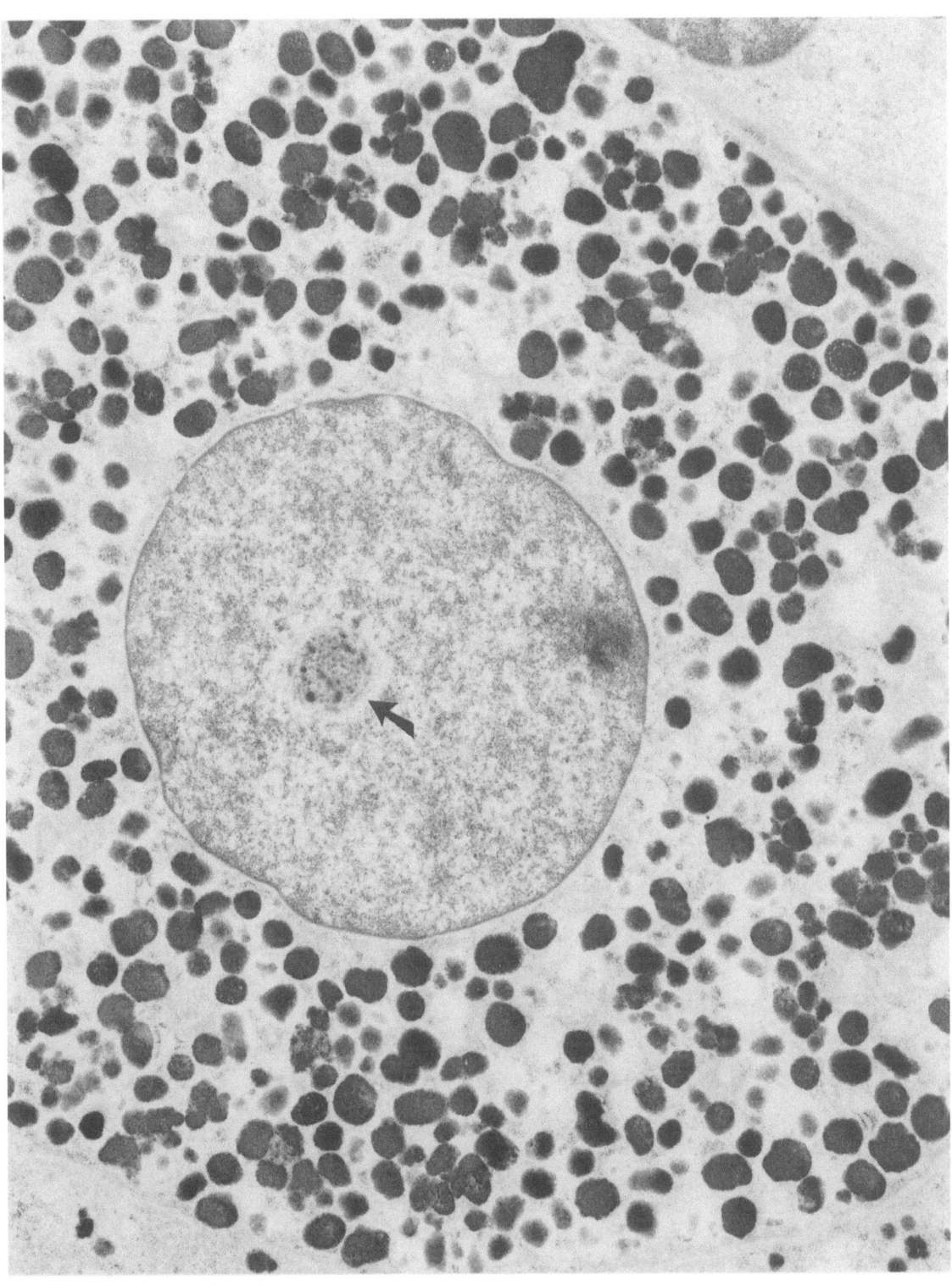

Fig. 24.3. Primary intracranial *malignant melanoma* (the same case as in Fig. 24.1). A malignant melanocyte contains abundant melanosomes, 300–750 nm in diameter. A nuclear body (*arrow*) is seen. × 14 000

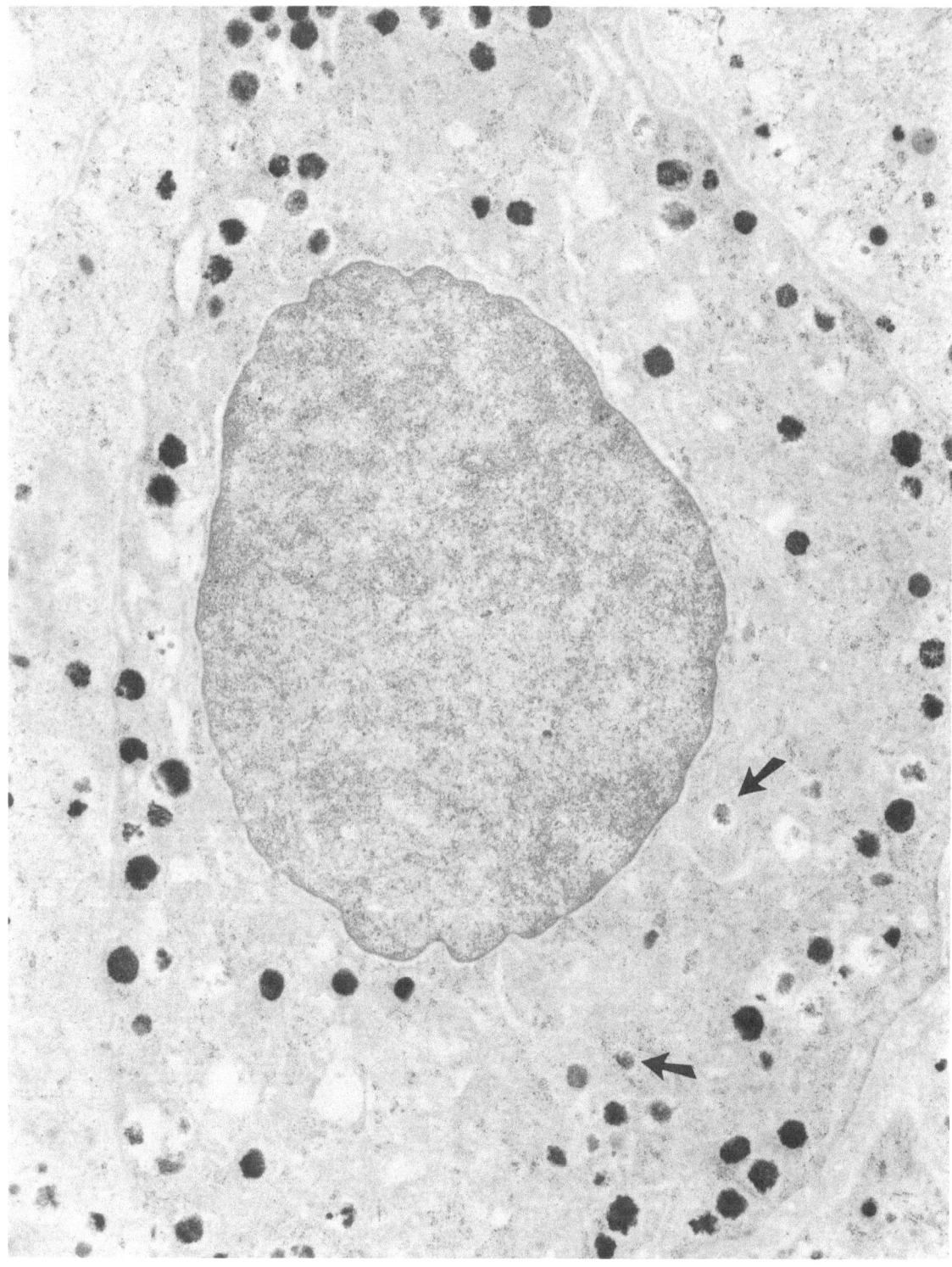

Fig. 24.4. Primary intracranial *malignant melanoma* (the same case as in Fig. 24.1). The melanosomes vary in the degree of melanization. Developing melanosomes (*arrows*) are sometimes difficult to recognize without melanization or the presence of nearby mature melanosomes. × 14 000

25. Malignant Lymphoma

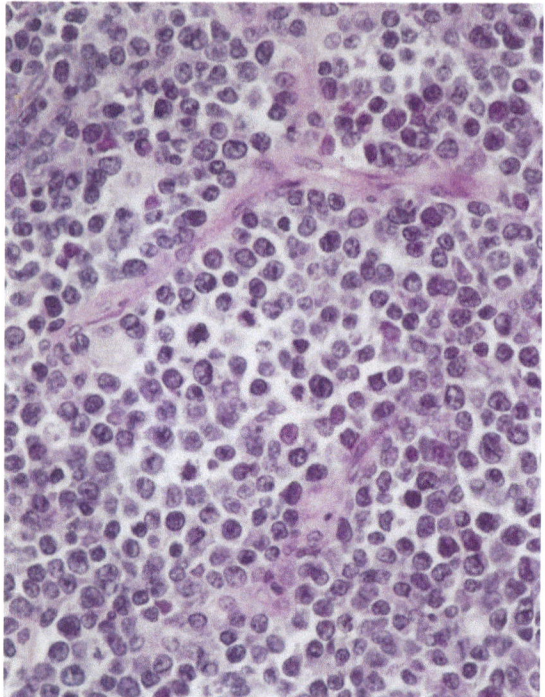

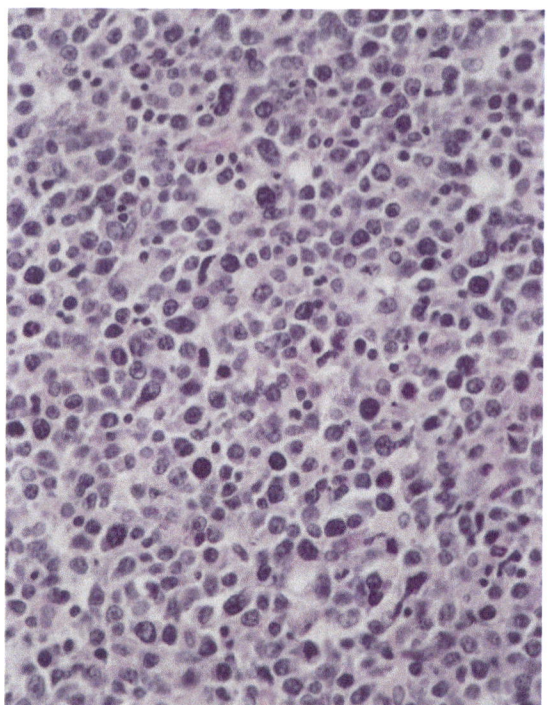

Fig. 25.1. Primary intracranial *malignant lymphoma* of the left frontal lobe in a 20-year-old man. A diffuse lymphoma of the medium-sized cell type shows a sheet of lymphoid cells without any particular architecture. H and E, × 180

Fig. 25.2. Primary intracranial *malignant lymphoma* of the right thalamus in a 49-year-old man. Diffuse lymphoma, mixed type. H and E, × 180

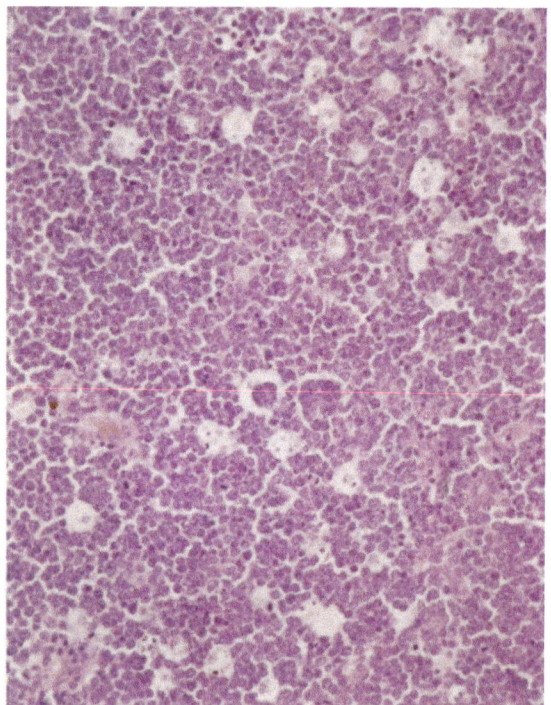

Fig. 25.3. Primary intracranial *malignant lymphoma* of the left frontal lobe in a 56-year-old woman. A diffuse lymphoma of the Burkitt type displays the starry sky appearance. H and E, × 60

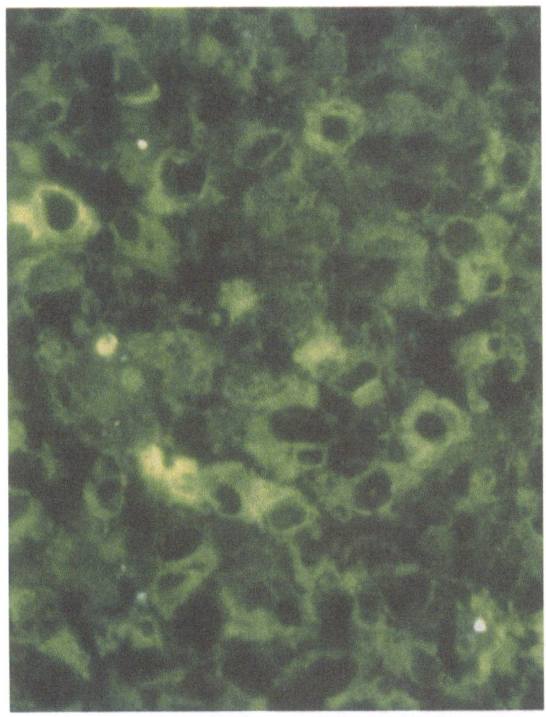

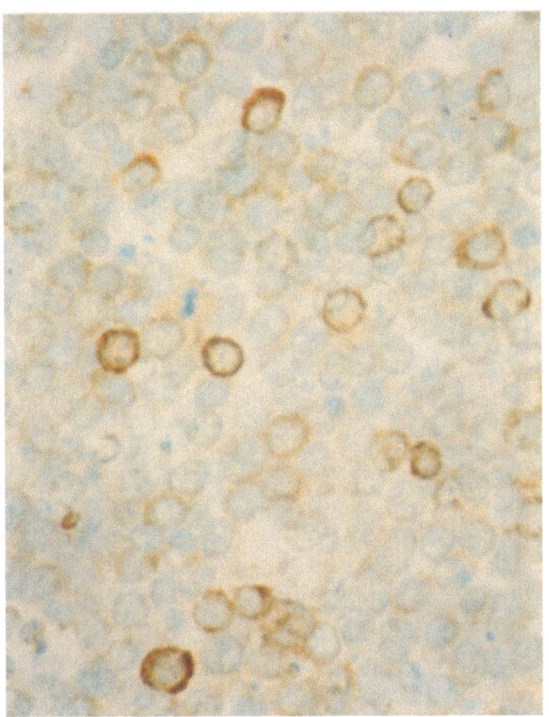

Fig. 25.4. *Malignant lymphoma* (the same case as in Fig. 25.1). Malignant lymphomas occurring in the central nervous system (CNS) are thought to be the morphological and functional counterparts of malignant lymphomas outside the CNS. Immunohistochemical examination is of great value in the classification of malignant lymphomas with respect to the nature of the cells they contain, e.g., T- or B-cell type. This frozen section stained for immunoglobulins reveals both cytoplasmic and surface IgM. Direct immunofluorescence method, × 360

Fig. 25.5. *Malignant lymphoma* (the same case as in Fig. 25.2). Many lymphoma cells demonstrate a positive reaction for monotypic (κ) IgM. Peroxidase antiperoxidase method counterstained with methyl green, × 360

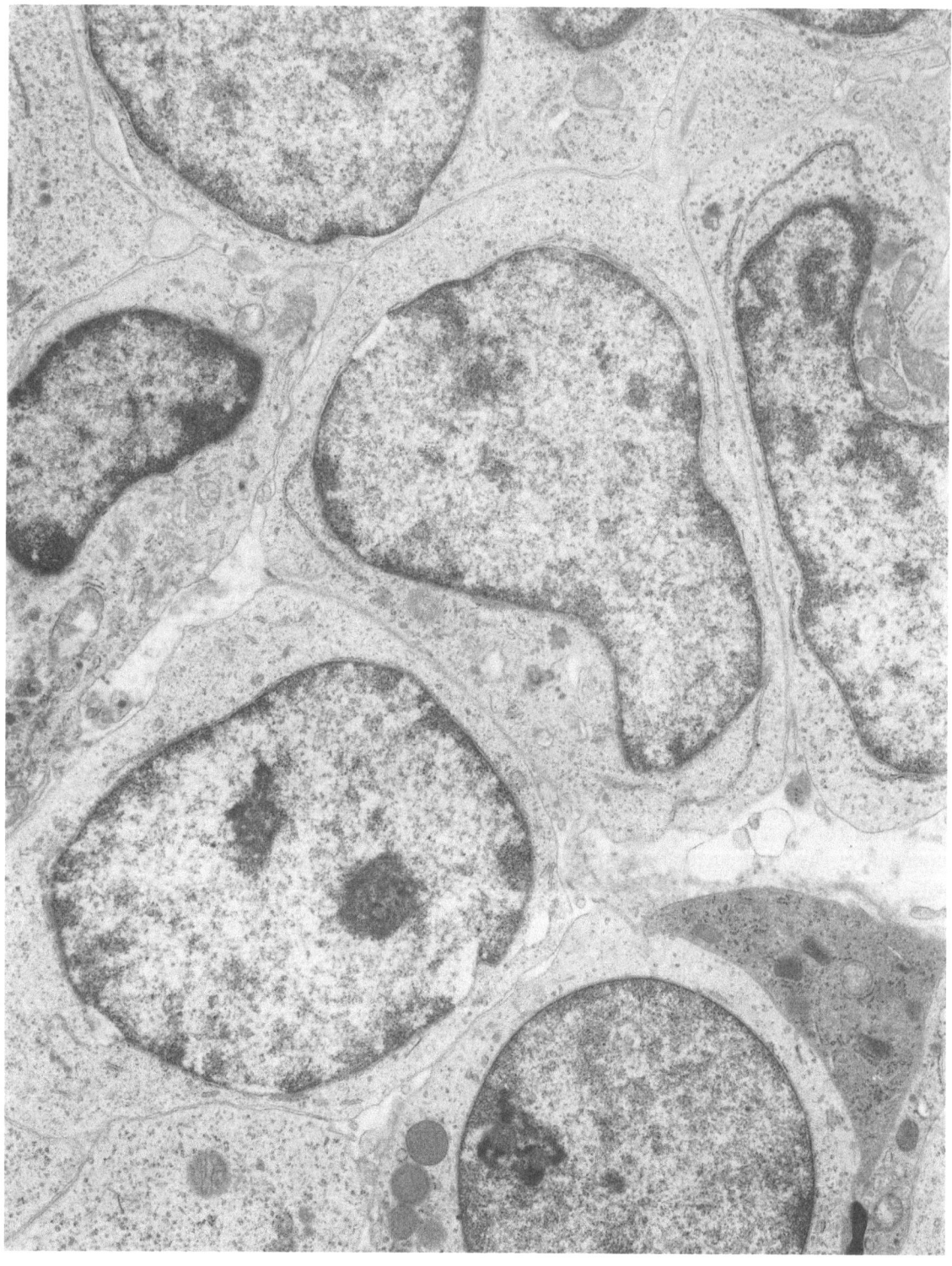

Fig. 25.6. *Malignant lymphoma* (the same case as in Fig. 25.1). Closely packed lymphoid cells have round, oval, or distorted nuclei, and the modest cytoplasm contains few organelles. Neither an intercellular junction nor basal lamina are seen. × 10 000

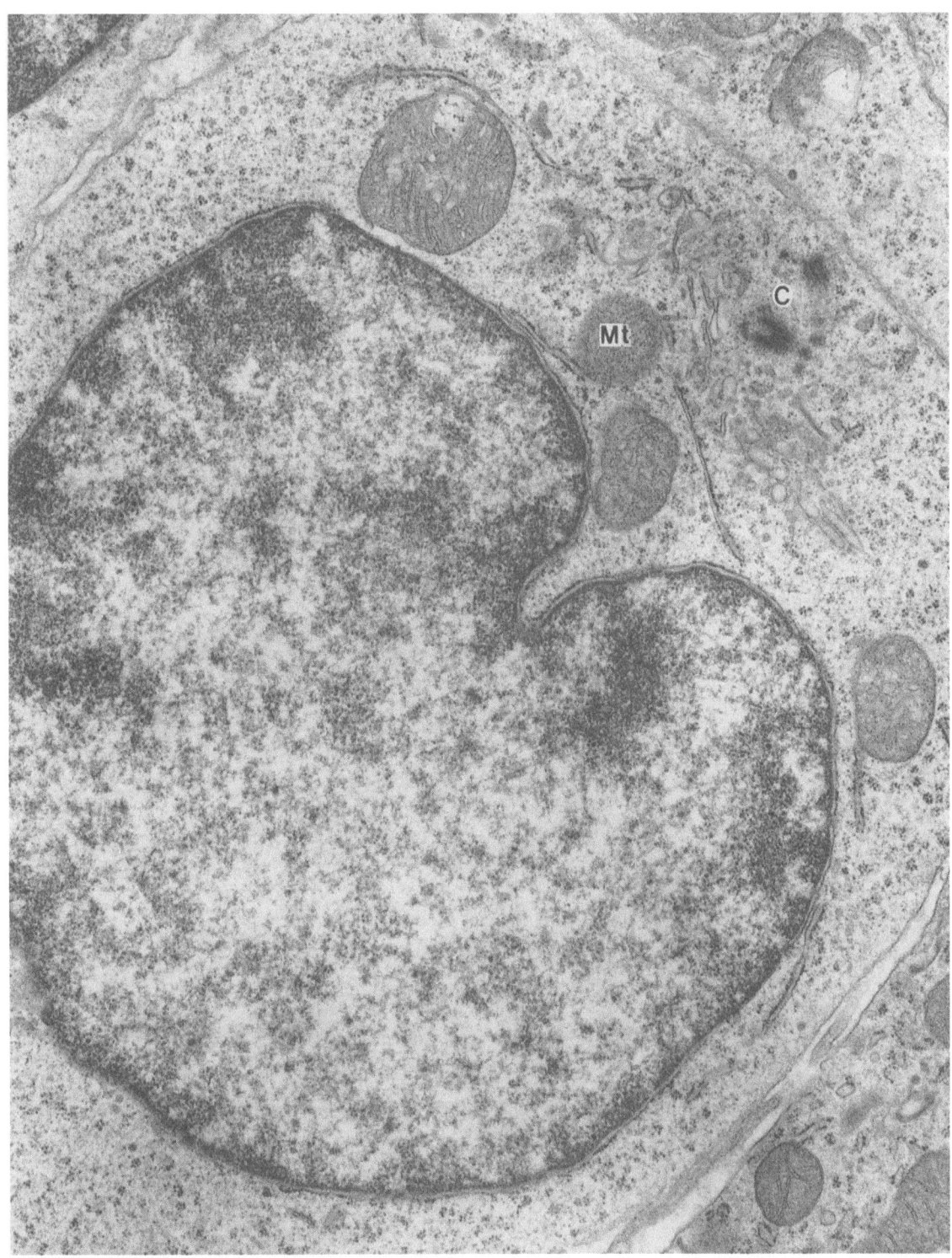

Fig. 25.7. *Malignant lymphoma* (the same case as in Fig. 25.1). The lymphoma cell with an indented nucleus is morphologically indistinguishable from its normal counterpart. *Mt* mitochondrion, *C* centriole. × 20 000

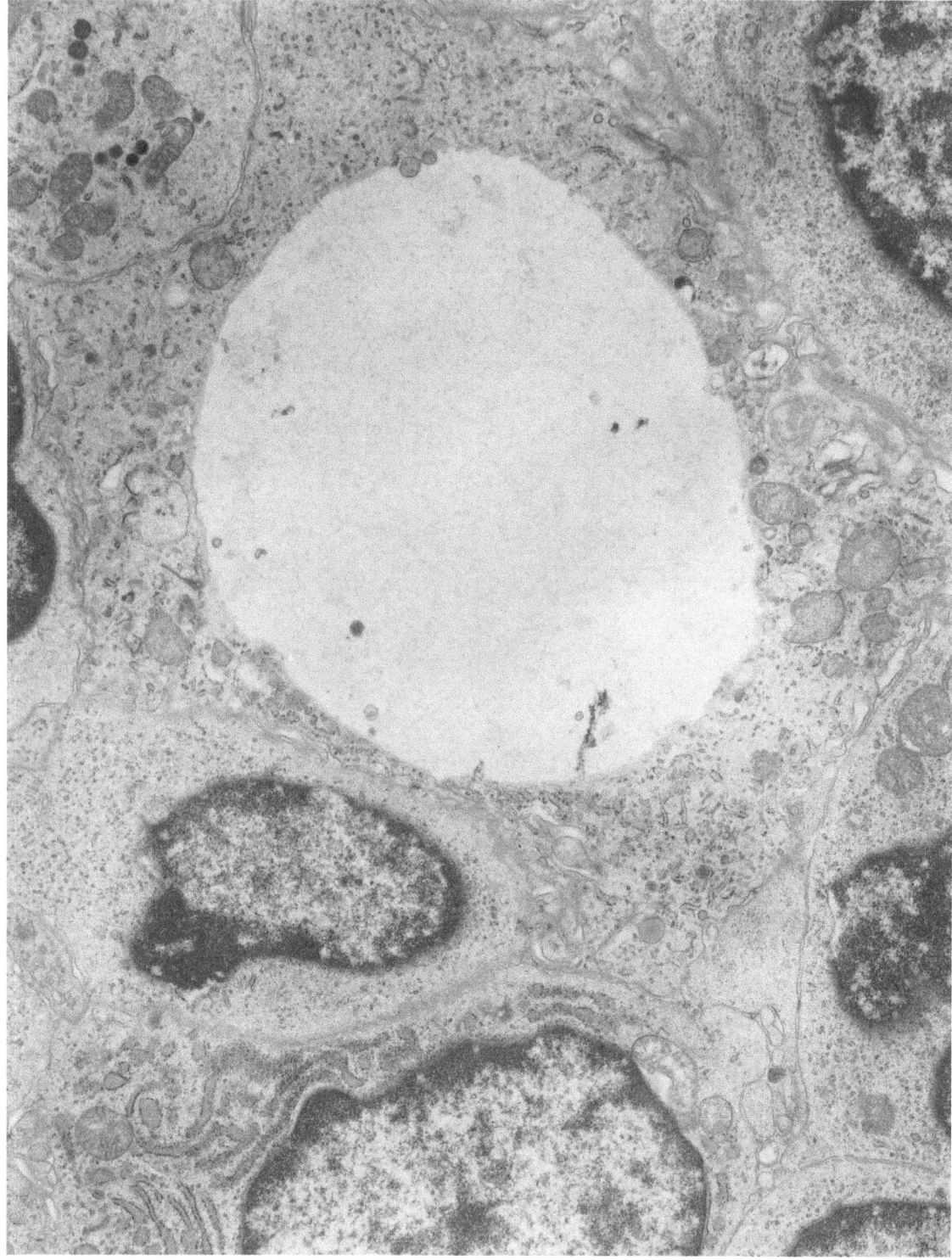

Fig. 25.8. *Malignant lymphoma* (the same case as in Fig. 25.1). The nucleus is absent from the lymphoma cell in the center and the cavity is replaced by a white-gray substance, probably proteinaceous fluid. × 10 000

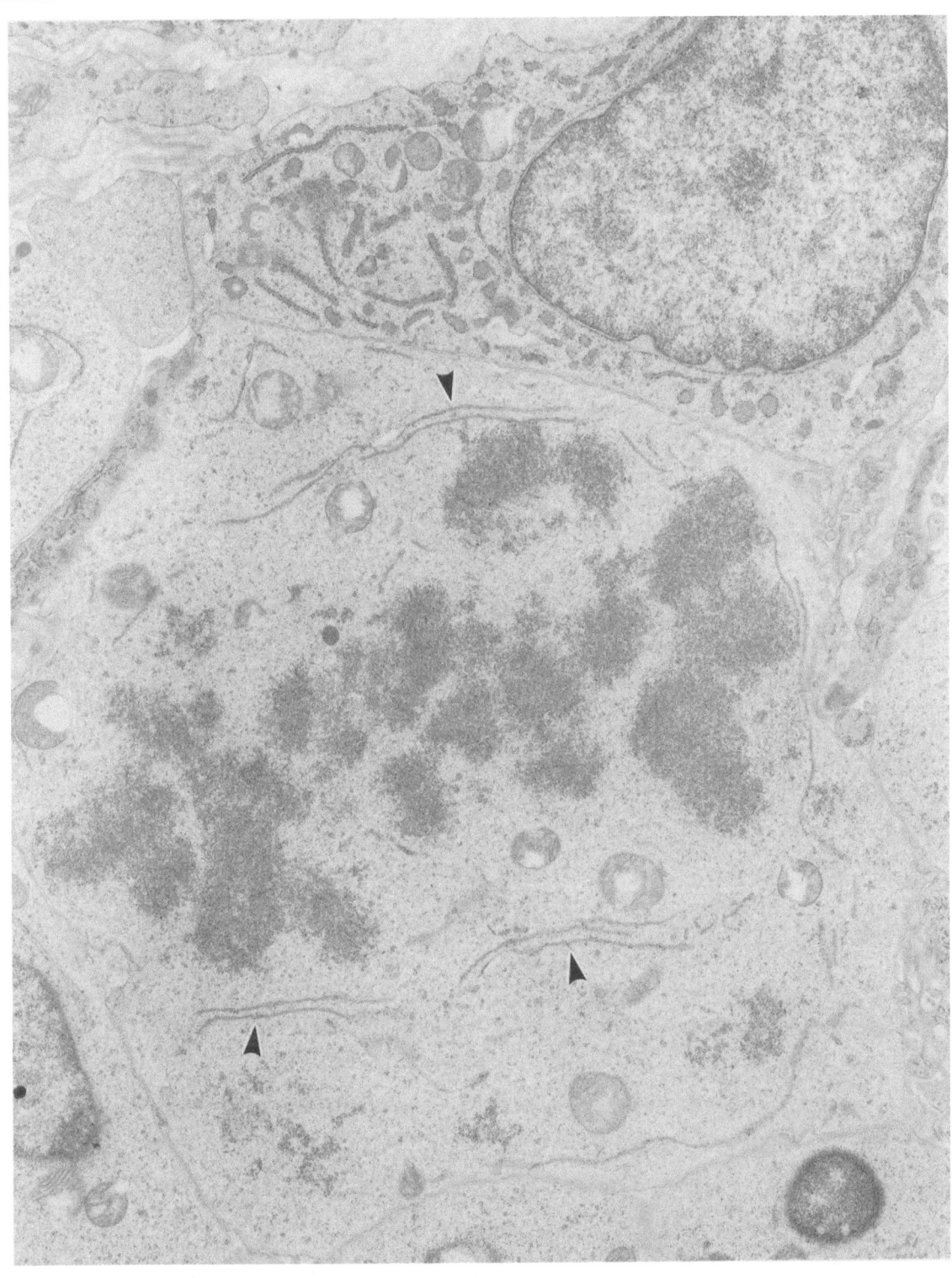

Fig. 25.9. *Malignant lymphoma* (the same case as in Fig. 25.1). A dividing cell in prometaphase demonstrates randomly placed chromosomes and the fragments of nuclear membranes (*arrowheads*). × 10 000

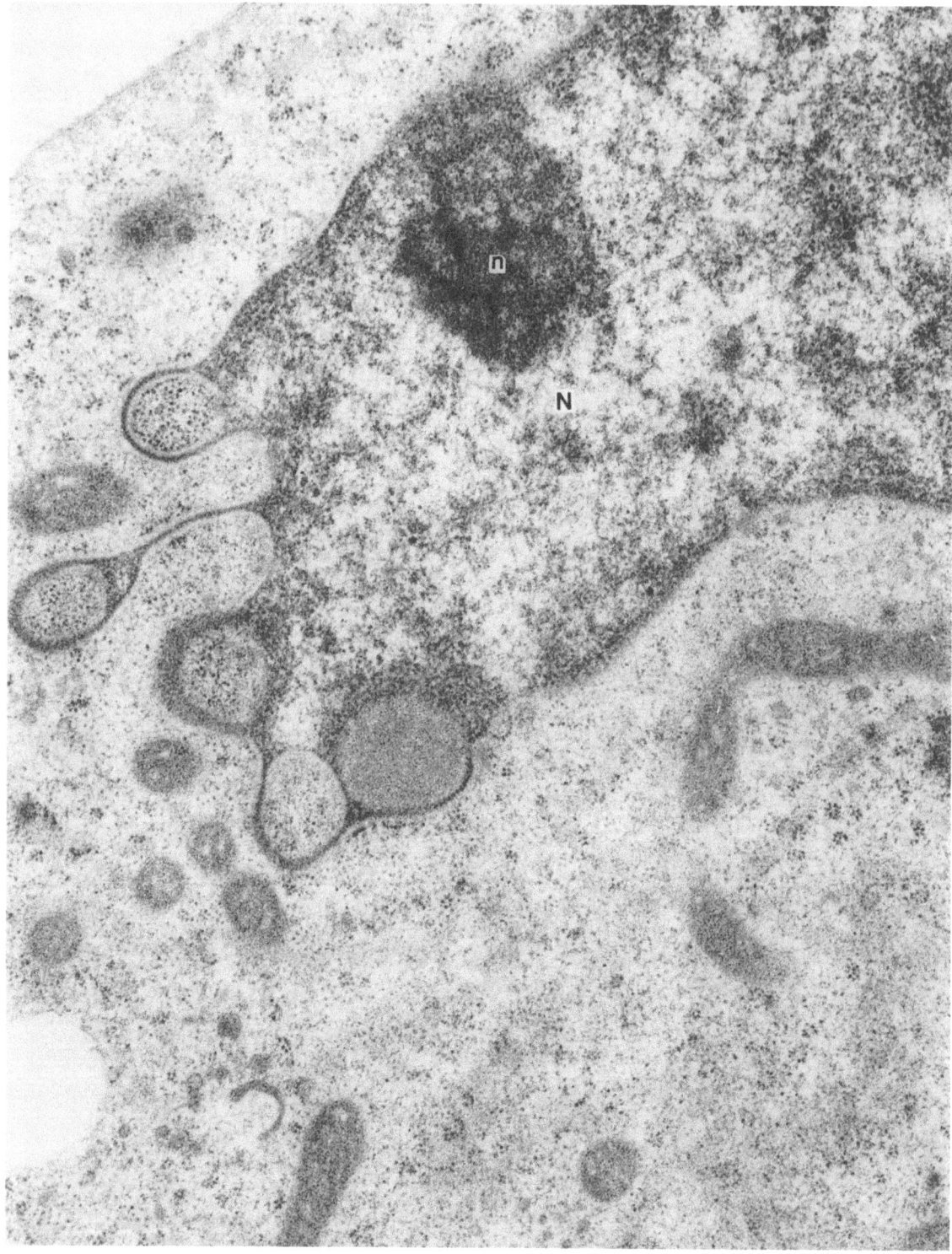

Fig. 25.10. *Malignant lymphoma* (the same case as in Fig. 25.1). The tumor cell often exhibits nuclear blebs, which are enclosed by nuclear membranes and whose electron density is basically identical with that of the cytoplasm. *N* nucleus, *n* nucleolus. × 31 000

26. Craniopharyngioma

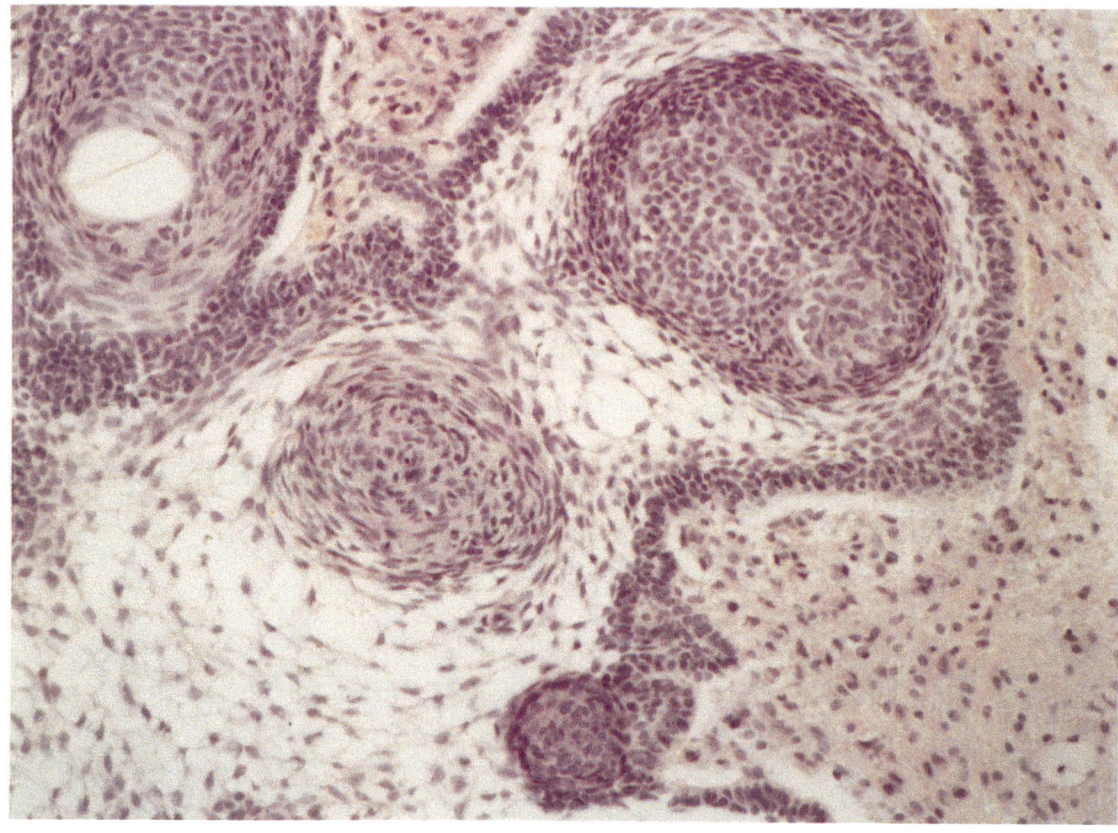

Fig. 26.1. *Craniopharyngioma* in a 44-year-old man. The tumor consists of islands of epithelial cells and palisaded columnar cells which merge into spidery cells. H and E, × 125

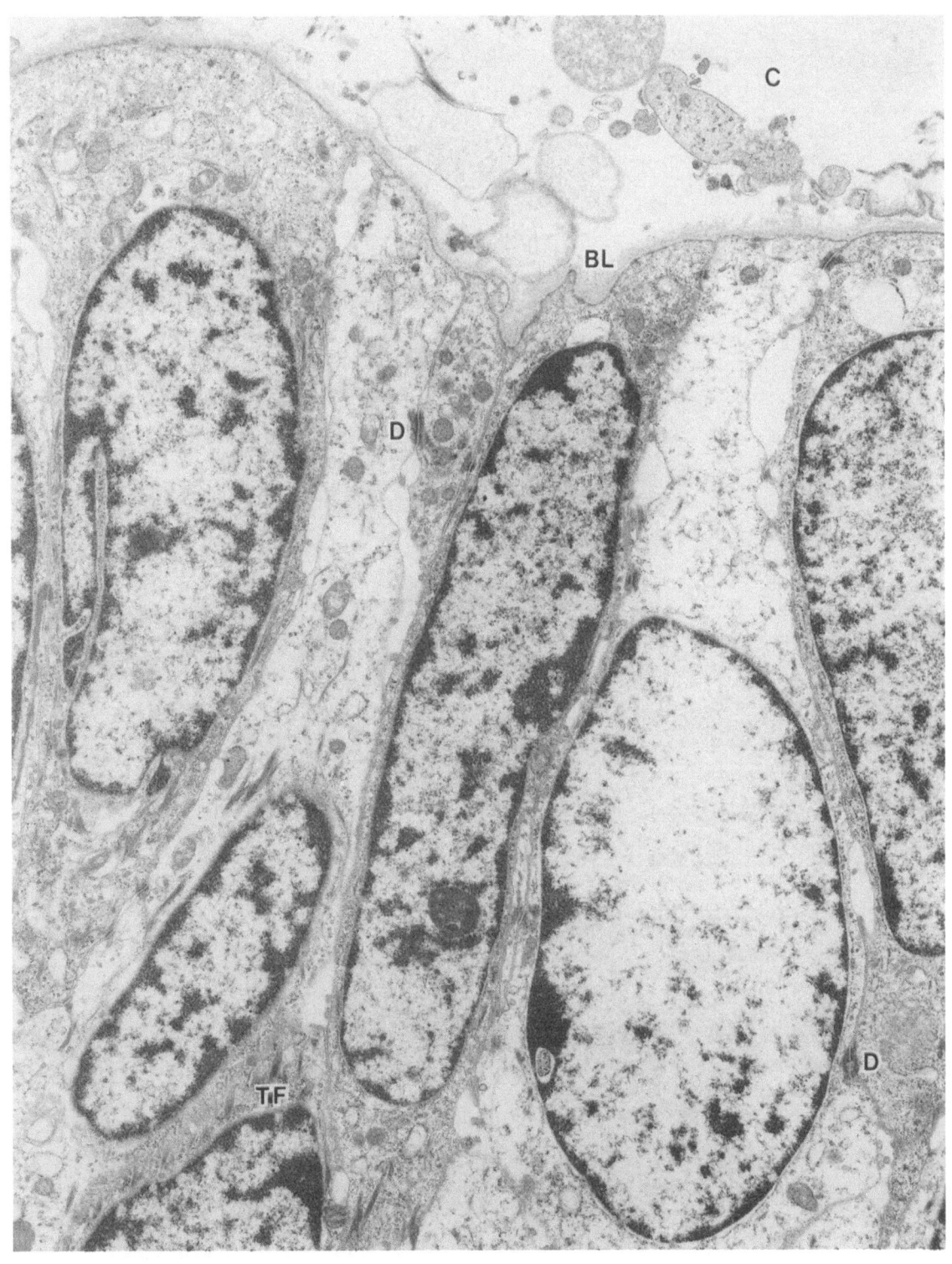

Fig. 26.2. *Craniopharyngioma* (the same case as in Fig. 26.1). Spindle-shaped tumor cells are apically arranged and have bundles of tonofilaments (*TF*) and desmosomes (*D*). A basal lamina (*BL*) is seen on the luminal surfaces of the tumor cells. *C* cyst cavity. × 10 000

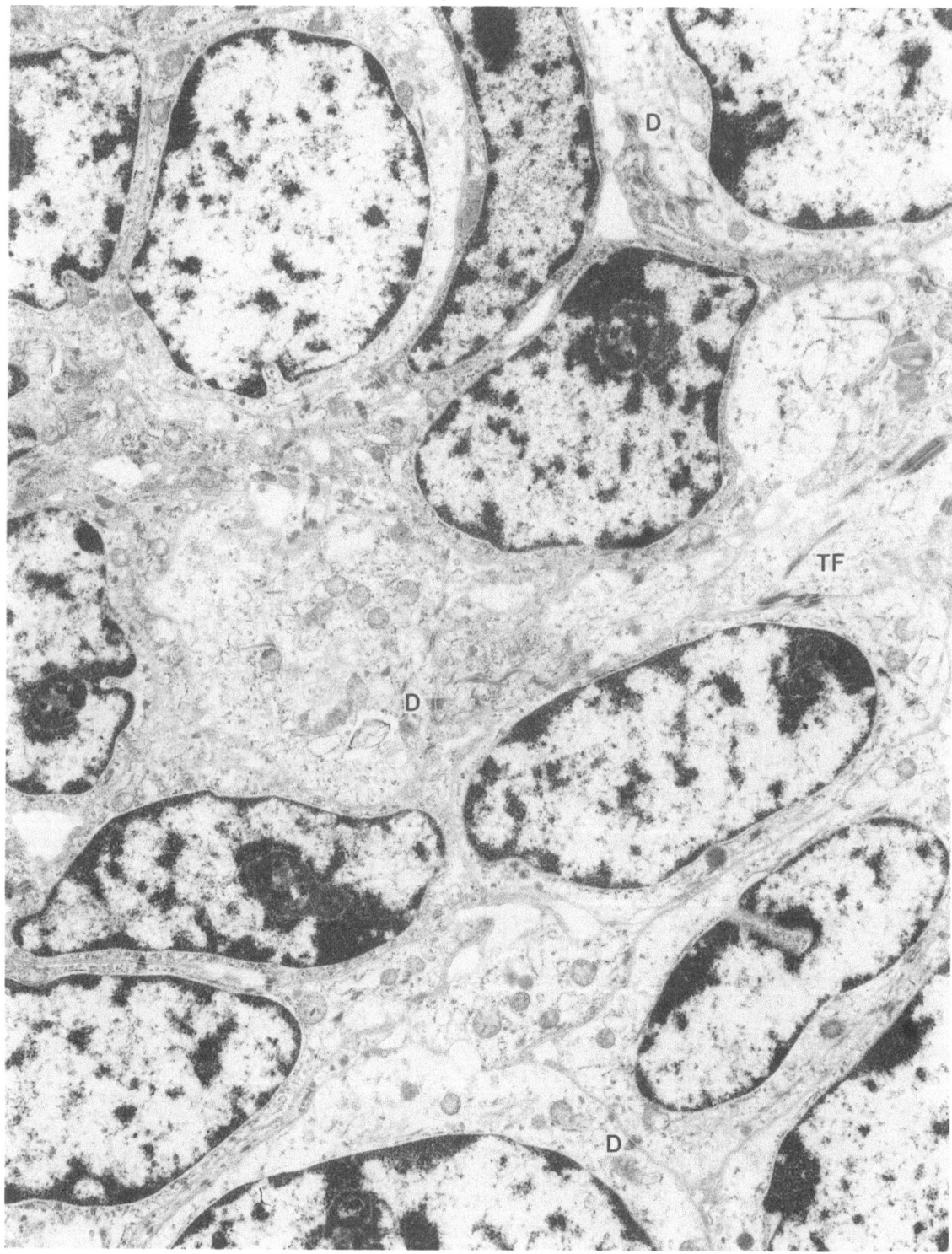

Fig. 26.3. *Craniopharyngioma* (the same case as in Fig. 26.1). The tumor is composed of compacted epithelial cells with tonofilaments (*TF*) and desmosomes (*D*), which are similar to the stratum spinosum of normal skin. × 10 000

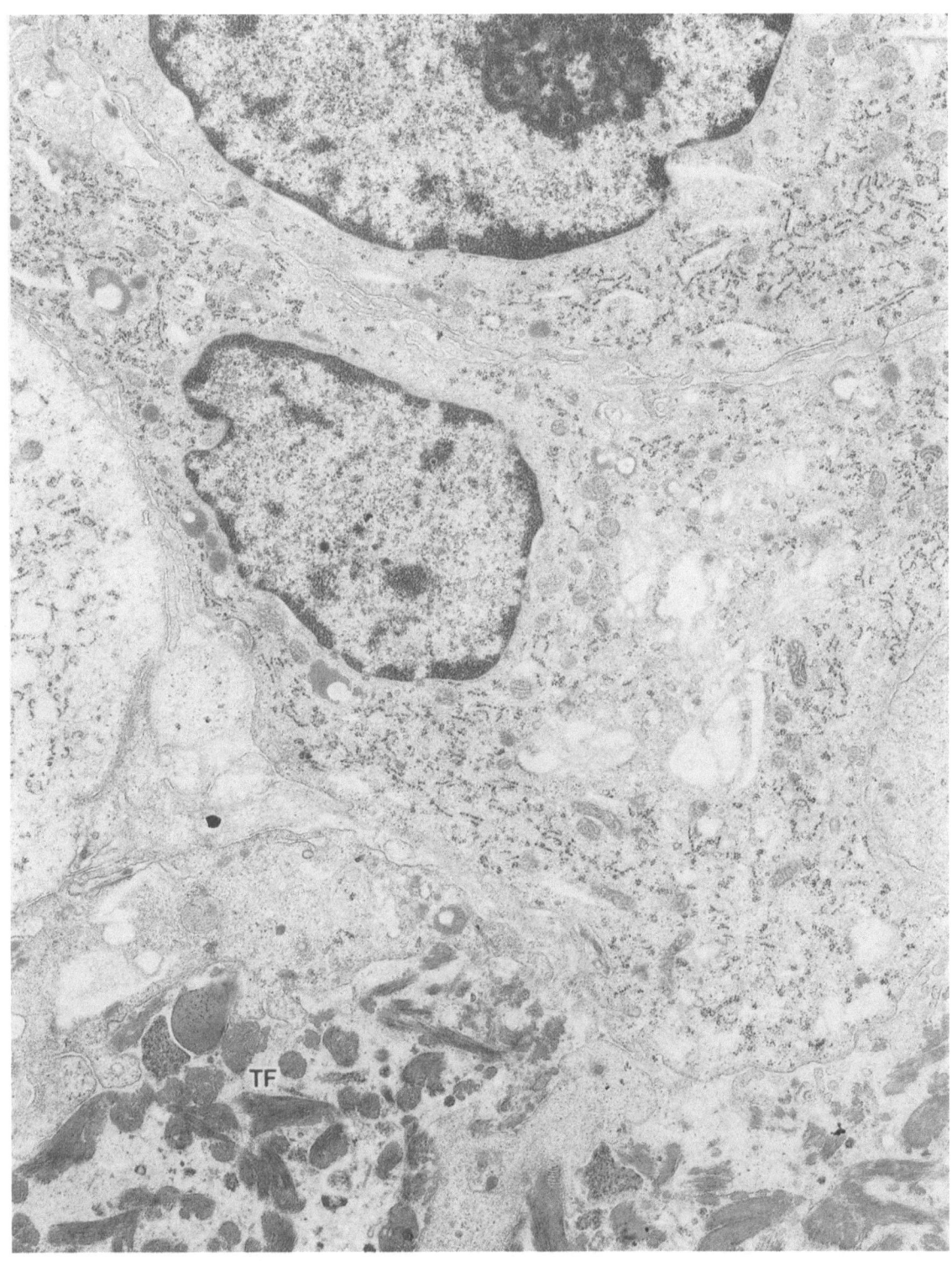

Fig. 26.4 *Craniopharyngioma* (the same case as in Fig. 26.1) The epithelial cells in the tumor vary in the number of bundles of tonofilaments (*TF*), which are visible as keratohyaline granules under the light microscope. × 14 000

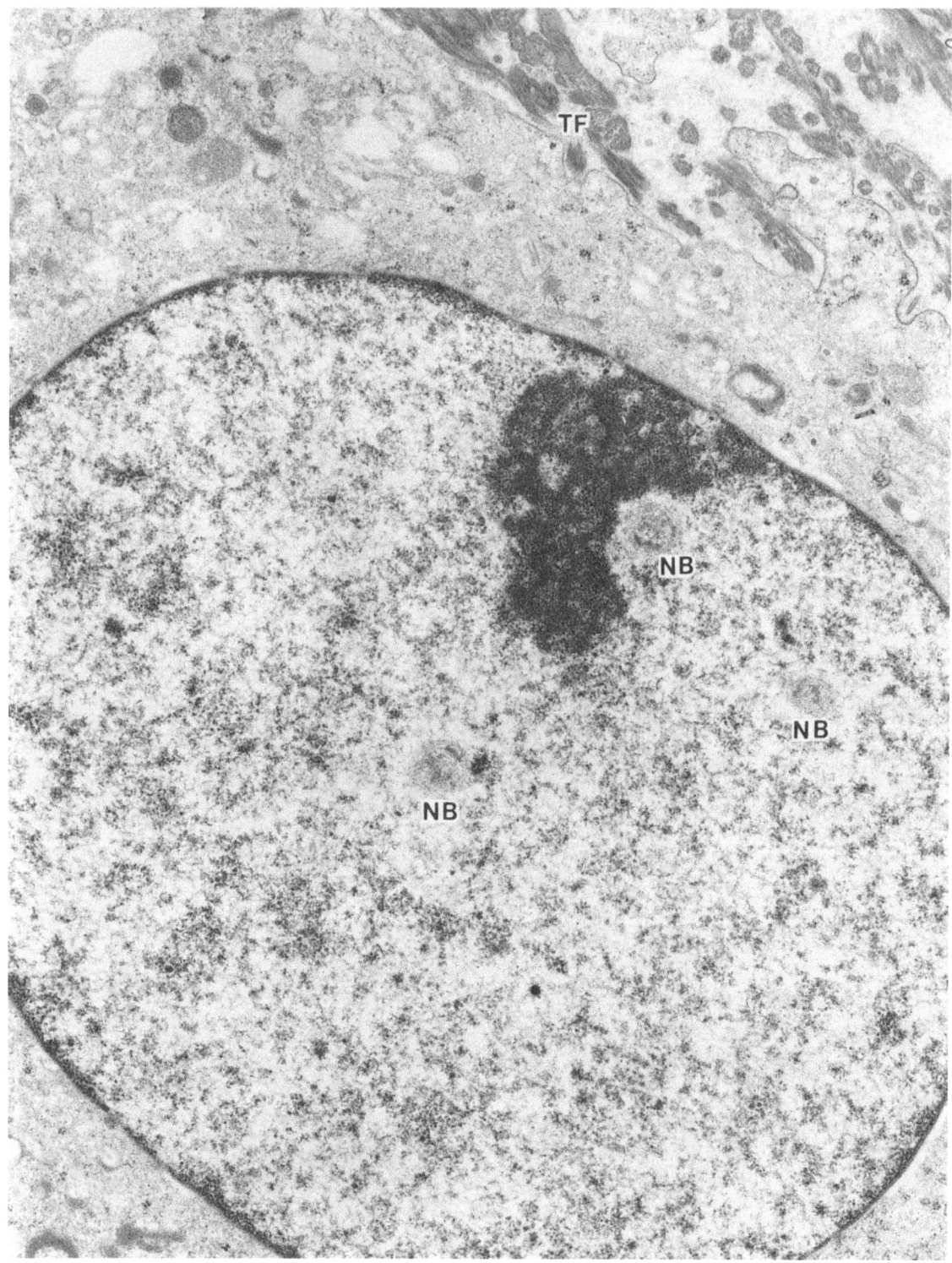

Fig. 26.5. *Craniopharyngioma* (the same case as in Fig. 26.1). An epithelial cell with a clear round nucleus has a few 7–8 nm intermediate filaments. *NB* nuclear bodies, *TF* tonofilaments. × 20 000

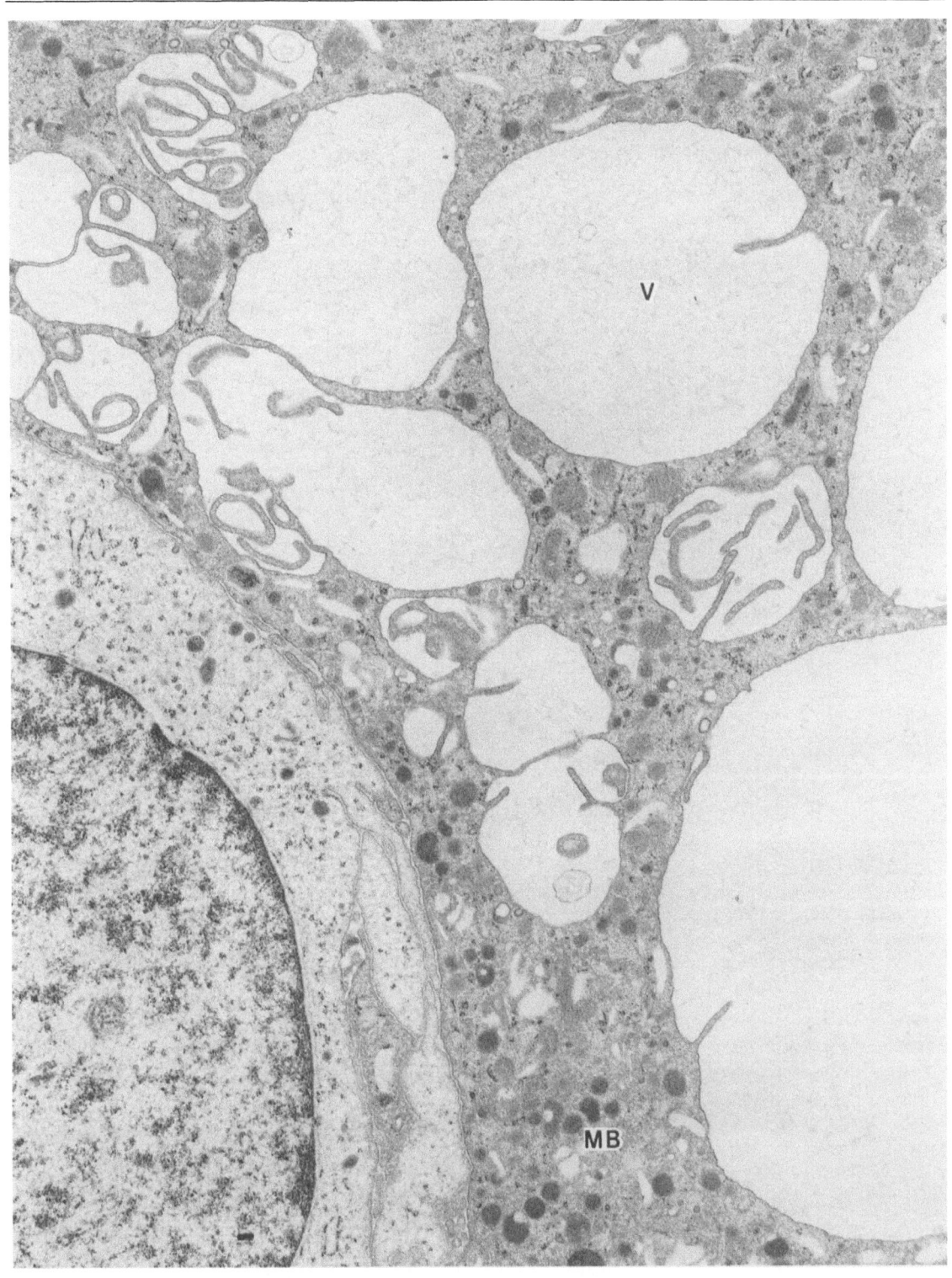

Fig. 26.6. *Craniopharyngioma* (the same case as in Fig. 26.1). Intracytoplasmic vacuoles (*V*) and microbodies (*MB*) are observed in an epithelial cell. × 15 000

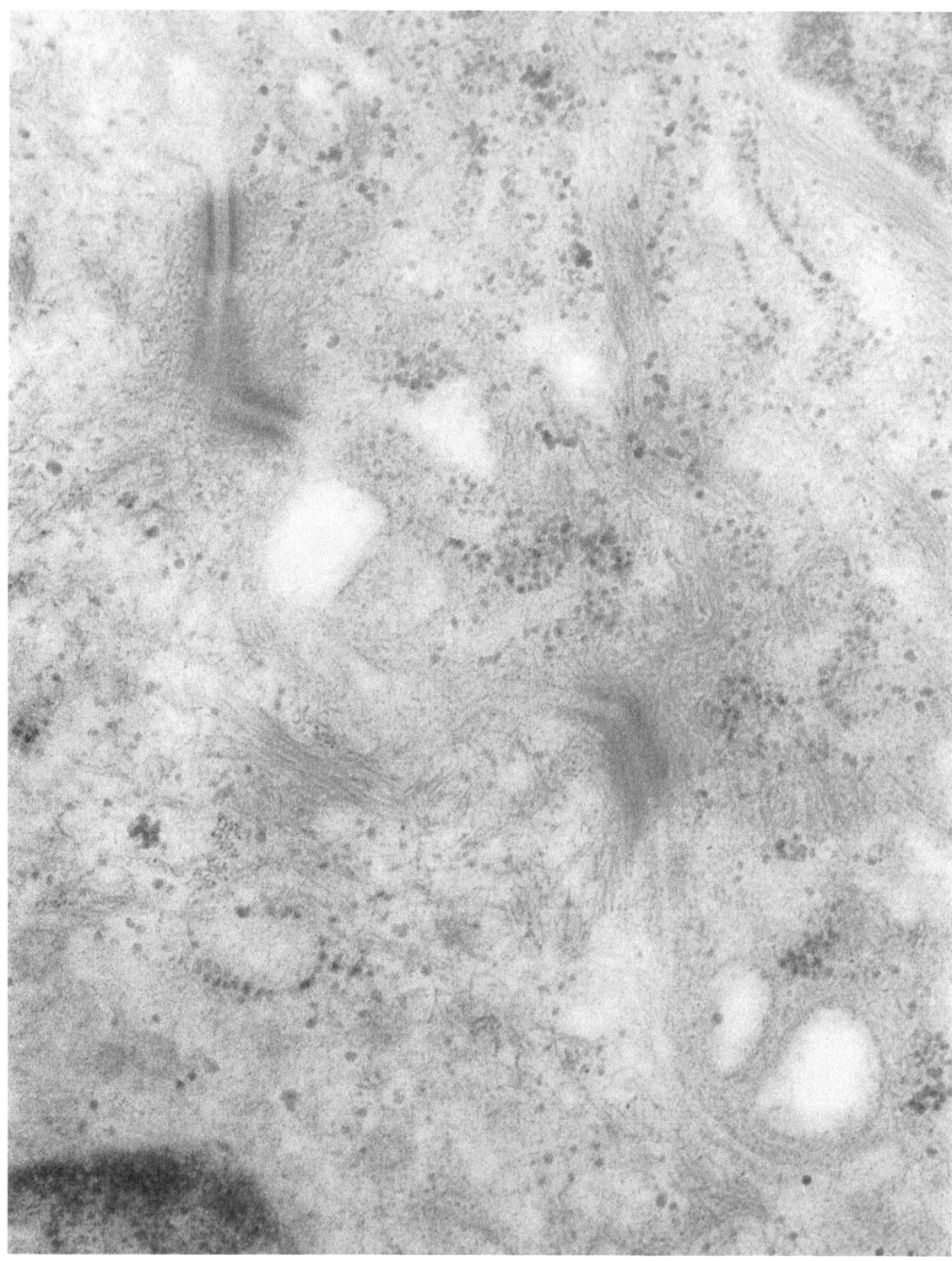

Fig. 26.7. *Craniopharyngioma* (the same case as in Fig. 26.1). High-power view of the tonofilaments and desmosomal structures in a craniopharyngioma. × 71 000

27. Chordoma

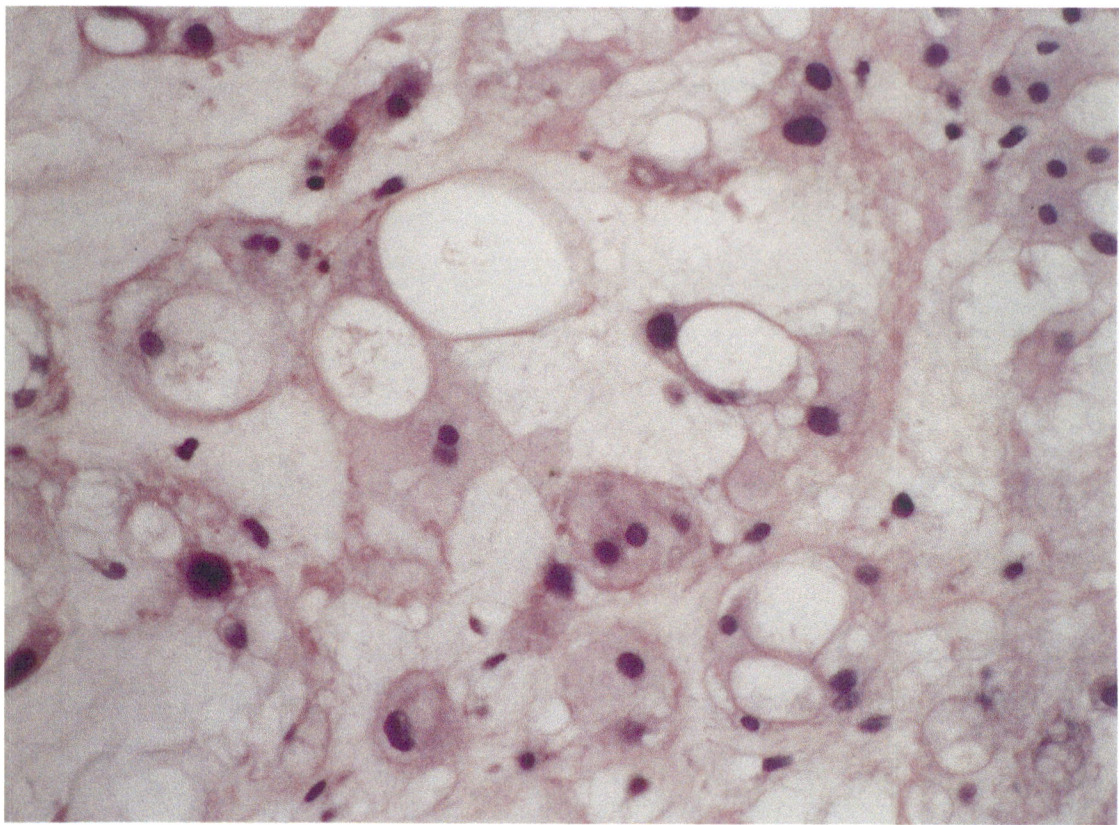

Fig. 27.1. *Chordoma* of the clivus in a 61-year-old man. The tumor consists of physaliphorous (containing vacuoles) cells with eosinophilic cytoplasm. The nuclei of the chordoma cells show marked pleomorphism and occasional mitotic figures. H and E, × 250

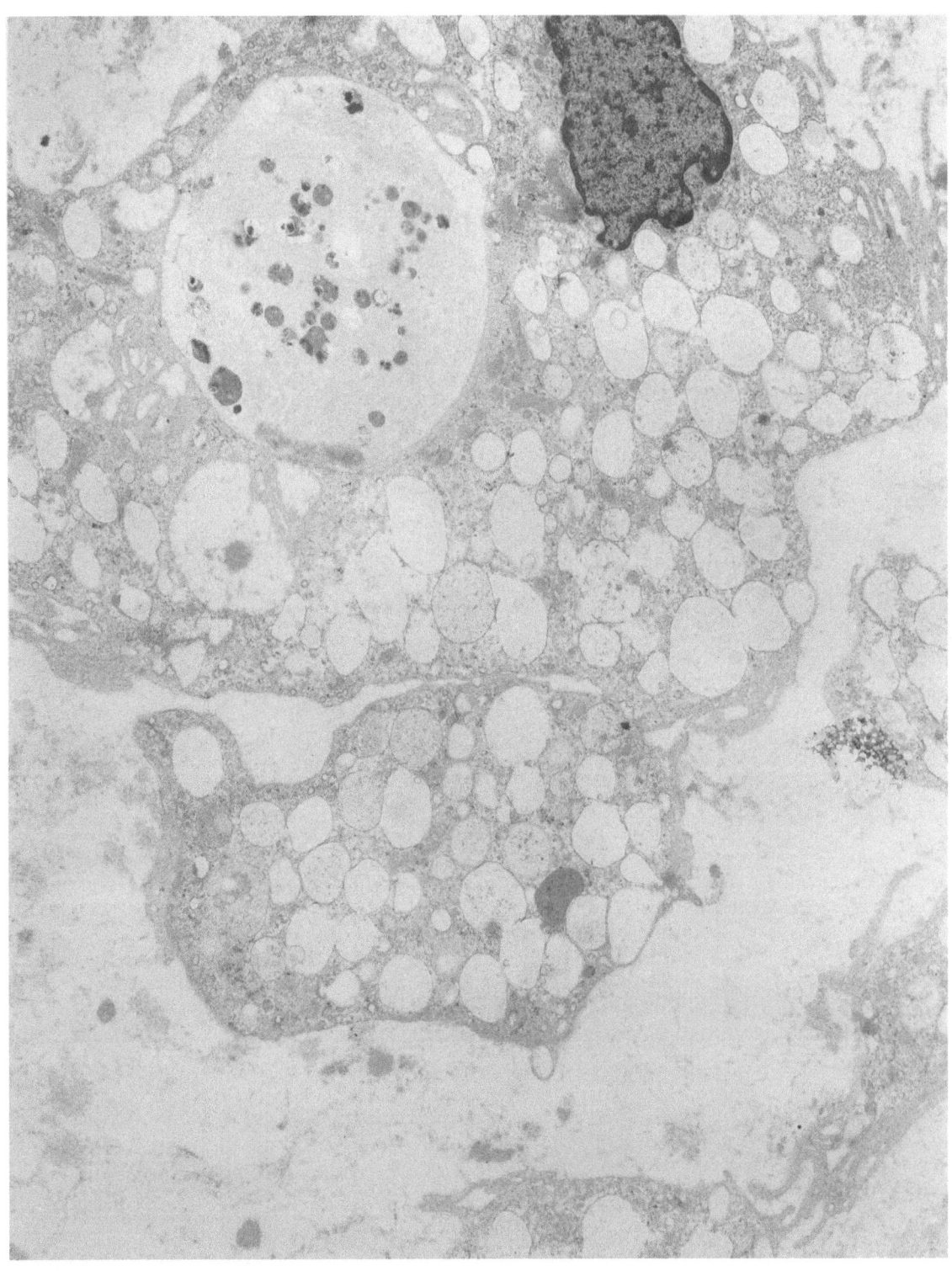

Fig. 27.2. *Chordoma* (the same case as in Fig. 27.1). The physaliphorous cell is characterized by numerous cytoplasmic vacuoles, which vary in size and contain an electron-lucent substance. × 8700

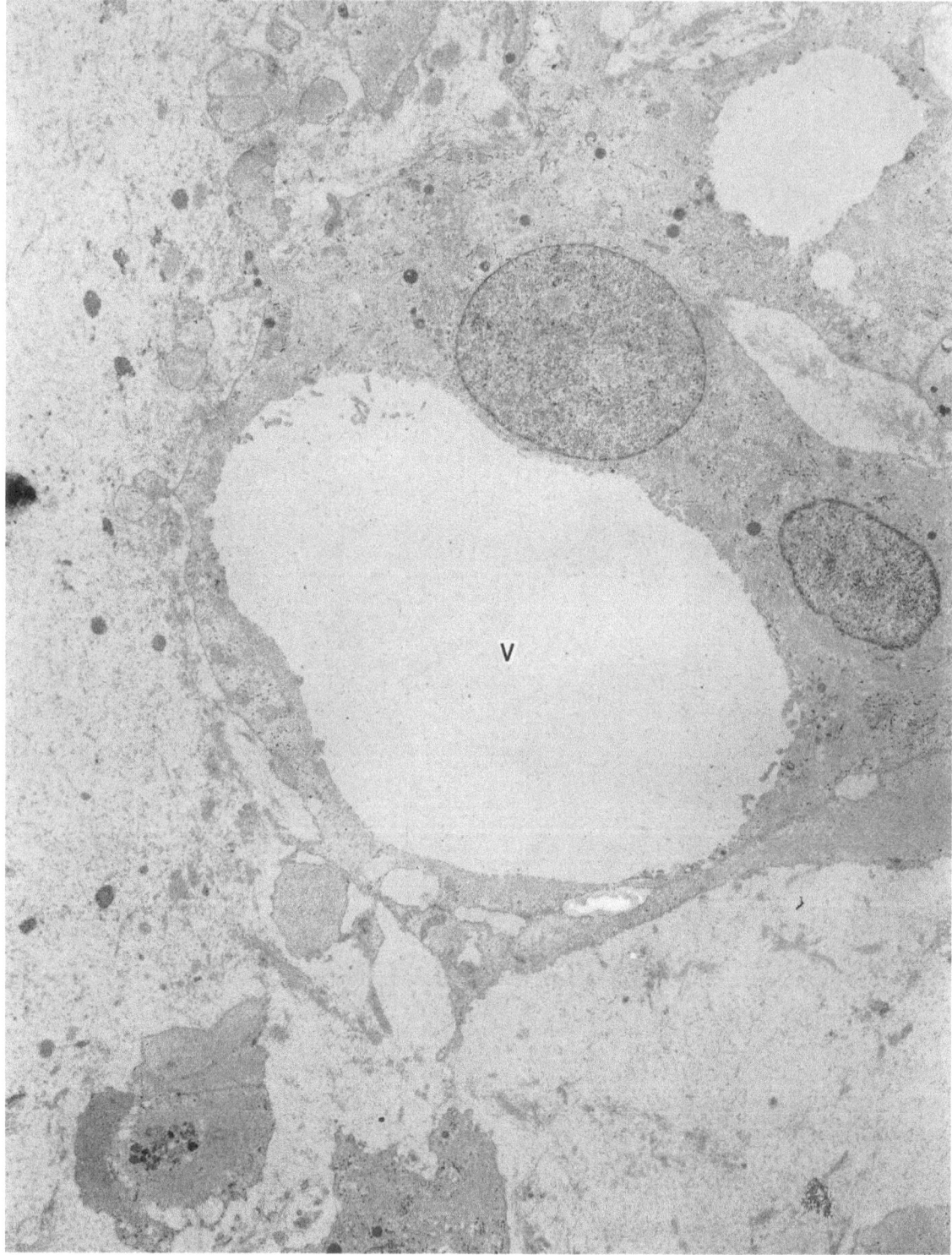

Fig. 27.3. *Chordoma* (the same case as in Fig. 27.1). The chordoma cell with a large cytoplasmic vacuole (*V*) appears to bear two nuclei. The electron-lucent extracellular matrix is considered to represent a mucinous substance. × 6400

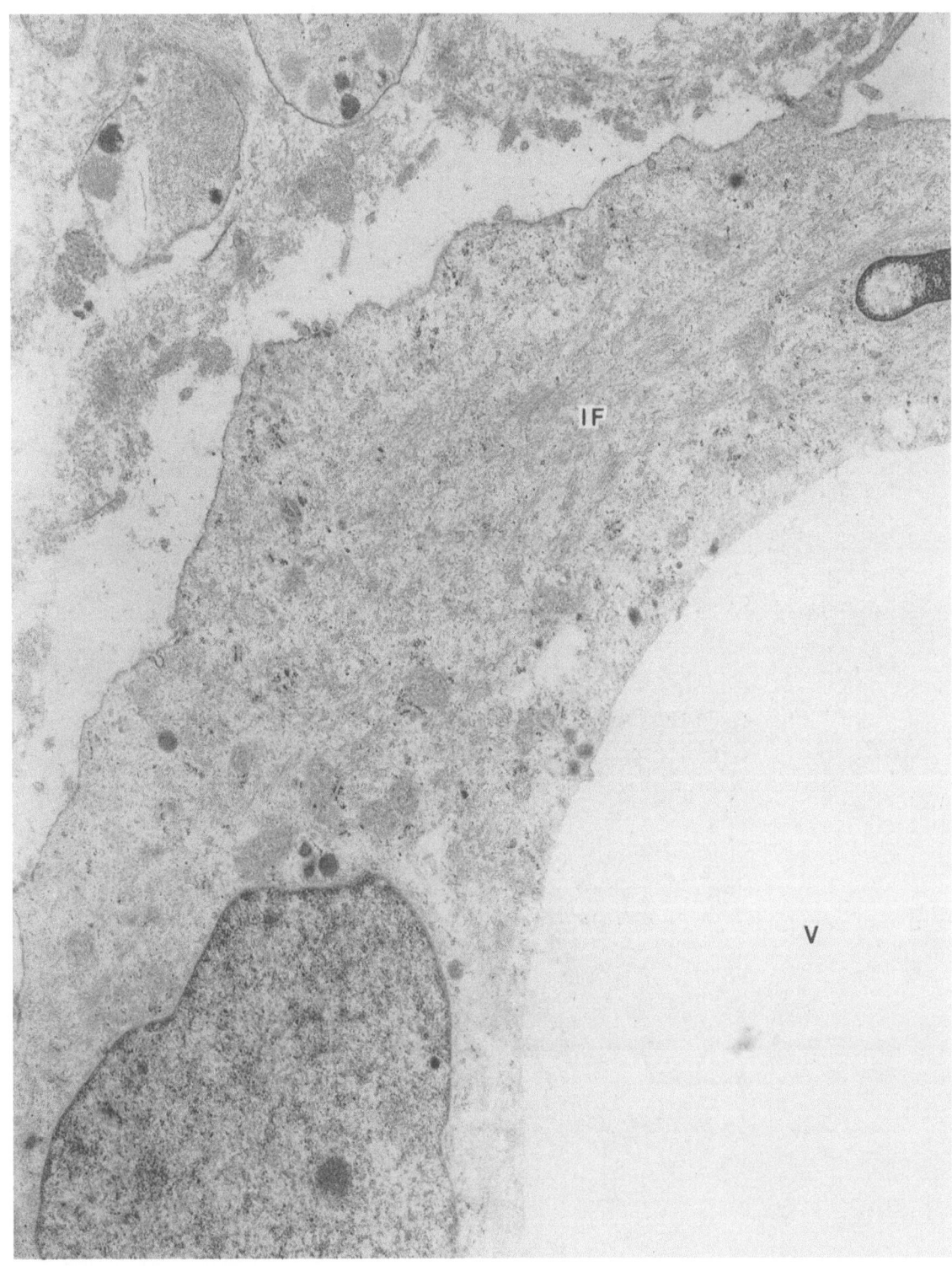

Fig. 27.4. *Chordoma* (the same case as in Fig. 27.1). Higher magnification reveals intermingled 8–10 nm intermediate filaments (*IF*). *V* intracytoplasmic vacuole. × 14 000

28. Metastatic Tumor

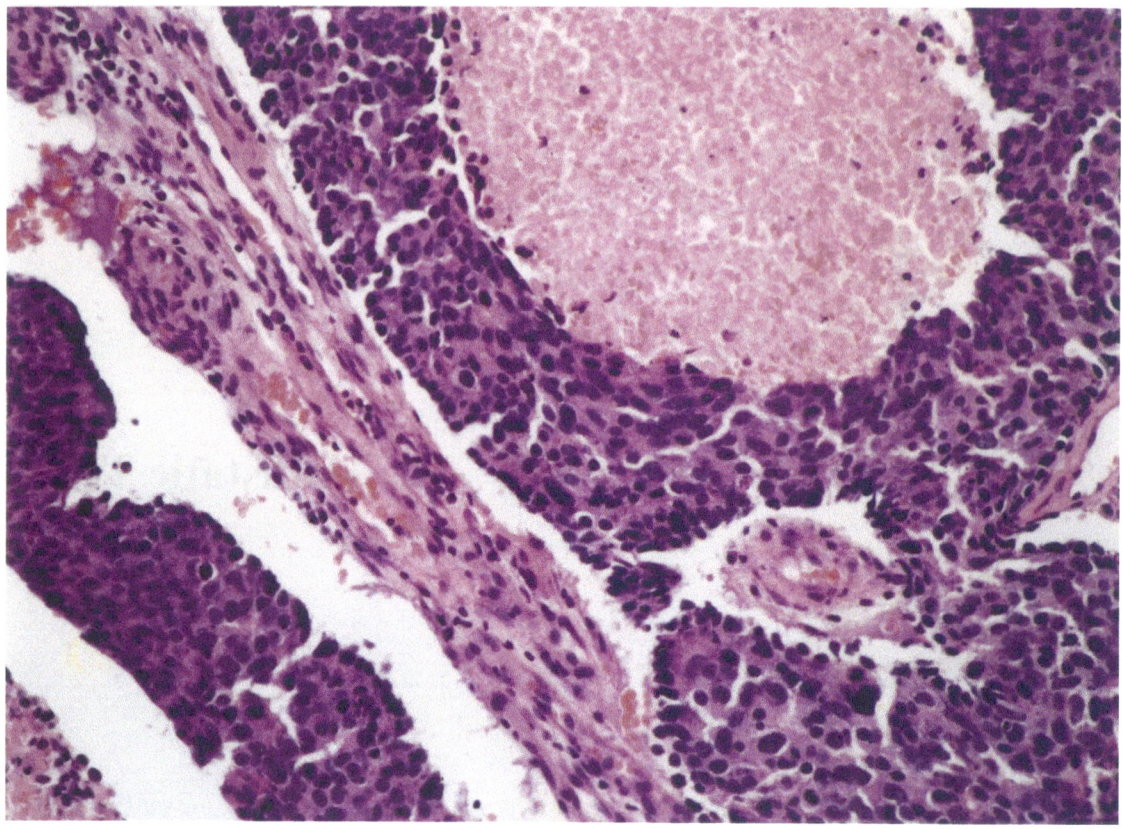

Fig. 28.1. Cerebral metastasis of *small-cell* (*oat-cell*) *carcinoma* of the lung in a 65-year-old man. The closely packed tumor cells with hyperchromatic nuclei are small, ovoid, and fusiform. Necrosis is present at the center of the cell mass. H and E, × 125

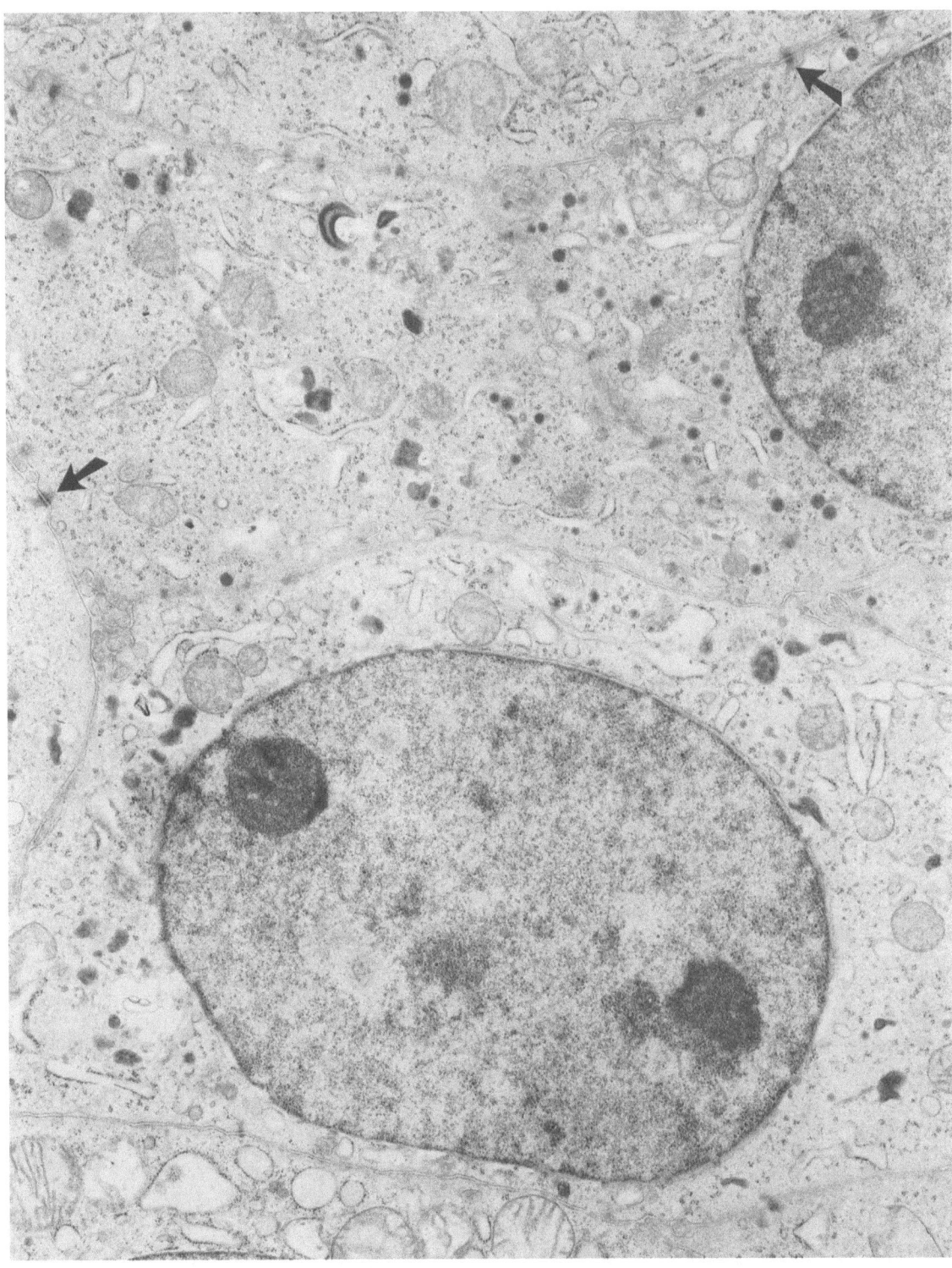

Fig. 28.2. Metastatic *small-cell carcinoma* (the same case as in Fig. 28.1). The tumor cell has an oval nucleus with two prominent nucleoli. The moderately developed cytoplasm contains occasional electron-dense (neurosecretory-like) granules, measuring 150–200 nm in diameter. Desmosomes (*arrows*) are also discernible. × 14 000

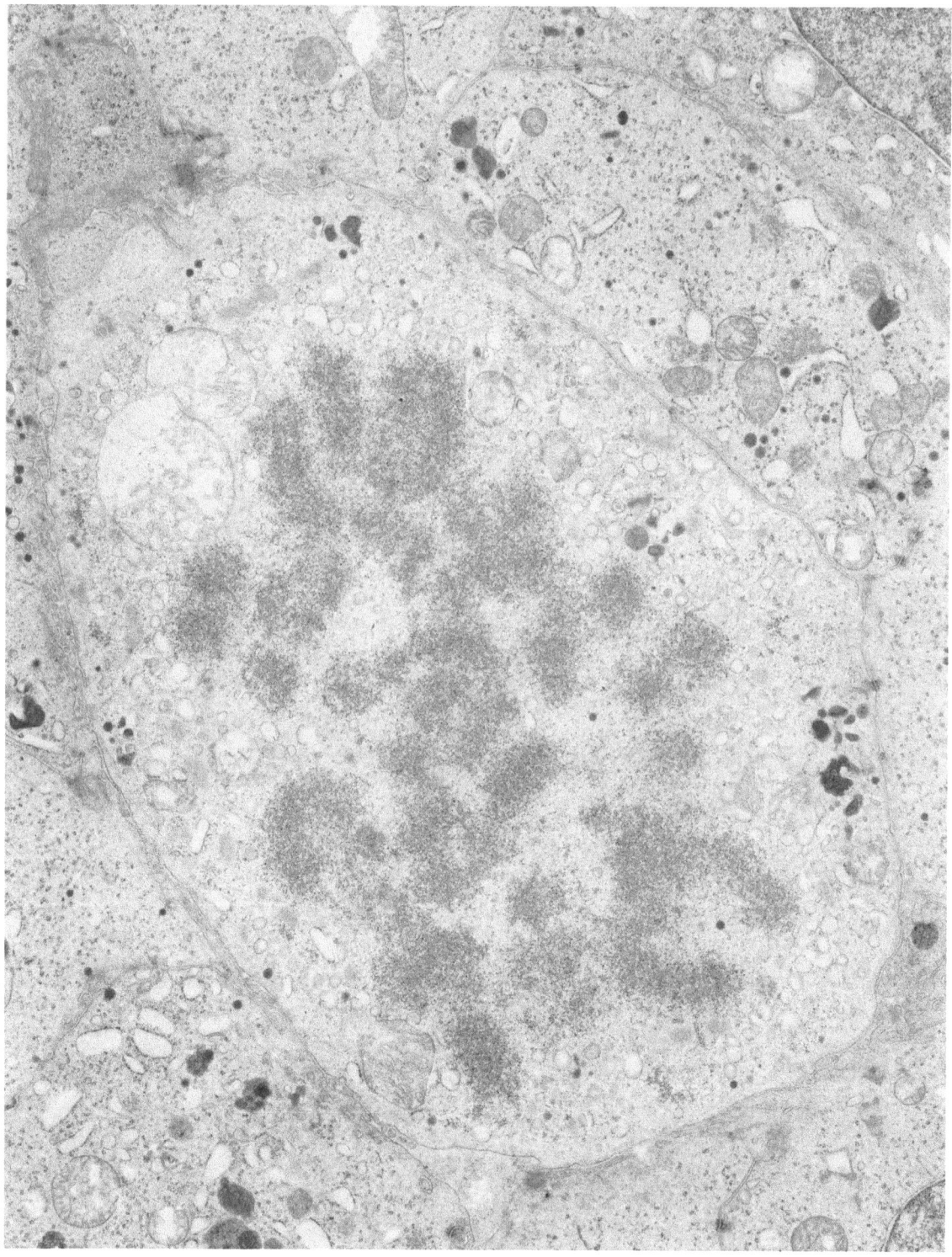

Fig. 28.3. Metastatic *small-cell carcinoma* (the same case as in Fig. 28.1). A mitotic cell, as shown here, is often encountered, indicating the high proliferative potential of this tumor. × 9900

References

General

Barnard RO, Logue V, Reaves PS (1976) An atlas of tumours involving the central nervous system. Bailliere. Tindall, London

Burger PC, Vogel FS (1982) Surgical pathology of the nervous system and its coverings, 2nd edn. Wiley, New York

Dolman CL (1985) Ultrastructure of brain tumors and biopsies, a diagnostic atlas. Praeger, New York

Duffy PE (1983) Astrocytes: normal, reactive, and neoplastic. Raven, New York

Ghadially FN (1975) Ultrastructural pathology of the cell and matrix. Butterworths, London

Henderson DW, Papadimitriou JM (1982) Ultrastructural appearances of tumours. A diagnostic atlas. Churchill Livingstone, Edinburgh

Hirano A, Iwata M. Llena JF, Matsui T (1980) Color atlas of pathology of the nervous system. Igaku-Shoin, Tokyo

Moss TH (1986) Tumours of the nervous system, an ultrastructural atlas. Springer, London Berlin Heidelberg New York Paris Tokyo

Poon TP, Hirano A, Zimmerman HM (1971) Electron microscopic atlas of brain tumors. Grune and Stratton, New York

Rubinstein LJ (1972) Tumors of the central nervous system. Atlas of tumor pathology, Second series, Fascicle 6, AFIP, Washington, DC

Russell DS, Rubinstein LJ (1977) Pathology of tumours of the nervous system, 4th ed. Arnold, London

Sternberger LA (1979) Immunocytochemistry. Wiley, New York

Tseng CH (1980) Atlas of ultrastructure. Ultrastructural features in pathology. Appleton-Century-Crofts, New York

Zülch KJ (1979) Histological typing of tumours of the central nervous system. WHO, Geneva

Zülch KJ (1986) Brain tumors. Their biology and pathology, 3rd ed. Springer, Berlin Heidelberg New York Tokyo

Astrocytoma

Duffell D, Farber L, Chou S, Hartmann JB, Nelson E (1963) Electron microscopic observations on astrocytomas. Subependymal glomerulate astrocytoma. Am J Pathol 43: 539–545

Ebhardt G, Cervos-Navarro J (1981) The fine structure of cells in astrocytomas of various grades of malignancy. Acta Neuropathol (Suppl) 7: 88–90

Hossmann KA, Wechsler W (1971) Ultrastructural cytopathology of human cerebral gliomas. Oncology 25: 455–480

Jones MC, Drut R. Raglia G (1983) Pleomorphic xanthoastrocytoma: A report of two cases. Pediatr Pathol 1: 459–467

Kepes JJ, Rubinstein LJ, Eng LF (1979) Pleomorphic xanthoastrocytoma: a distinctive menigocerebral glioma of young subjects with relatively favorable prognosis. A study of 12 cases. Cancer 44: 1839–1851

Kubota T, Hirano A, Sato K, Yamamoto S (1985) The fine structure of astroblastoma. Cancer 55: 745–750

Luse SA (1960) Electron microscopic studies of brain tumours. Neurology 10: 881–905

Sima AAF (1980) Peroxisomes (microbodies) in human glial tumors. A cytochemical ultrastructural study. Acta Neuropathol 51: 113–117

Sumi SM, Reifel E (1971) Unusual nuclear inclusions in astrocytoma. Arch Pathol 92: 14–19

Weldon-Linne CM, Victor TA, Groothuis DR, Vick NA (1983) Pleomorphic xanthoastrocytoma. Ultrastructural and immunohistochemimal study of a case with a rapidly fatal outcome following surgery. Cancer 52: 2055–2063

Zülch KJ, Wechsler W (1968) Pathology and classification of gliomas. In: Krayenbuhl H, Maspes PE, Sweet WH (eds) Progress in neurological surgery, vol 2. Karger, Basel, pp 1–84

Oligodendroglioma

Cervos-Navarro J (1981) Ultrastructure of oligodendrogliomas. Acta Neuropathol (Suppl) 7: 91–93

Garcia JH, Lemini H (1970) Ultrastructure of oligodendroglioma of the spinal cord. Am J Clin Pathol 54: 757–765

Hossmann KA, Wechsler W (1971) Ultrastructural cytopathology of human cerebral gliomas. Oncology 25: 455–480

Luse SA (1960) Electron microscopic studies of brain tumours. Neurology 10: 881–905

References

Meneses ACO, Kepes JJ, Sternberger NM (1982) Astrocytic differentiation of neoplastic oligodendrocytes. J Neuropathol Exp Neurol 41: 368

Robertson DM, Vogel FS (1962) Concentric lamination of glial processes in oligodendrogliomas. J Cell Biol 15: 313–334

Takei Y, Mino SS, Miles ML (1976) Eosinophilic granular cells in oligodendrogliomas. An ultrastructural study. Cancer 38: 1968–1976

Ependymoma

Goebel HH, Cravioto H (1972) Ultrastructure of human and experimental ependymomas. J Neuropathol Exp Neurol 31: 55–71

Hirano A, Ghatak NR, Wisoff HS, Zimmerman HM (1971) Comparative ultrastructural study of ependymoma and ependymal cyst. Am J Pathol 62: 11a

Hirano A, Ghatak NR, Zimmerman HM (1973) The fine structure of ependymoblastoma. J Neuropathol Exp Neurol 32: 144–152

Liu HM, McLone DG, Clark S (1977) Ependymomas of childhood. Child's Brain 3: 281–296

Rainmondi AJ, Mullan S, Evans JP (1962) Human brain tumours. An electron microscopic study. J Neurosurg 19: 731–753

Rawlinson DG, Herman MM, Rubinstein LJ (1973) The fine structure of a myxopapillary ependymoma of the filum terminale. Acta Neuropathol 25: 1–13

Rubinstein LJ (1970) The definition of the ependymoblastoma. Arch Pathol 90: 35–45

Tani E, Higashi N (1972) Intercellular junctions in human ependymomas. Acta Neuropathol 22: 295–304

Choroid Plexus Papilloma

Carter LP, Beggs J, Waggener JD (1972) Ultrastructure of three choroid plexus papillomas. Cancer 30: 1130–1136

Dohrman GJ, Bucy PC (1970) Human-choroid plexus: a light and electron microscopic study. J Neurosurg 33: 506–516

McComb RD, Burger PC (1983) Choroid plexus carcinoma. Report of a case with immunohistochemical and ultrastructural observations. Cancer 51: 470–475

Navas JJ, Battifora H (1978) Choroid plexus papilloma. Light and electron microscopic study of three cases. Acta Neuropathol 44: 235–239

Rubinstein LJ, Brucher JM (1981) Focal ependymal differentiation in choroid plexus papillomas. An immunoperoxidase study. Acta Neuropathol 53: 29–33

Stefanko SZ, Vazevski VD (1985) Oncocytic variant of choroid plexus papilloma. Acta Neuropathol 66: 160–162

Taratuto AL, Molina H, Monges J (1983) Choroid plexus tumors in infancy and childhood. Focal ependymal differentiation. Acta Neuropathol 59: 304–308

Wolfson WL, Brown WJ (1977) Disseminated choroid plexus papilloma. An ultrastructural study. Arch Pathol Lab Med 101: 366–368

Glioblastoma

Hadfield MG. Silverberg SG (1972) Light and electron microscopy of giant cell glioblastoma. Cancer 30: 989–996

Hossman KA, Wechsler W (1971) Ultrastructural cytopathology of human cerebral gliomas. Oncology 25: 455–480

Jellinger K (1978) Glioblastoma multiforme: morphology and biology. Acta Neurochir (Wien) 42: 5–32

Luse SA (1960) Electron microscopic studies of brain tumours. Neurology 10: 881–905

Robertson DM, MacLean JD (1965) Nuclear inclusions in malignant gliomas. Arch Neurol 13: 287–296

Vazquez JJ, Ortuno G, Cervos-Navarro J (1970) An ultrastructural study of spheroidal nuclear bodies found in gliomas. Virchows Arch 5: 288–293

Zülch KJ, Wechsler W (1968) Pathology and classification of gliomas. In: Krayenbuhl H, Maspes PE, Sweet WH (eds) Progress in neurological surgery, vol 2. Karger, Basel, pp 1–84

Medulloblastoma

Camins MB, Cravioto HM, Epstein F, Ransohoff J (1980) Medulloblastoma: an ultrastructural study—evidence for astrocytic and neuronal differentiation. Neurosurgery 6: 398–411

Hassoun J, Hirano A, Zimmerman HM (1975) Fine structure of intercellular junctions and blood vessels in medulloblastomas. Acta Neuropathol 33: 67–78

Matakas F, Cervos-Navarro J, Gullota F (1970) The ultrastructure of medulloblastomas. Acta Neuropathol 16: 271–284

Moss TH (1983) Evidence for differentiation in medulloblastomas appearing primitive on light microscopy: an ultrastructural study. Histopathology 7: 919–930

Rubinstein LJ, Herman MM, Hanberry JW (1974) The relationship between differentiating medulloblastoma and dedifferentiating diffuse cerebellar astrocytoma. Cancer 33: 675–690

Tani E, Takeuchi J, Ishijima Y, Higashi N, Fugihara E, Ametani T, Ando K (1971) Elongated nuclear sheet and intranuclear myelin figure of human medulloblastoma. Cancer Res 31: 2120–2129

Ganglioglioma

Lee JC, Glasauer FE (1968) Ganglioglioma: light and electron microscopic study. Neurochir (Stuttg) 11: 160–170

Robertson DM, Hendry WS, Vogel FS (1964) Central ganglioneuroma: a case study using electron microscopy. J Neuropathol Exp Neurol 23: 692–705

Rubinstein LJ, Herman MM (1972) A light and electron microscopic study of a temporal lobe ganglioglioma. J. Neurol Sci 16: 27–48

240

Cerebral Neuroblastoma and Central Neurocytoma

Azzarelli B, Richards DE, Anton AH, Roessmann U (1977) Central neuroblastoma. Electron microscopic observations and catecholamine determinations. J Neuropathol Exp Neurol 36: 384–397

Grisoli F, Vincentelli F, Boudouresques G, Delpuech F, Hassoun J. Raybaud C (1981) Primary cerebral neuroblastoma in an adult man. Surg Neurol 16: 266–270

Hassoun J, Gambarelli D, Grisoli F, Pellet W, Salamon G, Pellissier JF, Toga M (1982) Central neurocytoma. An electron-microscopic study of two cases. Acta Neuropathol 56: 151–156

Pearl GS, Takei Y, Bakay AE, Davis P (1985) Intra-ventricular primary cerebral neuroblastoma in adults: report of three cases. Neurosurg 16: 847–849

Rhodes RH, David RL, Kassel SH, Clague BH (1978) Primary cerebral neuroblastoma: a light and electron microscopic study. Acta Neuropathol 41: 119–124

Shin WY, Laufer H, Lee YC, Aftalion B, Hirano A, Zimmermann HM (1978) Fine structure of a cerebellar neuroblastoma. Acta Neuropathol 42: 11–13

Yagishita S, Itoh Y, Chiba Y, Yamashita T, Nakazima F, Kuwabara T (1980) Cerebellar neuroblastoma. A light and ultrastructural study. Acta Neuropathol 50: 139–142

Olfactory Neuroblastoma

Chaudhry AP, Haar HG, Koul A, Nickerson PA (1979) Olfactory neuroblastoma (esthesioneuroblastoma). A light and ultrastructural study of two cases. Cancer 44: 564–579

Taxy JB, Hidvegi DF (1977) Olfactory neuroblastoma. An ultrastructural study. Cancer 39: 131–138

Primitive Neuroectodermal Tumors

Boesel CP, Suhan JP, Bradel EJ (1978) Ultrastructure of primitive neuroectodermal neoplasms of the central nervous system. Cancer 42: 194–201

Hart MN, Earle KM (1973) Primitive neuroectodermal tumors of the brain in children. Cancer 32: 890–897

Rorke LB (1983) The cerebellar medulloblastoma and its relationship to primitive neuroectodermal tumors. J Neuropathol Exp Neurol 42: 1–15

Primary Pineal Tumors

Hassoun J, Gambarelli D, Peragut JC, Toga M (1983) Specific ultrastructural markers of human pinealomas. Acta Neuropathol 62: 31–40

Herrick MK, Rubinstein LJ (1979) The cytological differentiating potential of pineal parenchymal neoplasms (true pinealomas). A clinicopathological study of 28 tumours. Brain 102: 289–320

Kline KT, Damjanor I, Katz SM, Schmidek H (1979) Pineoblastomas: an electron microscopic study. Cancer 44: 1692–1699

Markesberry WR, Haugh RM, Young AB (1981) Ultrastructure of pineal parenchymal neoplasms. Acta Neuropathol 55: 143–149

Neuwelt EA, Glasbery M, Frenkel E, Clark WK (1979) Malignant pineal region tumors. A clinico-pathological study. J Neurosurg 51: 597–607

Nielson SL, Wilson BB (1975) Ultrastructure of a 'pineocytoma'. J Neuropathol Exp Neurol 34: 148–158

Germinoma

Cravioto H, Dart D (1973) The ultrastructure of "pinealomas" (seminoma-like tumour of the pineal region). J Neuropathol Exp Neurol 32: 552–565

Ramsey HJ (1965) Ultrastructure of pineal tumour. Cancer 18: 1014–1025

Tabuchi K, Yamada O, Nishimoto A (1973) The ultrastructure of pinealomas. Acta Neuropathol 24: 117–127

Wischnitzer S (1970) The annulate lamellus. Int Rev Cytol 27: 65–100

Schwannoma

Cravioto H (1969) The ultrastructure of acoustic nerve tumours. Acta Neuropathol 12: 116–140

Erlandson RA, Woodruff JM (1982) Peripheral nerve sheath tumours: an electron microscopic study of 43 cases. Cancer 49: 273–287

Luse SA (1960) Electron microscopic studies of brain tumours. Neurology 10: 881–905

Sian CS, Ryan SF (1981) The ultrastructure of neurilemmoma with emphasis on Antoni B tissue. Hum Pathol 12: 145–160

Waggener JD (1966) Ultrastructure of benign peripheral nerve sheath tumours. Cancer 19: 699–709

Teratoma

Afshar F, King TT, Berry CL (1982) Intraventricular fetus-in-fetu. J Neurosurg 56: 845–849

Lanuza M, Poon TP, Belmonte A (1985) Mixed teratoma and meningioma in the temporoparietal region. Surg Neurol 23: 399–402

Wakai S, Segawa H, Kitahara S, Asano T, Sano K, Ogihara R, Tomita S (1980) Teratoma in the pineal region in two brothers. J Neurosurg 53: 239–243

Pituitary Adenoma and Oncocytoma

Bauserman SC, Hardman JM, Schochet SS, Earle EM (1978) Pituitary oncocytoma. Indispensable role of electron microscopy in its identification. Arch Pathol Lab Med 102: 456–459

DeCicco A, Dekker A, Yunis EJ (1972) Fine structure of Crooke's hyaline change in the human pituitary gland. Arch Pathol 94: 65–70

Doniach I (1972) Cytology of pituitary adenomas. JR Coll Physicians 6: 299–308

References

Esiri MM, Adams CBT, Burke C, Underdown R (1983) Pituitary adenomas: immunohistology and ultrastructural analysis of 118 tumours. Acta Neuropathol 62: 1–14

Goebel HH, Schulz F, Rama B (1980) Ultrastructurally abnormal mitochondria in the pituitary oncocytoma. Acta Neurochir 51: 195–201

Horvath E, Kovacs K (1976) Ultrastructural classification of pituitary adenomas. Can J Neurol Sci 3: 9–21

Horvath E, Kovacs K (1978) Morphogenesis and significance of fibrous bodies in human pituitary adenomas. Virchows Arch (Zellpathol) 27: 69–78

Kalyanaraman UP, Halmi NS, Elwood PW (1980) Prolactin-secreting pituitary oncocytoma with galactorrhea-amenorrhea syndrome. A histologic, ultrastructural, and immunocytochemical study. Cancer 46: 1584–1589

Kovacs K, Horvath E (1973) Pituitary "chromophobe" adenoma composed of oncocytes. A light and electron microscopic study. Arch Pathol 95: 235–239

Landolt AM (1975) Ultrastructure of human sella tumours. Correlations of clinical findings and morphology. Acta Neurochir (Suppl) 22: 1–167

Landolt AM, Oswald UW (1973) Histology and ultrastructure of an oncocytic adenoma of the human pituitary. Cancer 31: 1099–1105

Schober R, Nelson D (1975) Fine structure and origin of amyloid deposits in pituitary adenoma. Arch Pathol 99: 403–410

Meningioma

Cervos-Navarro J, Vasquez JJ (1969) An electron microscopic study of meningiomas. Acta Neuropathol 13: 301–323

Copeland D, Bell SW, Shelburne JD (1978) Hemidesmosome-like intercellular specializations in human meningiomas. Cancer 41: 2242–2249

Gonatus NK, Besen M (1963) An electron microscopic study of three human psammomatous meningiomas. J Neuropathol Exp Neurol 22: 263–273

Humeau C, Vic P, Sentein P, Vlahovitch B (1979) The fine structure of meningiomas: An attempted classification. Virchows Arch (Pathol Anat) 382: 210–216

Kepes J (1961) Electron microscopic studies of meningiomas. Am J Pathol 39: 499–510

Kepes J (1982) Meningiomas, biology, pathology, and differential diagnosis. Masson, New York Masson Monographs in Diagnostic Pathology, vol 4

Kubota T, Hirano A, Yamamoto S, Kajikawa K (1984) The fine structure of psammoma bodies in meningocytic whorls. J Neuropathol Exp Neurol 43: 37–44

Napolitano L, Kyle R, Fisher ER (1963) Ultrastructure of meningiomas and the derivation and nature of their cellular components. Cancer 17: 233–241

Pena CE (1977) Meningioma and intracranial hemangiopericytoma. A comparative electron microscopic study. Acta Neuropathol 39: 69–74

Meningioangiomatosis

Kasantikul V, Brown WJ (1980) Meningioangiomatosis in the absence of von Recklinghausen's disease. Surg Neurol 15: 71–75

Kunishio K, Yamamoto Y, Sunami N, Satoh T, Asari S, Yoshino T, Ohtsuki Y (1987) Histopathologic investigation of a case of meningioangiomatosis not associated with von Recklinghausen's disease. Surgical Neurol 27: 575–579

Hemangioblastoma

Bonnin JM, Pena CE, Rubinstein JL (1983) Mixed capillary hemangioblastoma and glioma. A redefinition of the "angioglioma." J Neuropathol Exp Neurol 42: 504–516

Ceryos-Navarro J (1971) Elektronenmikroskopie der Hämangioblastome des ZNS und der angioblastischen Meningiome. Acta Neuropathol 19: 184–207

Deck JHN, Rubinstein LJ (1981) Glial fibrillary acidic protein in stromal cells of some capillary hemangioblastomas: Significance and possible implications of an immunoperoxidase study. Acta Neuropathol 54: 173–181

Ho KL (1985) Ultrastructure of cerebellar capillary hemangioblastoma: III. Crystalloid bodies in endothelial cells. Acta Neuropathol 66: 117–126

Kawamura J, Garcia JH, Kamijo Y (1973) Cerebellar haemangioblastoma: histogenesis of stromal cells. Cancer 31: 1528–1540

Kepes JJ, Rengachary SS, Lee SH (1979) Astrocytes in hemangioblastomas of the central nervous system and their relationship to stromal cells. Acta Neuropathol 47: 99–104

Shimura T, Hirano A, Llena JF (1985) Ultrastructure of cerebellar hemangioblastoma. Some new observations on the stromal cells. Acta Neuropathol 67: 6–12

Spence AM, Rubinstein LJ (1975) Cerebellar capillary haemangioblastoma: its histogenesis studied by organ culture and electron microscopy. Cancer 35: 326–341

Hemagiopericytoma

Pena CE (1975) Intracranial haemangiopericytoma. Ultrastructural evidence of its leiomyoblastic differentiation. Acta Neuropathol 33: 279–284

Popoff NA, Malinin TI, Rosomoff HL (1974) Fine structure of intracranial hemangiopericytoma and angiomatous meningioma. Cancer 34: 1187–1197

Ramsey HJ (1966) Fine structure of hemangiopericytoma and hemangio-endothelioma. Cancer 19: 2005–2018

Melanoma

Silbert SW, Smith KR Jr, Horenstein S (1978) Primary leptomeningeal melanoma. An ultrastructural study. Cancer 41: 519–527

Winston KR, Sotrel A, Schnitt SJ (1987) Meningeal melanocytoma. Case report and review of the clinical and histological features. J Neurosurg 66: 50–57

Primary Cerebral Malignant Lymphoma

Cravioto H (1975) Human and experimental reticulum cell sarcoma (microglioma) of the nervous system. Acta Neuropathol (Suppl) VI: 135–140

Henry JM, Heffner RR, Dillard SH, Earle KM, Davis RL (1974) Primary malignant lymphomas of the central nervous system. Cancer 34: 1293–1302

Hirano A, Ghatak NR, Becker NH, Zimmerman HM (1974) A comparison of the fine structure of small blood vessels in intracranial and retroperitoneal malignant lymphomas. Acta Neuropathol 27: 93–104

Ishida Y (1975) Fine structure of primary reticulum cell sarcoma of the brain. Acta Neuropathol (Suppl) VI: 147–153

Jellinger K, Slowick F, Sluga E (1979) Primary intracranial malignant lymphomas. A fine structural, cytochemical and CSF immunological study. Clin Neurol Neurosurg 81: 173–184

Johnson PC (1975) Ultrastructural study of two central nervous system lymphomas. Acta Neuropathol (Suppl) VI: 155–160

Mollo F, Monga G, Coda R, Palestro G (1975) Ultrastructural features of human lymphomas. Acta Neuropathol (Suppl) 6: 17–20

Schaefer HE, Kruger GRF, Fischer R (1975) Morphological classification of malignant lymphomas; ultrastructural, cytochemical and immunological results. Acta Neuropathol (Suppl) VI: 21–29

Craniopharyngioma

Ghatak NR, Hirano A, Zimmerman HM (1971) Ultrastructure of a craniopharyngioma. Cancer 27: 1465–1475

Landolt AM (1975) Ultrastructure of human sella tumours. Correlations of clinical findings and morphology: VII: Craniopharyngiomas. Acta Neuropathol (Suppl) 22: 104–119

Chordoma

Dolman CL (1984) Ultrastructure of brain tumours and biopsies. Praeger, New York, pp 85–105

Erlandson RA, Tandler B, Lieberman PM, Higinbotham NO (1968) Ultrastructure of human chordoma. Cancer Res 28: 2115–2125

Ho K-L (1985) Eccordosis physaliphora and chordoma: a comparative ultrastructural study. Clin Neuropathol 4: 77–86

Mikuz G, Mydla F, Gutter W (1977) Chordoma: Ultrastructural, biochemical and cytophotometric findings. Beitr Pathol 161: 150–165

Metastatic Brain Tumors

Ghadially FN (1980) Diagnostic electron microscopy of tumours. Butterworths, London, pp 51–57

Saba SR, Espinoza CG, Richman AV, Azar HA (1983) Carcinomas of the lung: An ultrastructural and immunoytochemical study. Am J Clin Pathol 80: 14–20

Trump BF, Jesudason ML, Jones RT (1978) Ultrastructural features of diseased cells: neoplasia. In: Trump BF, Jones RT (eds) Diagnostic electron microscopy, vol 1. Wiley, New York, pp 54–64

Immunohistochemistry

Bellon G, Gaulet T, Cam Y, Pluot M, Poulin G, Pytlinska M, Bernard MH (1985) Immunohistochemical localization of macromolecules of the basement membrane and extracellular matrix of human gliomas and meningiomas. Acta Neuropathol 66: 245–252

Bjornsson J, Scheithauser BW, Okazaki H, Leech RW (1985) Intracranial germ cell tumors: pathobiological and immunohistochemical aspects of 70 cases. J Neuropath Exp Neurol 44: 32–46

Bonnin JM, Rubinstein LJ (1984) Immunohistochemistry of central nervous system tumors, its contributions to neurosurgical diagnosis. J Neurosurg 60: 1121–1133

Bonnin JM, Rubinstein LJ, Papasozomenos SCH, Marangos PJ (1984) Subependymal giant cell astrocytoma. Acta Neuropathol 62: 185–193

Choi H-SH, Anderson PJ (1985) Immunohistochemical diagnosis of olfactory neuroblastoma. J Neuropath Exp Neurol 44: 18–31

Eng LF, Rubinstein LJ (1978) Contribution of immunohistochemistry to diagnostic problems of human cerebral tumors. J Histochem Cytochem 26: 513–522

Esiri MM, Adams CBT, Burke C, Underdown R (1983) Pituitary adenomas: immunohistology and ultrastructural analysis of 118 tumours. Acta Neuropathol 62: 1–14

Figols J, Iglesias JR, Kazner E (1985) Myelin basic protein (MBP) in human gliomas: a study of twenty-five cases. Clin Neuropathol 4: 116–120

Herpers MJH, Budka H (1984) Glial fibrillary acidic protein (GFAP) in obligodendroglial tumors: Gliofibrillary oligodendroglioma and transitional oligoastrocytoma as subtypes of oligodendroglioma. Acta Neuropathol 64: 265–272

Herpers MJHM, Ramaekers FCS, Aldeweireldt J, Moesker O, Slooff J (1986) Co-expression of glial fibrillary acidic protein- and vimentin-type intermediate filaments in human astrocytomas. Acta Neuropathol 70: 333–339

Hoshino T, Nagashima T, Murovic J, Levin EH, Levin VA, Rupp SH (1985) Cell kinetic studies of in situ human brain tumors with bromodeoxyuridine. Cytometry 6: 627–632

Ho-Soon HC, Anderson PJ (1985) Immunohistochemical diagnosis of olfactory neuroblastoma. J Neuropathol Exp Neurol 44: 18–31

Llena JF, Hirano A, Inoue A (1984) Vasoformative tumor of the brain—immunohistology and ultrastructure. Clin Neuropathol 3: 155–159

Mannoji H, Takeshita I, Fukui M, Ohta M, Kitamura K (1981) Glial fibrillary acidic protein in medulloblastoma. Acta Neuropathol 55: 63–69

McComb RD, Bigner DD (1985) Immunolocalization of laminin in neoplasms of the central nervous systems. J Neuropath Exp Neurol 44: 242–253

References

Naganuma H, Inoue HK, Nakamura M, Koizumi H (1985) Localization of carcinoembryonic antigen in mature intracranial teratomas. J Neurosurg 62: 870–873

Nakajima T, Kameya T, Tsumuraya M, Shimosato Y, Isobe T, Ishioka N, Okuyama T (1983) Immunohistochemical demonstration of neuron-specific enolase in normal and neoplastic tissues. Biomed Res 4: 495–504

Nakajima T, Kameya T, Tsumuraya M, Shiomosato Y, Kato K (1984) Enolase distribution in human brain tumors, retinoblastomas and pituitary adenomas. Brain Res 308: 215–222

Nakajima T, Kameya T, Watanabe S, Hirota T, Shimosato Y, Isobe T (1984) S-100 Protein distribution in normal and neoplastic tissues. In: DeLellis RA (ed) Advances in immunohistochemistry. Masson, New York, pp 141–158

Nakamura Y, Becker LE (1983) Subependymal giant-cell tumors: astrocytic or neuronal? Acta Neuropathol 60: 272–277

Nakamura Y, Becker LE, Marks A (1983) Distribution of immunoreactive S-100 protein in pediatric brain tumors. J Neuropath Exp Neurol 42: 136–145

Perentes E, Rubinstein LJ (1986) Immunohistochemical recognition of human neuroepithelial tumors by anti-Leu 7 (HNK-1) monoclonal antibody. Acta Neuropathol 69: 227–233

Roessmann U, Velasco ME, Gambetti P, Autilio-Gambetti L (1983) Neuronal and astrocytic differentiation in human neuroepithelial neoplasms. J Neuropath Exp Neurol 42: 113–121

Royds JA, Ironside JW, Taylor CB, Graham DI, Timperley WR (1986) An immunohistochemical study of glial and neuronal markers in primary neoplasms of the central nervous system. Acta Neuropathol 70: 320–326

Schiffer D, Giordana MT, Mauro A, Migheli A, Germano I, Giaccone G (1986) Immunohistochemical demonstration of vimentin in human cerebral tumors. Acta Neuropathol 70: 209–219

Shinoda J, Miwa Y, Sakai N, Yamada H, Shima H, Kato K, Takahashi M, Shimokawa K (1985) Immunohistochemical study of placental alkaline phosphatase in primary intracranial germ-cell tumors. J Neurosurg 63: 733–739

Smith DA, Lantos PL (1985) Immunocytochemistry of cerebellar astrocytomas: with a special note on Rosenthal fibres. Acta Neuropathol 66: 155–159

Strom EH, Skullerud K (1983) Pleomorphic xamthoastrocytoma: report of 5 cases. Clin Neuropathol 2: 188–191

Tabuchi K, Moriya Y, Furuta T, Ohnishi R, Nishimoto A (1982) S-100 protein in human glial tumors—Qualitative and quantitative studies. Acta Neurochir 65: 239–251

Tabuchi K, Ohnishi R, Furuta T, Moriya Y, Nishimoto A (1984) Immunohistochemical demonstration of S-100 protein in meningioma. Neurol Med Chir 24: 464–470

Tabuchi K, Ohnishi R, Nishimoto A (1985) Immunohistochemical evidence for the presence of S-100 protein in stromal cells of cerebellar hemangioblastomas. Neurol Med Chir 25: 522–527

Takahashi K, Isobe T, Ohtsuki Y, Akagi T, Sonobe H, Okuyama T (1984) Immunohistochemical study on the distribution of α and β subunits of S-100 protein in human neoplasm and normal tissues. Virchows Arch 45: 385–396

Taratuto AL, Molina H, Monges J (1983) Choroid plexus tumors in infancy and childhood. Focal ependymal differentiation: An immunoperoxidase study. Acta Neuropathol 59: 304–308

Trojanowski JQ, Lee VM-Y (1983) Anti-neurofilament monoclonal antibodies: reagents for the evaluation of human neoplasms. Acta Neuropathol 59: 155–158

Van der Meulen JDM, Houthoff HJ, Edels EJ (1978) Glial fibrillary acidic protein in human gliomas. Neuropathol Appl Neurobiol 4: 177–190

Velasco ME, Dahl P, Roessmann U, Gambetti PL (1980) Immunohistochemical localization of glial fibrillary acidic protein in human glial neoplasms. Cancer 45: 484–494

Velasco ME, Ghobrial MW, Ross ER (1985) Neuron-specific enolase and neurofilament protein as markers of differentiation in medulloblastoma. Surg Neurol 23: 177–182

Wai-Kwan AY, Luna M, Borit A (1985) Vimentin and glial fibrillary acidic protein in human brain tumors. J Neuro-oncol 3: 35–38

Subject Index

Adrenocorticotropic hormone 159
Anaplastic astrocytoma 18
Angiogenesis
  medulloblastoma 84
Anti-Leu 7 24, 34
Antoni's type A and Type B 150, 154
Astrocytes 2
Astrocytoma
  anaplastic 18
  fibrillary 2
  subependymal giant cell 14
Autophagic vacuoles
  oligodendroglioma 30
Axons
  glioblastoma 67

Basal body
  ependymoma 44
Basal lamina
  fibrillary astrocytoma 7
  ependymoma 48
  glioblastoma 73
  olfactory neuroblastoma 119
  teratoma and teratoid tumor 142, 145
  schwannoma 151, 153
  pituitary adenoma 163, 179
  craniopharyngioma 223
B cell
  malignant lymphoma 215
Bromodeoxyuridine
  glioblastoma 60
  medulloblastoma 76
Burkitt type 214

Calcification
  choroid plexus papilloma 57
Calcospherites
  ganglioglioma 88
  meningioma 187
  oligodendroglioma 33
Capillary
  anaplastic astrocytoma 19
  central neurocytoma 94, 96
  ependymoma 48

fibrillary astrocytoma 7
germinoma 137
glioblastoma 73
hemangioblastoma 200, 201
hemangiopericytoma 205
medulloblastoma 84
oligodendroglioma 40
olfactory neuroblastoma 119
pituitary adenoma 163
pituitary oncocytoma 179
Carcinoma
  small cell 236
Central neurocytoma 93
Centriole
  germinoma 133
  malignant lymphoma 217
  medulloblastoma 80
  oligodendroglioma 37
  pituitary adenoma 161
Cerebral neuroblastoma 109
Chondrocytes
  teratoma 140
Chordoma 229
Choroid plexus papilloma 49
Chromatin
  germinoma 133
Chromosome
  glioblastoma 72
  malignant lymphoma 225
  medulloblastoma 80
  primitive neuroectodermal tumor 125
Cilia
  choroid plexus papilloma 55
  ependymoma 43, 44
Collagen fibers
  hemangioblastoma 201
  meningioangiomatosis 197
  schwannoma 151
  teratoma 141
Craniopharyngioma 221
Cyst
  craniopharyngioma 223
  fibrillary astrocytoma 2

Dark cells

central neurocytoma 96
Daughter cells
  oligodendroglioma 37
Degenerating features
  medulloblastoma 83
Dense core vesicles
  central neurocytoma 97, 106
  cerebral neuroblastoma 111, 113, 114
  ganglioglioma 89, 92
  olfactory neuroblastoma 117, 118
Deoxyribonucleic acid (DNA)
  glioblastoma 60
Desmosomes
  craniopharyngioma 223, 224
  fibrillary astrocytoma 5
  germinoma 135
  meningioma 191
  primitive neuroectodermal tumor 121
  teratoma 139

Endothelial cells
  ependymoma 48
  fibrillary astrocytoma 7
  hemangioblastoma 200, 201
  glioblastoma 73
  medulloblastoma 84
  oligodendroglioma 40
  olfactory neuroblastoma 119
Endothelial fenestration
  olfactory neuroblastoma 119
  germinoma 137
  pituitary adenoma 163
  pituitary oncocytoma 179
Endothelial proliferation
  glioblastoma 63
Ependymoma 41
Esthesioneuroblastoma 115
Euchromatin
  medulloblastoma 78
  oligodendroglioma 29
Exocytosis 163
Extracellular space
  glioblastoma 61

Factor VIII-related antigen 200
Fibrillary astrocytoma 1
Follicle stimulating hormone (FSH) 174

Ganglioglioma 87
Ganglion cells
  teratoma 140
Germinoma 131
Giant cells
  glioblastoma 66
  subependymal giant cell astrocytoma 14
Glial fibrillary acidic protein (GFAP)
  central neurocytoma 103
  fibrillary astrocytoma 2
  ganglioglioma 88
  glioblastoma 70
  hemangioblastoma 200
  medulloblastoma 77
  oligodendroglioma 24, 34
  pineocytoma 128
  pleomorphic xanthoastrocytoma 10
  primitve neuroectodermal tumor (PNET) 122
Glial filaments
  anaplastic astrocytoma 20
  choroid plexus papilloma 54
  ependymoma 46
  fibrillary astrocytoma 3, 6
  ganglioglioma 91
  pleomorphic xanthoastrocytoma 12
Glioblastoma 59
Golgi apparatus
  anaplastic astrocytoma 20
  germinoma 133
  pituitary adenoma 160, 164
Growth hormone (GH) 159, 164, 169, 170
Glycogen
  germinoma 133, 134
  glioblastoma 65

Hemangioblastoma 199
Hemangiopericytoma 203
Heterochromatin
  glioblastoma 64, 71
Homer-Wright rosettes
  central neurocytoma 102

Immunoglobulins
  malignant lymphoma 215
Interchromatin granules
  glioblastoma 71
Intermediate filaments
  cordoma 233
  ganglioglioma 89
  medulloblastoma 86
  meningioma 185
  pituitary adenoma 157

Junctional apparatus

choroid plexus papilloma 51, 52
  ependymoma 43, 44
  medulloblastoma 82
  pituitary oncocytoma 182
  teratoid tumor 147

Keratohyaline granules 225

Laminated membraneous structure
  oligodendroglioma 32
Lipid droplets
  hemangioblastoma 202
  meningioma 194
  schwannoma 154
  subependymal giant cell astrocytoma 15
Luse body 151, 152
Luteinizing hormone (LH) 174
Lymphocytes 133, 136
Lysosomes
  anaplastic astrocytoma 19
  pituitary oncocytoma 178

Malignant lymphoma 213
Medulloblastoma 75
Melanoma 209
Melanosomes 211, 212
Meningioangiomatosis 195
Meningioma 185
Metaphase
  endothelial cell 73
Metaphase plate 73
Metastasis 236
Microbodies
  craniopharyngioma 227
Microfilaments
  corticotroph cell adenoma 172, 173
  growth hormone cell adenoma 165
Microtubules
  central neurocytoma 100, 106
  choroid plexus papilloma 55
  ependymoma 45
  ganglioglioma 90
  medulloblastoma 80
  pituitary oncocytoma 182
Microvilli
  choroid plexus papilloma 51, 54
  ependymoma 43, 44
  teratoma 142
Misplaced exocytosis 166
Mitochondria
  anaplastic astrocytoma 21
  choroid plexus papilloma 52
  germinoma 134
  pituitary oncocytoma 175, 178
Mitosis
  medulloblastoma 76
  oligodendroglioma 24
Mitotic figure
  glioblastoma 60
Myelin
  oligodendroglioma 26, 38
Myelin basic protein (MBP)
  oligodendroglioma 34
Myelinosome 126

Neuroblastoma
  cerebral 109
  olfactory 115
Neuron specific enolase (NSE)
  central neurocytoma 102
  ganglioglioma 88
  pineocytoma 128
Neuronal cells
  ganglioglioma 88
Neuropil
  central neurocytoma 100, 105
  medulloblastoma 85
Nuclear blebs 220
Nuclear bodies
  craniopharyngioma 226
  fibrillary astrocytoma 5
  hemangiopericytoma 206
  melanoma 211
  oligodendroglioma 29, 30
Nuclear inclusions
  choroid plexus papilloma 54
  hemangiopericytoma 207
  glioblastoma 70
  primitive neuroectodermal tumor 123
Nuclear membranes
  glioblastoma 71, 72
  pituitary adenoma 167, 183
  primitive neuroectodermal tumor 124
Nuclear pores
  pituitary adenoma 167
  pituitary oncocytoma 183
Nuclear pseudoinclusions
  cerebral neuroblastoma 112
  meningioma 190
  primitive neuroectodermal tumor 124
Nuclei
  anaplastic astrocytoma 20
  central neurocytoma 94
  ependymoma 42
  fibrillary astrocytoma 2, 3
  germinoma 132
  glioblastoma 61, 64
  malignant lymphoma 216
  meningioma 186
  oligodendroglioma 24, 28, 29, 34, 35
  pineocytoma 130
  pituitary adenoma 172
  small cell carcinoma 236
Nucleoli
  fibrillary astrocytoma 3
  ganglioglioma 89
  glioblastoma 71
  malignant lymphoma 220
  oligodendroglioma 35
  primitive neuroectodermal tumor 124
  small cell carcinoma 237
Nucleolonema 15, 133

Oat cell carcinoma 236

Olfactory neuroblastoma   115
Oligodendrocytes   39
Oligodendroglioma   23
Organelles
  anaplastic astrocytoma   19
  central neurocytoma   95
  choroid plexus papilloma   52
  fibrillary astrocytoma   4
  ganglioglioma   89
  germinoma   133
  medulloblastoma   78
  oligodendroglioma   27
  pineocytoma   130

Perichromatin granules
  glioblastoma   71
Pericytes
  fibrillary astrocytoma   7
  hemangioblastoma   200, 201
  oligodendroglioma   25
  pituitary oncocytoma   179
Perinuclear cytoplasmic halos   24, 98
Physaliphorous cells   230
Pineocytoma   127
Pinocytotic vesicles   163
Pituitary adenoma   157
Pituitary oncocytoma   174
Placental alkaline phosphatase
  germinoma   132
Plasmacyte   134
Pleomorphic xanthoastrocytoma   9
Primitive neuroectodermal tumor
  (PNET)   121
Processes
  central neurocytoma   95, 96, 100, 106
  ependymoma   46, 47
  fibrillary astrocytoma   7
  glioblastoma   67
  medulloblastoma   81, 82
  oligodendroglioma   35
  pineocytoma   128, 129
  schwannoma   151
Prolactin   159, 160, 169, 170
Psammoma bodies   187
Pseudorosettes
  ependymoma   42
Pyknosis

meningioma   192

Residual bodies   168
Reticular lamina   7
Ribosome granules
  glioblastoma   61
Rosenthal fibers
  fibrillary astrocytoma   2, 3, 6
  subependymal giant cell
    astrocytoma   16
Rosettes
  central neurocytoma   102
  ependymoma   43
  medulloblastoma   76
Rough endoplasmic reticulum
  (RER)
  anaplastic astrocytoma   21
  choroid plexus papilloma   56
  glioblastoma   61
  pituitary adenoma   160, 168

S-100 protein
  anaplastic astrocytoma   18
  central neurocytoma   94, 103
  cerebral neuroblastoma   110
  choroid plexus papilloma   50
  ependymoma   42
  fibrillary astrocytoma   2
  ganglioglioma   88
  glioblastoma   63, 70
  hemangioblastoma   200
  medulloblastoma   77
  meningioma   186
  oligodendroglioma   24, 34
  pleomorphic xanthoastrocytoma   10
  primitive neuroectodermal tumor
    (PNET)   122
  schwannoma   150
  teratoma   140
S phase
  glioblastoma   60
Satellite cells
  teratoma   140
Schwannoma   149
Secretory granules
  pituitary adenoma   160, 162, 164, 166, 172
  pituitary oncocytoma   175, 176
  small cell carcinoma   28

Smooth endoplasmic reticulum
  (SER)
  choroid plexus papilloma   7
  glioblastoma   62
  pituitary oncocytoma   175, 182
Starry sky appearance   214
Stratum spinosum   224
Stromal cells
  hemangioblastoma   200, 201
Subependymal giant cell
  astrocytoma   13
Synapse
  central neurocytoma   97, 99, 100, 106

T cell
  malignant lymphoma   215
Telophase
  glioblastoma   72
  primitive neuroectodermal tumor   125
Teratoid tumor   144
Teratoma   140
Tight junctions
  fibrillary astrocytoma   7
  oligodendroglioma   40
Tonofilaments
  craniopharyngioma   223, 228
Tuberous sclerosis   14

Vacuoles
  autophagic   30
  chordoma   230, 231
  craniopharyngioma   227
  pleomorphic xanthoastrocytoma   10, 11
Vescicles
  glioblastoma   68
Von Willebrand antigen   200

Weibel-palade bodies, endothelial
  cells
  medulloblastoma   84
Whorl formation   186

Xanthomatous cells
  meningioma   187

Zonula occludens
  pineocytoma   130